05-08

D0219100

# Skin Care

*Beyond the Basics*

## THIRD EDITION

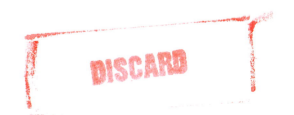

DISCARD

~~MANCOS~~
~~PUBLIC LIBRARY~~

# Skin Care

## Beyond the Basics

### THIRD EDITION

### MARK LEES

**THOMSON**

**DELMAR LEARNING**  Australia   Canada   Mexico   Singapore   Spain   United Kingdom   United States

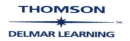

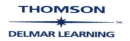THOMSON

DELMAR LEARNING

**Skin Care: Beyond the Basics, Third Edition**

Mark Lees

**President, Milday:**
Dawn Gerrain

**Managing Editor:**
Robert L. Serenka, Jr.

**Acquisitions Editor:**
Martine Edwards

**Product Manager:**
Jennifer Anderson

**Editorial Assistant:**
Falon Ferraro

**Director of Production:**
Wendy A. Troeger

**Production Manager:**
JP Henkel

**Senior Content Project Manager:**
Kathryn B. Kucharek

**Director of Marketing:**
Wendy Mapstone

**Marketing Manager:**
Sandra Bruce

**Marketing Coordinator:**
Nicole Riggi

**Cover Image:**
Getty Images Inc.

**Cover and Text Design:**
Judi Orozco

© 2007 Thomson Delmar Learning, a part of the Thomson Corporation. Thomson, the Star logo and Delmar Learning are trademarks used herein under license.

Printed in Canada
1 2 3 4 5 XXX 10 09 08 07 06

For more information contact Thomson Delmar Learning, 5 Maxwell Drive, PO Box 8007, Clifton Park, NY 12065-2919.

Or you can visit our Internet site at
http://www.milady.com.

ALL RIGHTS RESERVED. No part of this work covered by the copyright hereon may be reproduced or used in any form or by any means—graphic, electronic, or mechanical, including photocopying, recording, taping, Web distribution or information storage and retrieval systems—without written permission of the publisher.

For permission to use material from this text or product, submit a request online at http://www.thomsonrights.com
Any additional questions about permissions can be submitted by email to thomsonrights@thomson.com

Library of Congress Cataloging-in-Publication Data
Application submitted.

**NOTICE TO THE READER**

Publisher does not warrant or guarantee any of the products described herein or perform any independent analysis in connection with any of the product information contained herein. Publisher does not assume, and expressly disclaims, any obligation to obtain and include information other than that provided to it by the manufacturer.

The reader is expressly warned to consider and adopt all safety precautions that might be indicated by the activities herein and to avoid all potential hazards. By following the instructions contained herein, the reader willingly assumes all risks in connection with such instructions.

The Publisher makes no representation or warranties of any kind, including but not limited to, the warranties of fitness for particular purpose or merchantability, nor are any such representations implied with respect to the material set forth herein, and the publisher takes no responsibility with respect to such material. The Publisher shall not be liable for any special, consequential, or exemplary damages resulting, in whole or part, from the readers' use of, or reliance upon, this material.

## Dedication

*This book is dedicated to my parents, Richard and Virginia Lees.*
*Thank you for your lifelong encouragement.*

# CONTENTS

# ACKNOWLEDGMENTS

Very special thanks to the following people and organizations for contributing in many ways to this book.

Editors and Staff of Milady/Thomson Learning.

My wonderful staff, family, and friends who put up with me while I was writing this book.

The late Erica Miller.

Timothy Berger, M.D., Dermatologist, San Francisco, California.

Michael Bond, M.D., Dermatologist, Orlando, Florida.

Sophia Camejo, Encino, California.

*Dermascope* Magazine, Sunnyvale, Texas.

Melvin Elson, M.D., Dermatologist, Nashville, Tennessee.

George Fisher, M.D., Dermatologist, Hickory, North Carolina.

Rebecca James-Gadberry, Instructor of Cosmetic Science, UCLA Extension.

Derek Jones, M.D., Facial Plastic Surgeon, Pensacola, Florida.

Samuel J. LaMonte, M.D., Facial Plastic Surgeon, Pensacola, Florida.

Les Nouvelles Esthetiques—American Edition, Coral Gables, Florida.

Anne Martin, Seattle, Washington.

Marta Martine, Martine Business Development, Santa Barbara, California.

Charles Mizelle, Los Angeles, California.

Howard Murad, M.D., Dermatologist, Murad, Inc., Los Angeles, California.

National Rosacea Society.

Rube Pardo, M.D., Ph.D., Dermatologist, Coral Gables, Florida.

Skin, Inc., Carol Stream, Illinois.

Kirk Smith, M.D., Plastic Surgeon, Pensacola, Florida.

Sothys USA, Miami, Florida.

St. Tropez, Inc., Santa Clarita, California.

David Suzuki, Bio-Therapeutic, Inc., Seattle, Washington.

Thibiant International, Guinot-Paris, Beverly Hills, California.

Department of Dermatology, University of Miami.

David Wanetik, Skin Culture Institute, New York, New York.

Figures are reprinted from *Acne: Morphogenesis and Treatment* by Gerd Plewig, M.D., and Albert M. Kligman, M.D., Ph.D.; permission of publishers, Springer-Verlag, New York, USA, Heidelberg, Berlin, Germany.

# ABOUT THE AUTHOR

Dr. Mark Lees is recognized as one of the world's renowned skin-care specialists, is an award-winning speaker and product developer, and has been actively practicing clinical skin care for more than 20 years at his multi-award winning CIDESCO-accredited Florida salon, which has won multiple awards for "Best Day Spa on the Coast," and "Best Skin Care Center on the Coast" from the *Independent Florida Sun*.

His professional awards are numerous and include *American Salon* Magazine Esthetician of the Year, the Les Nouvelles Esthetiques Crystal Award, the Dermascope Legends Award, the Rocco Bellino Award for outstanding education from the Chicago Cosmetology Association, and Best Educational Skin Care Classroom from the Long Beach International Beauty Expo. Dr. Lees has recently been inducted into the National Cosmetology Association's Hall of Renown.

Dr. Lees has been interviewed and quoted by NBC News, The Associated Press, The Discovery Channel, *Glamour, Self, Teen, Shape*, and many other publications. Dr. Lees is co-founder of the Institute of Advanced Clinical Esthetics in Seattle, a special science-based advanced training program for clinical estheticians.

Dr. Lees is former chairman of EstheticsAmerica, the esthetics education division of the National Cosmetology Association. He currently serves on the Board of Directors of the National Cosmetology Association. He has also served as an affiliate officer for NCA and has served as a CIDESCO International Examiner.

Dr. Lees is former chairman of the Board of the Esthetics Manufacturers and Distributors Alliance and is a member of the Society of Cosmetic Chemists. Dr. Lees is an accomplished writer, having published dozens of skin-care, technical, and business articles for almost every major beauty and esthetics trade publication. He serves on the editorial advisory board of *Les Nouvelles Esthetiques—American Edition*. He is a contributing author of *Milady's Standard Comprehensive Training for Estheticians*. He holds a Ph.D. in Health Sciences, a Master of Science in Health, and a CIDESCO International Diploma. He is licensed to practice in both Florida and Washington State.

His company, Mark Lees Skin Care, Inc., specializes in the development of products for acne-prone, sensitive, and sun-damaged skin. His products are available at finer salons and clinics throughout the United States.

# LETTER TO THE READER

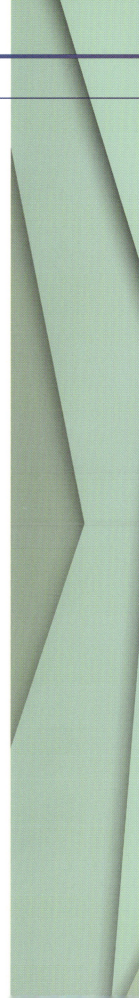

Skin-care professionals are living in a very exciting time. There is an incredible amount of new technology, new ingredients that produce wonderful appearance changes for the skin, new methods for anti-aging, and many new medical procedures that help the appearance of the aging skin. Every day, the scientific community understands more about how the skin functions.

It has been very exciting for me to revise this book. I have tried to include the latest information on many phases of skin treatment in easy-to-understand language. New chapters on rosacea and skin analysis and expanded new information on ingredients and medical procedures are a few of the many changes you will find.

I want to thank so many teachers, students, and skin-care professionals who tell me they always keep this book within reach.

Whether you are a skin-care student, practicing esthetician, medical professional, or simply wanting to understand the skin and its treatment, I sincerely hope you find this new edition of *Skin Care: Beyond the Basics* helpful.

*Mark Lees, Ph.D.*
CIDESCO Diplomate
Pensacola, Florida

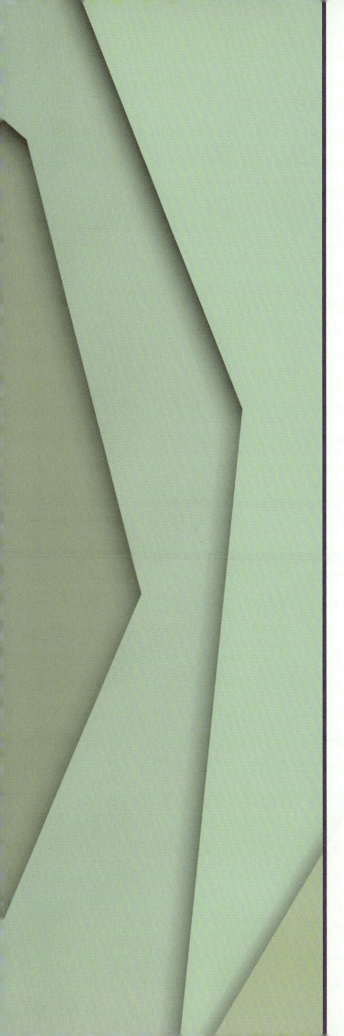

# CHAPTER 1

# Advanced Anatomy and Physiology of the Skin

## OBJECTIVES. . .

In this chapter you will learn about the anatomy and functions of cells. You will also recognize different types of tissues and their functions. You will learn, in detail, about the different layers of the skin and functions of various reactions that take place in the different layers of the skin. Skin penetration will be studied, as well as some techniques for better penetrating, moisturizing, and conditioning treatments for the skin.

Before we can fully understand how to treat cosmetic disorders of the skin, we must first fully understand the functions and activities of the body, more specifically, the cell. The cell is almost a self-contained factory of life. Cells are the building blocks of the human body. Within each cell, many chemical and physical processes constantly take place. To simplify, let's think of the cell as a very, very small living body. This is, of course, an oversimplification, but it will help us understand the many miraculous functions that happen inside each cell of the human body.

**Cell** is a very small, self-contained unit of life. Within the human body, cells specialize in individual functions.

**Cell membrane** gives the cell structure and shape and contains the many internal parts of the cell.

**Selective permeability** means that the cell membrane can let substances into the cell, such as food, water, and oxygen. It can also let substances out of the cell, such as waste and carbon dioxide.

**Receptor sites** are small structures on the cell membrane that are "docking stations" for hormones and other chemicals. Receptor sites receive chemical messages from other cells or organs that cause the cell to behave in a certain way.

**Cytoplasm** is a fluid inside cells that is made of water and other substances.

# THE STRUCTURE OF THE CELL

Much like the skin that covers our bodies, the **cell** is protected by an outer shell known as the **cell membrane** (Figure 1-1). The cell membrane gives the cell structure and shape and contains the many internal parts of the cell. The cell membrane is made of a network of lipids (fatty matter) and protein. The cell membrane possesses a function known as **selective permeability**. Selective permeability means that the cell membrane can let substances into the cell, such as food, water, and oxygen. It can also let substances out of the cell, such as waste and carbon dioxide. The cell is furnished food, water, and oxygen by the blood. Blood is also the vehicle that carries waste materials and carbon dioxide away from the cell membrane and eventually out of the body. Blood itself is made up of cells.

Located on the cell membrane are special structures called **receptor sites**. Receptors are the communication system between different cells, tissues, organs, and parts of the body. Each tissue has cells with unique receptor sites that carry out the activity of a particular type of cell. Receptors receive messages from hormones and other chemical messengers made by other cells. Receptor sites work with these chemical messengers like a "lock and key" system. The receptor site is the "lock," and the chemical it comes in contact with is the "key." When a chemical comes in contact with its specific special receptor, a message is sent to the cell, which carries out specific functions. A good example of this is sebaceous gland activity. Production of sebum in the sebaceous gland is stimulated by male hormones that are received by the receptor sites in the cells of the sebaceous gland. The sites are like "switches" that are "turned on" when a male hormone stimulates the receptor site.

Inside the cell is a fluid called **cytoplasm**. Cytoplasm is made of water and other substances. It has a gel-like consistency. Cytoplasm allows other structures to move around inside the cell. If you think of the cell as a human body, the cytoplasm would play the part of the blood, allowing transportation within the cell.

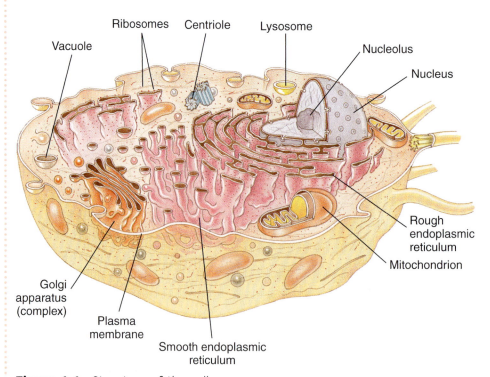

**Figure 1-1** Structure of the cell

# Organelles

**Organelles** are small structures within the cell that each have their own function. You can think of organelles as being miniature body organs in the cell. For many years, scientists did not know about the existence of organelles. But as science progressed, these super-small structures were discovered.

Inside the cell cytoplasm, there is a structure that is formed like a maze, sort of like a house of mirrors at a carnival. This maze is called the **endoplasmic reticulum**. This network of material forms little canals within the cytoplasm that allow substances and other organelles to move around. Think of the endoplasmic reticulum as blood vessels within the body.

The **mitochondria** are the "lungs" and the "digestive system" of the cell. The mitochondria can be thought of as the cell's nutritionist. They convert oxygen and nutrients so that they can be used as energy by the cell. The mitochondria are also responsible for converting oxygen to carbon dioxide, which is an essential part of the oxygen usage system within the body. The mitochondria have "departments" that also control the amount of water and other substances that are allowed into the cytoplasm at particular times. As a "digestive factory" they help to break down simple sugars, fats, and parts of proteins called **amino acids**. Mitochondria take nutrients such as proteins, fats, and carbohydrates and manufacture a substance called **adenosine triphosphate**, better known as **ATP**. You can think of ATP as a ready-to-use energy packet that can be used by any organelle in the cell. Some skin treatments have been shown to increase production of ATP, making skin healthier. These will be discussed later in this book. The **Golgi apparatus** is a storage mechanism that helps store proteins for later conversion to manufacture other necessary chemicals when the cell needs them. Think of the Golgi apparatus as a tiny "silo" storing fuels for a future date.

**Ribosomes** are very small organelles that help build protein structures that the cell needs. They are the protein "construction division" of the cell.

**Lysosomes** are the "demolition crew" of the cell. They manufacture enzymes that help break apart large molecules entering the cell so that they can be more easily converted to other necessary chemicals and substances. Lysosomes also are the "self-destruct" mechanism for the cell. When a cell dies, the lysosome releases enzymes that help destroy the cell membrane.

**Vacuoles** are often one of the biggest organelles. They are the "storage vats" for waste and excess food supplies.

## A DAY IN THE LIFE OF A CELL

Let's go through an oversimplified yet representative "day in the life of a cell." The blood cells deliver foods for the cells that have already been substantially broken down by the digestive system, absorbed through the intestinal wall, and absorbed by the blood. The blood also delivers fresh oxygen from the lungs. First the cell membrane acts as a "guard," allowing certain substances into the cytoplasm. Once inside, they may be guided to their destination by the canals of the endoplasmic reticulum. The lysosomes start breaking down the large protein molecules. The ribosomes are building or "rebuilding" the proteins that the cell needs at the time. The mitochondria serve as a "power plant" making usable energy for the cell from the variety of proteins, sugars, oxygen, and fats that have arrived. Excess food product and waste from production are stored in the vacuoles. The Golgi apparatus stores proteins to use later for manufacturing enzymes and hormones. After production is over, waste materials and carbon dioxide are released by the cell membranes to the blood. The blood takes the waste away to the lungs, where the carbon dioxide is breathed out, and to the kidneys, which filter out the other waste.

**Organelles** are small structures within the cell that have their own function.

**Endoplasmic reticulum** is a structure inside cells that is formed like a maze. This network of material forms little canals within the cytoplasm that allows substances and other organelles to move around.

**Mitochrondria** are the "lungs" and "digestive system" of the cell.

**Amino acids** are proteins that help break down simple sugars, fats, and parts of proteins.

**Adenosine triphosphate**, also known as ATP, is a substance produced in the mitochondria as an energy source for the cell.

**Golgi apparatus** is a storage mechanism that helps store proteins for later conversion to manufacture other necessary chemicals when the cell needs them.

**Ribosomes** are very small organelles that help build protein structures that the cell needs.

**Lysosomes** manufacture enzymes that help break apart large molecules entering the cell so that they can be more easily converted to other necessary chemicals and substances.

**Vacuoles** are the "storage vats" for waste and excess food supplies.

## THE NUCLEUS

We have discussed some of the respiratory, digestive, and synthesis functions of the cell. But what controls these many functions? Where is the "brain" of the cell? Centered in the cytoplasm is a large structure called the **nucleus**. The nucleus of the cell is made largely of protein and is also responsible for building certain proteins. It contains fibers called **chromatin**. Chromatin is largely responsible for cell division, which will be discussed later. The chromatin is made of a mixture of protein and special chemicals called **nucleic acids**. The most important of these acids is deoxyribonucleic acid, better known as DNA. DNA is a long, spiral-shaped molecule that looks like a twisted ladder. The DNA has the power to duplicate itself, and within it are the "directions" for running the cell operations. Therefore, it may pass on instructions to new cells as it duplicates, ensuring that each type of cell will know the "blueprint" for life.

Cells divide and reproduce by a process known as mitotic division, or **mitosis**. Hereditary traits for the cell are found in small structures in the DNA called **genes**. When the cell divides, the chromatin fibers line up and are seen as **chromosomes**. The entire "blueprint" is duplicated in the DNA, and the cell splits into two separate cells, both containing the exact same DNA, and genes (Figure 1-2). By this process cells are constantly reproducing themselves, carrying out the same functions.

## CELL SPECIALIZATION

Many types of cells are found within the human body. Groups of cells that perform the same function are called **tissues**. There are many different types of tissue.

**Nucleus** of the cell is made largely of protein and is also responsible for building certain proteins.

**Chromatin** is largely responsible for cell division.

**Nucleic acids** are a mixture of protein and special chemicals that make up chromatin.

**Mitosis** is the division and reproduction of cells.

**Genes** are small structures that contain hereditary traits.

**Chromosomes** are chromatin fibers.

**Tissues** are groups of cells that perform the same function.

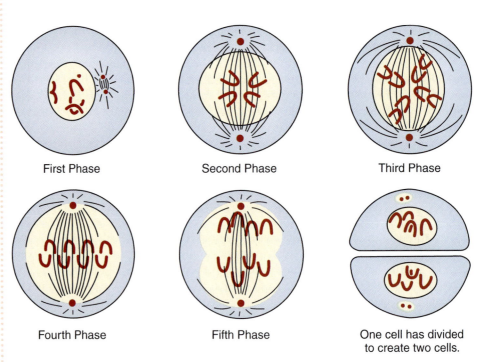

First Phase       Second Phase       Third Phase

Fourth Phase       Fifth Phase       One cell has divided
to create two cells.

**Figure 1-2**  Indirect division of the human cell.
First phase—Chromosomes begin to line up in the center of cell.
Second phase—Chromosomes duplicate themselves.
Third phase—New structures begin migrating to opposite ends of the cell.
Fourth phase—Nucleus of the cell begins dividing.
Fifth phase—Nucleus breaks into two identical nuclei.
Sixth phase—Cell forms two identical cells.

**Muscular tissue** is of three types, which include visceral muscle, skeletal muscle, and cardiac muscle.

**Visceral muscle** is responsible for involuntary muscle actions. Involuntary muscle actions are movements that happen subconsciously. Movement of the lungs expanding and contracting, muscles of the intestines, and muscles of the digestive system are involuntary muscles. In other words, these muscle structures operate on "automatic pilot." Involuntary muscles are also known as smooth muscle tissue.

**Skeletal muscles** are responsible for the movement of the bones and the body's physical motion. Because these muscle cells have stripes, or **striations**, they are also known as striated muscles. Skeletal muscles are responsible for voluntary movement and therefore are known as voluntary muscles. These muscles are controlled by the conscious brain, which means the brain directly controls their movement. Walking across a room to pick up an object is a motion in which the brain has complete control and is an example of a voluntary muscle action.

**Cardiac muscle tissue** used to be considered an involuntary smooth muscle, but it has since been established that this tissue is also striated, so it is classified in a separate category. Cardiac muscle is both striated and involuntary.

**Connective tissue** is a group of cells that specialize in providing support and cushioning for the body. **Cartilage** and **ligaments** are examples of connective tissue. They help to connect bones to each other and bones to muscle. The ear and nose are made of cartilage.

**Skeletal tissue** makes up the bones in the body.

**Nerve tissues** are cells that control the brain and the nerves. Nerve cells transmit messages to all parts of the body. There are many types of nerve cells in the skin, which will be discussed later in this chapter. Think of the nerves as a long line of dominoes that possess the ability to transmit messages by touching one another. This "domino effect" enables the nerves to transport commands from the brain and information to the brain. Let's pretend that you accidentally touch a hot stove. The heat and pain nerve cells in the skin transmit the feeling up the body to the brain in a split second. The brain, in turn, sends a response in another split second, telling your arm muscles to immediately remove your hand from the hot stove.

**Liquid tissue** includes blood and lymph. The blood is responsible for carrying oxygen and food to all the cells in the body and for carrying waste and carbon dioxide away from the cells. Blood is mostly made of a substance called **plasma**. Plasma makes up the liquid part of the blood. Floating in the plasma are red blood cells, or **red corpuscles**, whose function is to complete oxygen–carbon dioxide transport to and from all the cells. The other main type of blood cells are white blood cells, or **white corpuscles**, which are largely responsible for defending the body against bacterial invasion. Much more about the white blood cells will be discussed in Chapter 3, The Immune System.

Lymph is a liquid that bathes all the tissues of the body and helps filter wastes from the bloodstream and the body. Filters in the lymph system are present in many areas of the body such as the armpits, groin, and neck. These filters are called **lymph nodes**. When you are sick, sometimes you will have swollen areas in your neck or other areas. This is because the lymph is filtering debris and dead bacteria from the body, attempting to rid the body of these wastes. The lymph nodes swell when they are filtering lots of debris.

**Adipose tissue** is fat tissue. Fat, although it has a bad reputation, contributes to many functions within the body. It helps cushion all the other types of tissue. Imagine sitting on a sofa that had no cushions. It would be very hard and would break more easily if it was dropped or damaged. Fat helps the body in the same way, helping to soften injuries and protect the organs. Fat also is needed to produce hormones and other chemicals necessary for life.

**Endothelial tissue** refers to inner tissues that line the walls of the intestines, lungs, and other internal organs.

**Muscular tissue** is of three types, which include visceral muscle, skeletal muscle, and cardiac muscle.

**Visceral muscle** is responsible for involuntary muscle actions.

**Skeletal muscles** are responsible for the movement of the bones and the body's physical motion.

**Striations** are stripes on skeletal muscles that control body movement. These muscles are known as striated muscles.

**Cardiac muscle tissue** is both striated and involuntary.

**Connective tissue** is a group of cells that specialize in providing support and cushioning for the body.

**Cartilage** is a type of tough connective tissue that helps form structures in the body.

**Ligaments** are connective tissues that connect the bones of the body.

**Skeletal tissue** makes up the bones of the body.

**Nerve tissue** is a group of cells that control the brain and nerves.

**Liquid tissue** includes blood and lymph.

**Plasma** makes up the liquid part of the blood.

**Red corpuscles** complete oxygen–carbon dioxide transport to and from the cells.

**White corpuscles** are responsible for defending the body against bacterial invasion.

**Lymph nodes** are filters in the lymph system.

**Adipose tissue** is fat tissue.

**Endothelial tissue** refers to inner tissues that line the walls of the intestines, lungs, and other internal organs.

**Epithelial tissue** refers to outer tissues that line the outer and exposed body surfaces.

**Subcutaneous layer** is the most internal layer of the skin.

**Lamellated corpuscles** are nerve endings in the subcutaneous skin layer.

**Dermis**, often called the "live layer of the skin," lies next to the subcutaneous skin layer.

**Papillary layer** is the upper part of the dermis.

**Dermal papillae** attach to the epidermis.

**Epidermis** is the outermost layer of the skin and is made up of five layers.

**Meissner's corpuscles** are nerves located in the papillary layer that are sensitive to firm touch.

**Reticular layer** is the lower, more internal area of the dermis.

**Collagen** are large, long-chain molecular proteins that lie on the top of the skin and bind water, also helping to prevent water loss.

**Elastin fibrils** intertwine throughout the reticular layer and give the skin firmness and elasticity.

**Epithelial tissue** refers to outer tissues that line the outer and exposed body surfaces. The skin is an example of epithelial tissue.

## PHYSIOLOGY OF THE SKIN

The skin is comprised of three major layers (Figure 1-3). The **subcutaneous layer** is the most internal layer of the skin. It contains large layers of fat to provide cushion for the internal organs, as previously discussed. Winding through the subcutaneous layer are blood vessels and lymph vessels, again insulated by fat tissue. The subcutaneous layer also contains nerve endings called **lamellated corpuscles**, which are responsive to pressure.

The **dermis** is the next layer toward the skin surface. The dermis is often called the "live" layer of the skin. The upper part of the dermis is called the **papillary layer**, containing the **dermal papillae**. Think of the dermal papilla as a "handlike" structure that attaches to the **epidermis**, the outermost of the three layers. The dermal papillae look like fingers "holding" the two layers together. Inside the papillae are many small blood vessels called capillaries, spiraling through the papillae. Also found in the papillary layer are some nerves sensitive to firm touch, called **Meissner's corpuscles**. These nerves sense deep touch. As an experiment, gently touch your hand. Next, exert more pressure on your hand. Doesn't it have a completely different feeling? This is because deeper nerves are stimulated when the skin is touched or pushed in a firmer manner.

The lower, more internal area of the dermis is called the **reticular layer**. The reticular layer contains a multitude of structures and activity. **Collagen** and **elastin fibrils** intertwine throughout the reticular layer. Both of these fibers are made of protein and are examples of connective tissue. They give the skin firmness and elasticity. Collagen is not flexible and gives skin its firmness and inability to stretch very much.

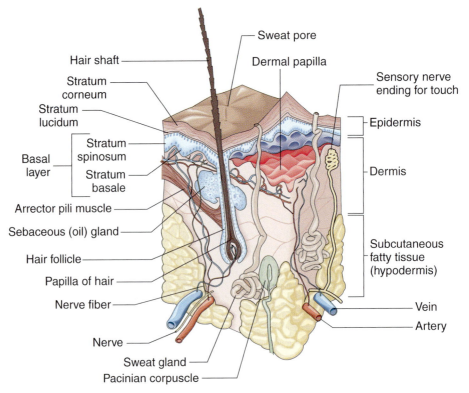

**Figure 1-3**  Histology of the skin, hair, and glands

Next to water, collagen is the most abundant substance in the skin. There are about 16 different types of collagen. The two types that are most important to the skin are Type I, which makes up most of the fibrils in the reticular dermis, and Type IV, which is present in the area between the dermis and the epidermis. Collagen is manufactured by **fibroblasts**, specialized cells that produce these long molecules of amino acids. Elastin is the fibrous structure that gives skin elasticity and the ability to "bounce back." The elastin and collagen fibrils are immersed in a jelly-like fluid called **ground substance**, which is made of **glycosaminoglycans (GAGs)**. Glycosaminoglycans are carbohydrate chains known as polysaccharides. One of these components very familiar to the esthetician is **hyaluronic acid**. Hyaluronic acid has a tremendous ability to bind water, holding up to 1,000 times its own weight in water. This gives more structure and stability to the dermis and cushions the fibrils, and the high water content allows for better communication between cells. Fat globules are also in this layer, as well as numerous blood vessels (arteries and veins), lymph vessels, and nerve endings that are sensitive to pain, heat, cold, and pressure. The base or bottom part of the hair follicle is also found in the reticular layer, as well as the **sudoriferous glands**, or sweat glands, and the **sebaceous (oil) glands**.

The sebaceous glands secrete an oily mixture of fatty materials known as **sebum**. Sebum's main functions are to protect the surface of the corneum against dehydration, and to provide an acid barrier against outside bacterial invasion.

The sudoriferous glands produce sweat. There are two kinds of sweat glands: the **apocrine glands** and the **eccrine glands**. The apocrine glands are present in the groin area and the armpits. They produce a thicker form of sweat and are basically responsible for producing the substance that, when in contact with bacteria, produces body odor.

The eccrine glands are abundant on the face and other parts of the body. They are present in extremely large numbers in the palms of the hands and the soles of the feet.

Sweat is a mixture of water, salt, urea, uric acid, ammonia, broken-down proteins (amino acids), simple sugars, and vitamins. Sweat is a function of the body that controls temperature. As sweat evaporates, it helps to cool the surface of the skin. Some wastes are excreted by sweat, but body temperature regulation is its major function. When looking through a microscope, eccrine glands take the form of a spiral tube, much like the inside of a refrigerator. Apocrine glands are branched, appearing more like blood vessels off a major artery.

**Fibroblasts** are specialized cells that produce collagen.

**Ground substance** is a jelly-like fluid in the dermis that cushions and helps with moisture retention.

**Glycosaminoglycans** are carbohydrate chains that help to bind water in the dermis.

**Hyaluronic acid** is a molecule that helps to bind water in the dermis. Also used in skin care products to bind water to the skin surface.

**Sudoriferous glands**, or sweat glands, are found in the reticular layer.

**Sebaceous (oil) glands** are found in the reticular layer.

**Sebum** is an oily substance secreted onto the skin surface by the sebaceous gland in the dermis that helps prevent dehydration of the corneum cells.

**Apocrine glands** are present in the groin area and armpits. They produce a thicker form of sweat and are responsible for producing the substance that, when in contact with bacteria, produces body odor.

**Eccrine glands** are sweat glands found in the face and other parts of the body.

## THE EPIDERMIS

The outermost major layer of the skin is known as the epidermis (Figure 1-4). This is the part of the skin the esthetician directly treats. The epidermis is located just above and is attached to the papillary dermis. This area is known as the **epidermal–dermal junction**.

The epidermis is very thin. To show how thin the epidermis is, think of a paper cut on your finger. A paper cut is a very shallow cut but deep enough to go through the epidermis. The reason we know this is that there are no blood vessels or nerve endings in the epidermis, and when you bleed or hurt from a paper cut, the cut has gone through to the papillary dermis, where there are nerve endings and small blood capillaries.

The epidermis is the layer of the skin that is constantly being replaced by new cells. Old cells shed off the skin in a process known as **desquamation**. The lower level cells are constantly dividing and pushing the old cells toward the skin surface, where they will shed. The cells are actually dying as they migrate toward the skin surface. Although the epidermis is mostly dead and dying cells, there is a tremendous amount of biochemical activity within this layer, and science is constantly realizing that many reactions within the epidermis influence how the dermis behaves.

**Epidermal–dermal junction** is where the epidermis and dermis are connected.

**Desquamation** is the process of dead cells shedding off the skin.

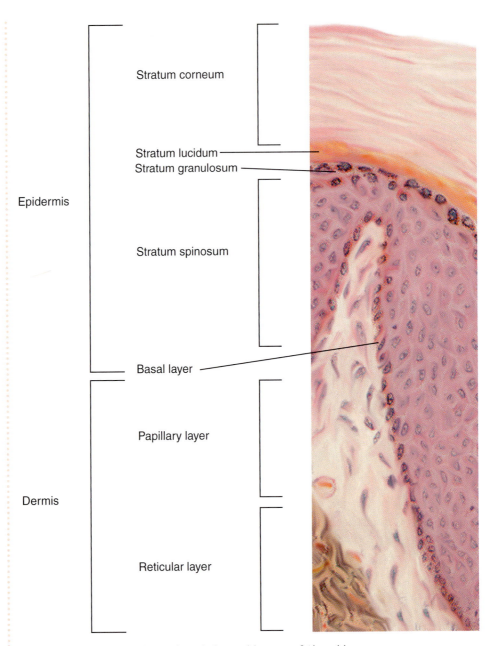

**Figure 1-4** The epidermal and dermal layers of the skin

**Strata** are skin layers.

**Basal cells** are the cells that make up the innermost layer of the epidermis, where the epidermal skin cells form.

**Basal layer** is the innermost layer of the epidermis.

**Keratin** is a protein that helps protect the skin against invasion.

**Lipids** are fats that occur naturally in the barrier function of the skin.

The epidermis is made of five basics layers, or **strata**. One layer is called a stratum.

The **basal cells** in the **basal layer**, formerly known as the germinative layer or stratum germinatavum, make up the innermost layer of the epidermis. The basal cells are the only truly live layer in the epidermis.

The basal cells are constantly dividing through mitosis, constantly pushing upward to the outside of the skin. As they divide and move toward the surface, the intercellular structures discussed earlier begin to change. They produce a protein called **keratin**, which is the "magic" that helps protect the skin against invasion. All of the cells in the epidermis are known as keratinocytes, which means cells full of keratin. As the cells change they also produce a variety of fats, or **lipids**, which help hold the keratinized cells together, much the way mortar holds a brick wall together.

Protein keratin synthesis begins in the basal layer, where fibrils of keratin begin to form out of the cytoplasm in the cell. As the cells move up from the basal layer, they start to form the next cellular layer, or **stratum**. The spiny layer, or **stratum spinosum**, is so called because the cells appear to have little spines or thorns on the outside of the cell membranes. In this layer, the cells change shape from cubelike to multisided.

The next layer is the **stratum granulosum**, or granular layer. The granular looking cells are filled with a substance called **keratohyalin**, which helps to form keratin from the microtubule structures first formed in the basal cell layer. Keratohyalin is produced by the endoplasmic reticulum, as previously discussed. The nuclei of the dying cells are breaking down, and the cell is dying. In the granular stage new lipids are formed, which will again help to serve as a medium or "mortar" for the outer cell layer.

It is this group of lipid substances that forms the "mortar" of the epidermis. They include triglycerides, sphingolipids, and glycolipids, also known as ceramides, cholesterol, phospholipids, waxes, and fatty acids.

The next layer of the skin is the **stratum lucidum**, or clear layer, so called because it appears lucid or clear on microscopic examination. It is filled with a substance called **eleidin**, which is produced from keratohyalin, and will eventually form keratin.

The outermost layer of the epidermis is called the **stratum corneum**, or "horny" layer, so called because the cells are piled up on top of one another in layers and have a horny appearance on the microscopic surface. Cells in this layer are referred to as **corneocytes**. In the "mortar" of the "bricks" in this layer are small structures called **lamellar bodies**. Lamellar bodies are thought to be produced during the stage of keratinization in the granular layer of the skin. Their function is to produce more lipids, which will serve to permit certain substances in and out of the corneum. In other words they will permit certain substances into the "mortar" of the cell layer and will allow certain gases and toxins produced by the skin to escape through the same pathway. The fats formed by the lamellar bodies serve almost the same purpose as the cell membrane discussed earlier. They possess the characteristic of selective permeability.

Let's take a minute to review the process of keratinization. The epidermis is divided into five layers:

1. The basal layer, which is a live layer, where the cells are dividing and constantly pushing upward. The melanocytes are also present in this layer. As cells drift upward through the five layers, they die. In the process of dying, they form keratin, a resilient protein that will eventually serve to protect the skin from invasion.

2. The spiny layer, where the shapes of the cells have changed.

3. The granular layer, where keratin continues to form and where fats that will make up the "mortar" begin to form.

4. The clear layer, where the process of keratinization continues.

5. Ultimately, the cells reach the top of the skin in the horny layer or stratum corneum, where they become the "bricks" in the outer, protective layer of skin. The cells are filled with keratin protein. The lamellar bodies are small "fat factories" and help produce "mortar" to seal between the cellular "bricks" but have the unique ability to allow certain substances in and out of the skin.

## SPECIALIZED CELLS AND PIGMENTATION

There are two types of specialized cells in the epidermis that should be discussed. One is the **Langerhans cell**, an immune "guard" cell that "patrols" the epidermis looking for foreign invaders. Much more on the immune system can be found in Chapter 3.

The second important specialized cell in the epidermis is the **melanocyte**. Melanocytes are cells that are the "pigment factories" for the skin. Melanocytes are

---

**Stratum** is a layer of the skin or epidermis.

**Stratum spinosum** is so called because the cells appear to have little spines or thorns on the outside of the membrane.

**Stratum granulosum** is the layer where cells are filled with keratohyalin, which helps form keratin.

**Keratohyalin** helps form keratin.

**Stratum lucidum**, or clear layer, is filled with a substance called eleidin.

**Eleidin** is a substance produced from keratohyalin and will eventually form keratin.

**Stratum corneum** is the outermost layer of the epidermis.

**Corneocytes** are cells of the stratum corneum.

**Lamellar bodies** are thought to be produced during the stage of keratinization in the granular layer of the skin. Their function is to produce lipids.

**Langerhans cell** is an immune cell that "patrols" the epidermis looking for foreign invaders.

**Melanocytes** are cells that are "pigment factories" for the skin.

located at the basal cell layer and also can be present in the upper papillary dermis (Figure 1-5). Different color skin types have the same number of melanocytes, but people of certain races and ethnic backgrounds simply carry genes that make the melanocytes produce more **melanin** or pigment. Sunlight, injuries to the skin, and hormones can stimulate melanin production.

**Melanin** is the pigment of the skin.

It is melanin that causes a tan to develop. The primary function of melanin is to shield and protect the skin from damaging sunrays or injury. It is the body putting up a "parasol" to deflect ultraviolet rays. Essentially a "healthy-looking" tan is actually an immune function, the body defending itself from something unhealthy!

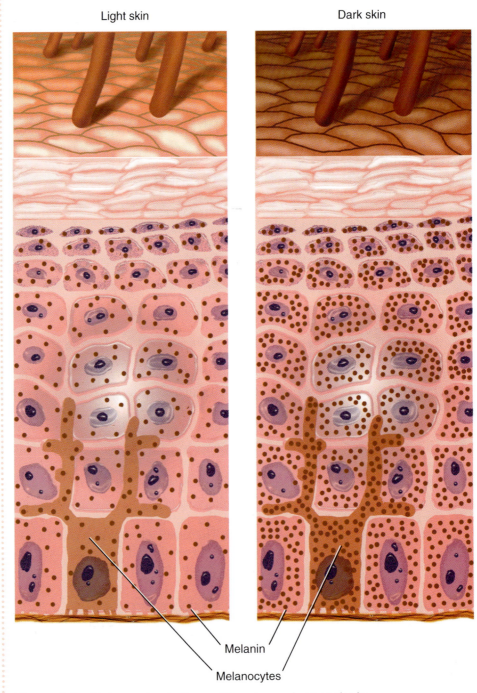

Light skin

Dark skin

Melanin

Melanocytes

**Figure 1-5** Melanocytes in the epidermis produce melanin

Melanocytes are **dendritic** cells, which means one end of the cell resembles a tree branch. The melanin is present in the **dendrites**, or branches. The melanocytes use their dendrites to "inject" melanin into the cells at the basal layer, and as they drift upward toward the surface, the cells are eventually shed from the surface through normal desquamation. This is what causes tans to fade and eventually disappear.

**Dendritic** describes cells that have one end with branches.

**Dendrites** are the branch-like structures on the end of certain cells, such as nerve cells and melanocytes.

## BARRIER FUNCTION OF THE SKIN

Dr. Peter Elias, a dermatologist at the University of California at San Francisco, created the "brick and mortar" concept of the skin. The cells are "bricks" and the lipids between the cells are the "mortar," forming a "brick wall" to the outside environment (Figure 1-6).

The **intercellular cement** or **interstitial lipid matrix** is the substance found between the cells in the epidermis, especially the stratum corneum. It is the "mortar between the bricks" and is referred to by scientists and dermatologists as the **barrier function** of the skin. The barrier function of the skin is an extremely important function to understand. It is responsible for binding water between the cells of the epidermis, helping the skin look smooth and firm, and maintaining the skin health. The barrier function lipids prevent **transepidermal water loss (TEWL)**, which dehydrates the skin surface, interferes with proper functioning of cells, and can lead to irritation or inflammation.

The barrier function also prevents irritants from entering the skin, helping the skin resist invasion by foreign objects or irritating substances or chemicals. A brick wall that is new has an even layer of mortar between the bricks. The top of the wall is even and smooth. The wall does not leak or allow rain or weather inside. An old or poorly maintained brick wall, however, is missing mortar, or the mortar is crumbling, allowing air inside the building to escape or rain or wind to enter the structure.

Keeping the barrier function healthy makes a huge difference in the way the skin looks and feels. If the lipid barrier is injured or damaged, it is said to be **impaired**. A skin with impaired barrier function looks dry, rough, and flaky. Wrinkles will be more apparent. The skin is irritated much easier than normal skin.

Let's look at an example. If your barrier function on the skin of your hand is healthy, you can get lemon juice on your hand and not feel anything. However, if your hands are chapped and rough, that lemon juice can burn and inflame the skin. The healthy barrier function stops the lemon juice from entering the epidermis. An impaired barrier function allows the lemon juice to enter between the cells, and the low pH of the lemon juice irritates nerve endings under the epidermis. If enough lemon juice gets through, redness can also appear as blood rushes to the scene with immune cells to check out the "invasion."

**Intercellular cement**, or **interstitial lipid matrix**, is the cushion of lipid substance between the cells of the corneum that keeps the skin from dehydrating and helps protect the skin from irritative substances.

**Barrier function** refers to the protective barrier furnished by the corneum and intercellular cement. This protects against dehydration of the epidermis and exposure to irritative substances.

**Transepidermal water loss (TEWL)** is the evaporation of excess intercellular water.

**Impaired** means there is damage in the barrier function of the skin.

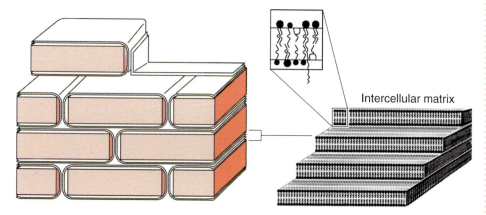

Intercellular matrix

**Figure 1-6**  The brick and mortar concept of the outermost layer of skin

**Petrolatum** is an occlusive agent that is used to prevent water loss and irritants from entering the skin.

**Natural moisturizing factors (NMFs)** is a group of substances produced in the interstitial layer that help to attract and retain moisture in the skin.

**Keratinization** is the process in which the epidermal cells fill with keratin protein as they approach the surface if the epidermis.

**Sodium PCA** is a humectant that helps to bind water in the epidermis.

**Sphingolipids**, also known as ceramides, are fatty substances that help hold water in the epidermis's barrier function.

**Glycosphingolipids**, also known as ceramides, are fatty substances that help hold water in the epidermis' barrier function.

**Fatty acids** are another component of the fatty materials in the barrier function.

**Triglycerides** are fatty materials that make up part of the barrier function.

**Cholesterol** is another component of the fatty materials in the barrier function.

**Transdermally** means to penetrate the epidermis and the dermis and then be absorbed in the bloodstream.

Another good example is the petroleum (**petrolatum**) jelly used on a baby's bottom. Petroleum jelly, in this case, is like a fake barrier function. The petrolatum prevents drying out of the skin and also prevents urine from irritating the baby's skin. The lipids that make up the barrier function are a variety of substances that help to both attract and retain moisture. These substances are known as **natural moisturizing factors (NMFs)**. NMFs are produced during the **keratinization** process as the cells fill with keratin on their way to the corneum. **Sodium PCA**, a strong humectant, **sphingolipids** and **glycosphingolipids** (also known as ceramides), **fatty acids**, **triglycerides**, and **cholesterol** are all components of the barrier function.

## SKIN PENETRATION

Not long ago, scientists and physicians believed that the skin was a barrier to almost everything. Now we know that a number of substances could indeed penetrate the skin. Drugs were developed that were absorbed **transdermally**, which means that these drugs penetrate the epidermis and the dermis and then are absorbed into the bloodstream. This discovery opened new pathways for many treatments, including treatment of heart irregularities and motion sickness, and now include nicotine and even hormone patches.

One of the first signs that the skin is more penetrable than first thought was an incident in which hexachlorophene, an antimicrobial, which at the time was available in an over-the-counter cleanser, was found to penetrate the skin readily and hence was taken off the over-the-counter market and is now only available by prescription.

A variety of tests have been developed to measure skin penetration of substances, using techniques involving dyes and substances that have been "labeled" with radioactive compounds. These radioactive substances can be measured in the tissue or the blood to determine the amount and level of penetration.

### Routes of Penetration

The investigation of skin penetration is still largely theoretical. Although we know that many substances can penetrate the skin to varying degrees, we know that many cannot. The issue of drug claims versus cosmetic claims influences the following few paragraphs. Please be careful with the claims you make for cosmetics. For more information on this issue, please read Chapter 12, Claims in Cosmetics.

It is generally accepted that there are four means of penetrating the skin (Figure 1-7). Certain substances can penetrate the skin through the following routes:

1. The hair follicle, which is essentially a hollow tube that begins with its opening at the epidermis and ends with its root in the dermis. It is theoretically possible that small enough substances could go into the hair follicle and end up a lot closer to the blood vessels because the hair follicle extends into the dermis. The inner walls of the follicle are lined with epidermal cells. The layers of the epidermis basically dip into the follicle. The problem here is that the space is relatively limited because the hair follicles occupy a relatively small proportion of the entire epidermis.

2. The sebaceous glands may also provide a pathway for certain substances. Many of these glands empty directly into the hair follicle; however, some of the apocrine glands may not be associated with a hair follicle.

3. The sudoriferous duct, which is relatively small compared with the size of a follicle (pore) opening, may provide a pathway.

4. The intercellular ("mortar") fluids are probably the best vehicle for penetration of the epidermis. Its surface area is large. But how do we penetrate the stacks of

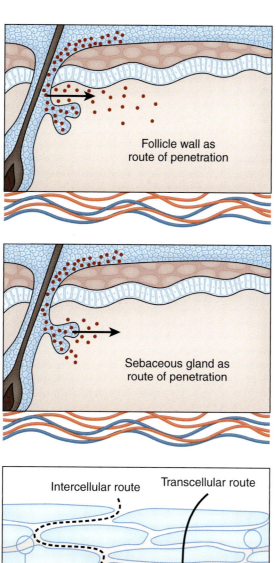

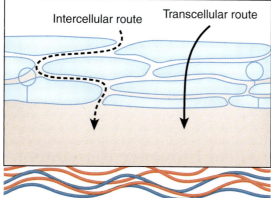

**Figure 1-7** Various routes of skin penetration: through the follicle wall, the sebaceous glands, and intercellular and transcellular routes.

keratinized corneocytes, which are impermeable to many substances? The fatty fluid holding the cells together is actually permeable by certain substances.

Remember that earlier in the chapter we discussed how cells migrate from the basal layer to the corneum. In this process they die and form keratin but also manufacture new lipids, along with the lamellar bodies that secrete more lipids into the intercellular cement.

These lipids in the intercellular cement will accept similar substances. In other words, theoretically, if we can make substances that are similar to the lipids in the intercellular cement, these substances may be readily accepted by the intercellular cement.

Other factors that affect skin penetration include the specific area where penetration is attempted. The order of permeability of various areas of the body are, in descending order: the genitals, head, trunk, and finally the arms and legs. So the face is generally more accepting of skin penetration than the back, and so forth. The forehead seems to be the most penetrable area of the skin on the face.

The size of the corneocytes may play an important role in penetration potential. The forehead's corneocytes are smaller than other areas on the face. The thickness of the stratum corneum may also be a factor. Another issue is the condition of the skin being treated. Torn or injured tissue, or skin that has a rash or abrasion, may be more easily penetrated. This is simply explained. Skin that is injured or suffering from a rash, eczema, or abrasion is said to have a **compromised** barrier function, which means that the barrier function is not working like it should because of the injury or disorder. A compromised barrier function will enable the skin to be more permeable by sometimes nondesirable materials such as allergens and irritants. Barrier function can be injured or decreased by exposure to detergents, acids, alkaline substances, keratolytics, or injuries. Even overexposure to an alphahydroxy acid could interfere with barrier function by exposing lipids to chemicals that loosen or dissolve the lipids within the intercellular fluids. The corneocytes are not as thick in such areas.

The size of the molecule being penetrated has a big effect on its permeability. Large proteins like collagen are not permeable. They are simply too big to go between the cells. However, smaller molecules with more affinity for lipids like sodium PCA (a humectant), retinoids, squalane, and fat-soluble vitamins such as vitamins A, D, and E seem to have good permeability. Some large molecules such as collagen do not need to penetrate the skin to be useful cosmetically. Collagen is a substantive, which means that it adheres readily to the surface of the corneum, helping to bind water and reduce water loss from within the epidermis. Cleansers, sunscreens, and makeup foundations are other examples of substances that should not be penetrated. They totally lose their cosmetic effectiveness at lower levels, assuming they could be penetrated at all. Keratolytics like salicylic acid need to stay on the surface because they work solely on the corneum; we do not want to dissolve other layers. However, for medicinal purposes, we would obviously want to penetrate the full epidermis in many cases. Cosmetically, moisturizers will work better and hold moisture for longer periods of time if they are able to penetrate deeper into the corneum.

## Other Factors That Influence Penetration

The thickness of the stratum corneum will obviously have an effect on skin permeability. If there is a large buildup of dead cells on the surface, penetration is hindered. When applying a moisturizer, for example, an excessively thick corneum will not absorb the moisturizer as well. The buildup of cells is usually dry and brittle, due to the large amount of keratin present within each cell, and will "grab" the moisture from the moisturizer. Therefore, the lower corneum is less likely to benefit from the moisture treatment.

Excessively oily skin will have a layer of excess sebum on the surface, further slowing penetration. Doctors often apply a strong solvent such as acetone before applying chemical peel solutions. This is to cut the excess sebum on the surface, so that the chemical peeling solution can better adhere to and affect the desired area. This, of course, is for a medical procedure and not recommended for salon services.

Temperature of the skin also influences its acceptance of preparations. Warm skin is generally more accepting. Heat causes activity within molecules, kind of "stirring up" the molecules in the intercellular cement and the cell activity itself.

---

**Compromised** is to be impaired or injured, not completely functional.

However, certain substances such as hydrocortisone are known to absorb better when cold compresses are applied to the area.

Wet skin is more receptive to penetration than dry skin. In addition, wet skin has water on the surface that can become trapped by moisturizers or other products applied over wet (damp) skin. This helps the skin increase its water content. This is why dermatologists tell patients to apply moisturizers immediately after a shower or bath.

## Salon Application Techniques for Good Absorption of Topical Preparations

Because some routes of penetration are more effective than others, some techniques can be used in the salon to get products to penetrate better. Moisturizing and conditioning treatments will be more effective if they can get deeper into the corneum.

## Preparing the Skin for Treatment

Cleansing the skin helps rid the surface of dirt, dust, pollutants, makeup, and excess secretions such as sweat and sebum. Some dead keratinocytes (corneal cells) are removed during basic cleansing.

Using toners, fresheners, and astringents helps to remove more excess sebum on the surface. Using these products both in the salon and at home will help to better prepare the surface for penetration of appropriate cosmetic treatment preparations.

The amount of alcohol, propylene glycol, and other solvents will have a direct effect on the amount of sebum removed. The oilier the skin is, the more solvent should be present in the toner. This process can work against us as well. For example, if you use a strong astringent on dry, dehydrated, thin, sensitive skin and then apply a treatment that is too strong, it can irritate the skin instead of helping it. In this type of incidence, the chemicals will dissolve part of the lipid barrier, reducing the barrier function. A toner for oily skin is often not appropriate for dry skin. Be careful to choose the appropriate cleanser and toner for the skin type you are treating.

Removing cellular buildup—for skin types with excess corneum the use of mechanical, enzyme, or cosmetic peeling or other exfoliating treatments—will help remove excess corneocytes. Removing these dead cells will help improve the appearance of the skin in four ways.

1. Removing these dead keratinized cells will immediately improve the skin's surface appearance, making it look smoother and clearer. Removing the cells that surround wrinkles will make wrinkles look less apparent. If you think of a wrinkle as a ditch, a mound of dead cells on either side of the ditch will make the ditch look deeper. Removing the mounds will reduce the space between the bottom of the wrinkle and the skin surface, making it look less obvious.

2. Makeup will apply more evenly to a smoother surface. Clients report that makeup applies much easier for up to two weeks after a good exfoliation.

3. Removal of the cells increases the cell turnover rate, stimulating the division of cells and the production of intercellular lipids, therefore improving the barrier function. The improved barrier function and increased intercellular lipids make the skin look healthier and smoother, with improved circulation and glow.

4. Removing the cells increases physical penetration of moisture treatments or other preparations applied after the exfoliation.

We must remember that too much exfoliation disturbs the barrier function, causing skin irritation and making the skin more susceptible to inflammation and irritation from topical substances, allergens, and the environment. It can also cause redness and scaling, and cause skin to look less smooth and less firm.

## Types of Exfoliation

Mechanical exfoliation means that the cells are mechanically removed by physically removing them from the skin. They are actually being "bumped" from the surface of the skin. Good examples of mechanical exfoliation are the use of a brushing machine or granulated scrub. "Peel-off" masks and drying preparations that are rubbed off are also good examples of mechanical exfoliation.

Enzyme treatment uses **proteolytic**, or protein dissolving, enzymes that actually dissolve the excess corneocyte buildup. Enzyme "peeling" is a common salon treatment that will be discussed in more detail in Chapter 21, Chemical Peeling and Exfoliation Procedures.

Chemical solvents and light chemical peeling are used to reduce excess corneocytes on the surface. Glycolic acid, resorcinol, salicylic acid, and lactic acid are chemicals used in this type of procedure, which will be discussed in more detail in Chapter 21.

Another relatively new mechanical exfoliation technique is **microdermabrasion**. This procedure uses **corundum**, or aluminum oxide crystals, to "sandblast" the skin. This procedure will be further discussed in Chapter 21.

## Increasing Physical Absorption of Moisture Treatments

Besides improving the surface permeability by the skin preparation techniques we have just discussed, using various techniques or tools to increase absorption can make penetration of treatment preparations more likely.

Massage stimulates the skin both physically and thermostatically, meaning that the heat generated by friction with the skin actually warms the surface as well as warms the preparation you are using. A good but gentle massage with the appropriate moisturizer will increase its penetration and effectiveness.

Use the knowledge you obtain in this book to help select the right preparation. Manufacturers now develop preparations that are more readily accepted by the lipids in the intercellular cement. Examples are lipid-containing moisture products and liposome treatments. Creams that are very heavy or greasy may be less permeable due to the large size of the molecules in their base formulations. Classic "massage creams,"

**Proteolytic** means protein dissolving.

**Microdermabrasion** uses a pump-driven machine to exfoliate the skin by propelling small particles onto the skin surface.

**Corundum** is an aluminum oxide crystal powder often used in microdermabrasion.

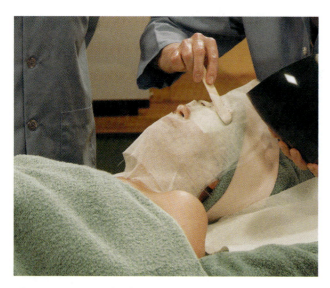
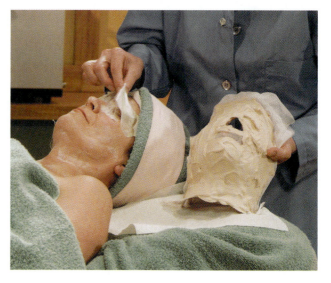

**Figure 1-8** Occlusive mask

usually based with petrolatum or mineral oil, are good examples of nonpermeable creams.

Use of heat and cold will increase cream penetration. Infrared lamps and infrared "skin irons" release heat, which aids absorption. Heat masks and paraffin treatments produce similar results. Warning! Do not use direct heat on sensitive skin; red, irritated skin; rosacea; or skin with enlarged or distended capillaries!

Cold penetration with cold "globes" may be more appropriate for sensitive skin. Globes are glass or plastic balls that contain cryogenic (extremely cold) liquids. You can cut irritation from globes by placing a large piece of gauze over the face after applying the treatment and before using the cold therapy. Cold globes are also very helpful in reducing redness and irritation.

**Occlusion** is the process of covering the skin with a heavy substance such as a mask (Figure 1-8). Applying a hydrating fluid, serum, or ampoule and then applying a mask will **occlude** the skin, forcing more penetration of the product. Occlusion also traps already existing moisture in the corneum. Examples of occlusive masks include alginate (seaweed type) "rubberized" masks and mineral masks that harden, such as plaster of paris.

**High-frequency treatment** releases heat deeper into the skin layers, helping to stimulate the skin and increase product absorption.

**Iontophoresis** or **ionization** uses electrical current to polarize preparations into the skin (Figure 1-9). Ions are repelled into the skin by use of galvanic current. See *Milady's Standard Comprehensive Training for Estheticians* for further instructions on machine usage.

Use of masks over creams restricts evaporation of the creams, therefore increasing penetration.

**Occlusion** means covering the skin with some sort of impermeable substance, which helps to improve moisturization of the skin and block moisture evaporation.

**Occlude** is the process of covering the skin with some sort of substance, helping to improve moisturization of the skin and block moisture evaporation.

**High-frequency treatment** releases heat deeper into the skin layers, helping to stimulate the skin and increase product absorption.

**Iontophoresis** uses electrical current to polarize preparations into the skin.

**Ionization** uses electrical current to polarize preparations into the skin.

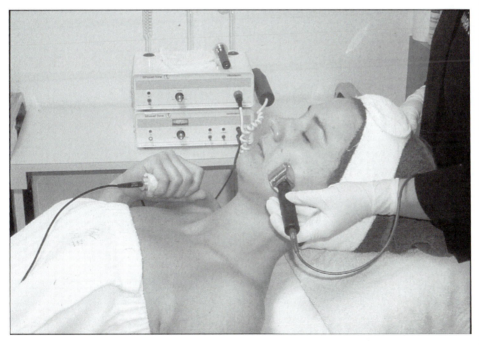

**Figure 1-9** The electrode on the client's face is the positive pole. The current flows to the negative pole in the client's hand. Positively charged, water-based materials are repelled by the positive pole and attracted to the negative pole, increasing absorption of material into the skin surface. Desincrustation, using negatively charged alkaline liquids, is performed by switching the electrodes—using negative on the face while the client holds the positive electrode. (Courtesy Mark Lees Skin Care, Inc.)

Warning! Some types of treatments should not be used with these penetration techniques and certain individuals are not good candidates for some of these techniques. Use common sense and follow manufacturers' instructions for all treatments, preparations, and devices.

## TOPICS FOR DISCUSSION

1. What is the function of the cell membrane?
2. What is selective permeability?
3. Why is the nucleus of the cell so important?
4. What is the difference between involuntary and voluntary muscles?
5. Discuss the three major layers of skin and the structures contained in each.
6. Discuss in detail methods for helping creams penetrate the skin better in the salon.
7. What is a receptor site?
8. What is barrier function and why is it important?
9. Why should estheticians be careful with exfoliation procedures?

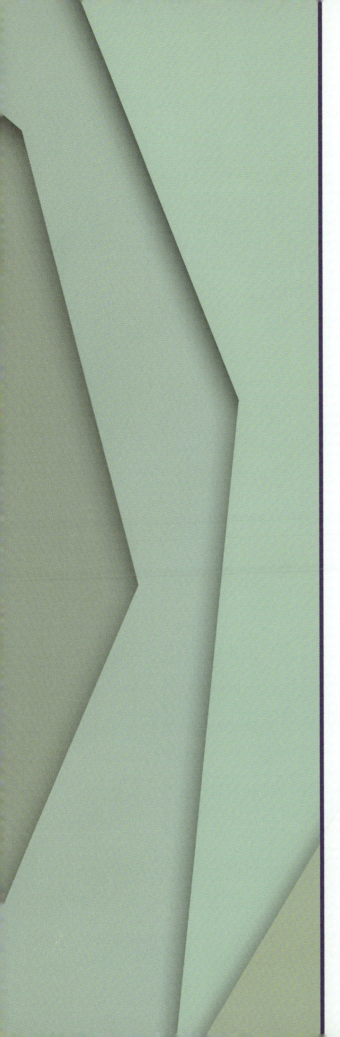

# CHAPTER 2

# Hygiene and Sterilization Techniques

## OBJECTIVES. . .

Sterilization, aseptic techniques, good hygiene, and disinfection methods are essential for every health and personal care practice. Esthetics is no exception. You will learn techniques for disinfecting many salon implements, as well as the importance of aseptic techniques. You will learn to protect yourself and your clients from exposure to pathogenic organisms.

Germs are microorganisms that literally cover almost every surface, including the skin of the human body. Because this is true, it is important that we learn how to control microorganisms through proper sanitation and sterilization.

Let's take a minute to review some of the various types of microorganisms. Bacteria are one-celled microorganisms. There are both **pathogenic** (disease-causing) and **nonpathogenic** (non-disease–producing) bacteria. In fact, our bodies need certain types of bacteria to help process foods. However, this chapter will not focus on "good guy" bacteria. We are concerned here about disease-producing, pathogenic bacteria (Figure 2-1).

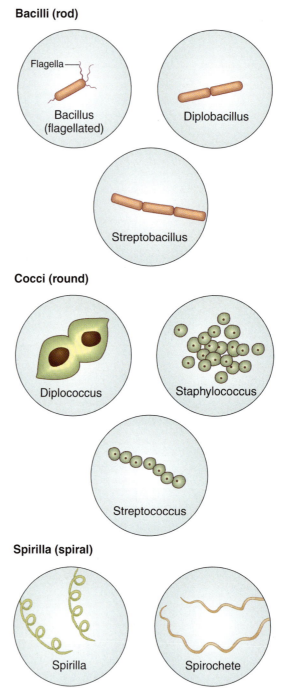

**Figure 2-1** Bacterial shapes

**Pathogenic** means disease-causing.

**Nonpathogenic** means non-disease–producing.

**Bacilli** are rod-shaped bacteria that cause a variety of diseases, including tuberculosis and tetanus.

**Cocci** are round bacteria that often occur in groups.

There are basically three types of bacteria:

1. **Bacilli** are rod-shaped bacteria that cause a variety of diseases. Among these diseases are tuberculosis and tetanus.

2. **Cocci** are round bacteria that often occur in groups. There are three types of cocci. Staphylococci grow in small groups. Pustules are an example of an infection caused by staphylococci. Staphylococci can produce various systemic infections, which are those that affect the entire body. Localized infections are

confined to one area. A pustule is an example of a localized infection. If an infection spreads into the bloodstream, then it is said to be systemic. Staphylococci infections are sometimes called staph ("staff") infections. Streptococci infections cause strep throat. They are another form of cocci. Diplococci, still another form of cocci, cause pneumonia.

3. **Spirilla** are a third form of bacteria. Spirilla are also called spirochetes. They are spiral in shape. Syphilis is probably the best known disease caused by spirilla.

> **Spirilla** are spiral in shape. Syphilis is the best known disease caused by spirilla.

Bacteria can be active or inactive. In their inactive stage, they form cocoon-like shells called spores. Spores are much harder to kill than active bacteria. This is important to know when we discuss sterilization later in the chapter.

**Viruses** are another form of microorganism. Viruses are not really cells, in that they do not have membranes. They are more like pieces of DNA proteins and are very small.

There are various types of fungi. Mold and mildew are examples of fungi. Fungal infections in humans are known as **mycoses**. Many, many illnesses are caused by microorganisms. The variety of bacteria, viruses, and fungi, and the various diseases they can cause, is much too extensive to discuss in this book. We touch on the basics in order to understand the importance of hygiene and sterilization.

> **Mycoses** are fungal infections.

## STERILIZATION

**Sterilization** is the process of killing all microorganisms, including good and bad ones. Sterilization also kills spores—bacteria that are in their inactive stage.

True sterilization is performed by a process called autoclaving. An **autoclave** is a machine that sterilizes equipment, utensils, and other materials through a combination of steam heat and pressure. It works similarly to a pressure cooker. Microorganisms cannot survive in an autoclave (Figure 2-2).

Autoclaves have a large metal chamber in which can be placed metal surgical instruments, sponges, gauze, and other materials. After the chamber is filled with the materials to be sterilized, a heavy-duty door is shut, locking and forming an air-tight seal.

> **Sterilization** is the process of killing all microorganisms, including good and bad ones. Sterilization also kills spores—bacteria that are in their inactive phase.
>
> **Autoclave** is a machine that sterilizes equipment, utensils, and other materials through a combination of steam heat and pressure.

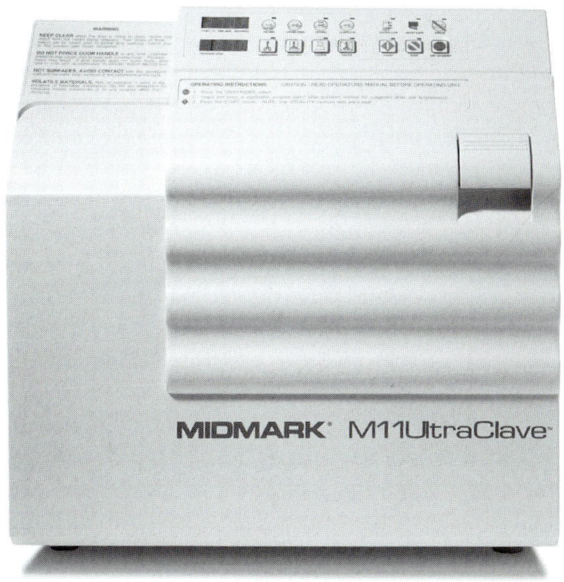

**Figure 2-2** Example of an autoclave

The autoclave then heats up, at the same time building pressure inside the chamber. The temperature of the heat goes above the boiling point of 212°F. Articles are sterile when they have been exposed to very high heat (usually about 260°) and sufficient pressure has built up inside the autoclave. Once the autoclave has reached a sufficient temperature and pressure, materials are left to sterilize for about 20 minutes. The autoclave is then vented, allowing the pressure and temperature to drop. The pressure is so high that it is impossible to open an autoclave during the sterilization cycle.

Items placed in the autoclave are placed in sealed special plastic or paper envelopes so they remain sterile once the autoclave has completed sterilizing. It is important to read the manufacturer's instructions well before operating an autoclave, because different manufacturers will have different instructions for sterilizing procedures.

Some materials cannot be autoclaved. Glass, for example, cannot withstand the high pressure. Check manufacturers' instructions to see what items cannot be autoclaved.

An autoclave is a very important tool for the esthetician as well as any other personal care or health care professional. In this age of AIDS, it is very important to protect your clients and yourself from exposure to any pathogenic microorganisms. The AIDS epidemic brought great attention to sterilization procedures. However, the AIDS virus is relatively easy to kill through sterilization. Hepatitis viruses, tuberculosis bacteria, and other microorganisms actually pose a much greater health risk in terms of sterilization procedures.

**Disinfection** is the process of killing the majority of pathogenic microorganisms. Disinfection is the general procedure that is usually followed in the cosmetology industry. Because we do not perform **invasive procedures**, or procedures that enter the body, we do not have to concern ourselves with the types of sterilization that are used in hospitals. However, we do perform procedures such as extraction, waxing, and tweezing that sometimes expose blood on the surface of the skin. Because of this exposure to blood, we must be very careful to use excellent hygiene and sterile or disinfected materials.

**Disinfectants** are chemicals that kill pathogenic microorganisms. The most popular disinfectant chemical used in the cosmetology industry is quaternary ammonia. Seventy percent isopropyl alcohol is another commonly used disinfectant for surface disinfecting.

Disinfectants are also used in maintenance, such as disinfectant floor detergents and aerosol sprays, to kill bacteria in the air and control the odors they cause.

**Antiseptics** are a weaker form of disinfectant. They are usually mild enough to use on the skin. Hydrogen peroxide and other first-aid chemicals are examples of antiseptics.

**Aseptic procedure** is the term scientists use to describe proper handling techniques of sterilized and disinfected equipment. Placing a sterile comedone extractor on a dirty towel is a violation of aseptic procedure. Handling sterile equipment with other sterile materials is good aseptic procedure.

Theoretically, nothing is completely sterile once a seal has been broken on an envelope of an autoclaved utensil. Because bacteria, viruses, and other microorganisms are in the air, they land on the sterile equipment. But we cannot sterilize a building or a room, so we must do the next best thing in handling disinfected and sterile equipment with the best hygienic techniques possible.

Some hospital disinfectants are somewhat stronger than quaternary ammonia and are being used more frequently in salons, particularly in esthetics and electrolysis practices.

Popular stronger disinfectants are glutaraldehyde, formaldehyde solutions, benzalkonium chloride, and sodium hypochlorite (household bleach). These types of

---

**Disinfection** is the process of killing the majority of pathogenic microorganisms.

**Invasive procedures** are procedures that enter the body.

**Disinfectants** are chemicals that kill pathogenic microorganisms.

**Antiseptics** are a weaker form of disinfectant. They are usually mild enough to use on the skin.

**Aseptic procedure** is the term scientists use to describe proper handling techniques of sterilized and disinfected equipment.

disinfectants are very strong. If they are not thoroughly removed by lots of rinsing, the residue can cause allergic and irritating reactions to the skin.

Glutaraldehyde solutions are excellent for disinfecting mask brushes, metal instruments such as tweezers, and other implements that cannot be autoclaved. Glutaraldehyde is available from medical and esthetic supply houses under a variety of trade names.

Glutaraldehyde often comes in concentrated form. It is mixed with water to form a solution that is potent in killing many microorganisms for three weeks. Read the label well and follow all manufacturer's instructions. Household bleach can be diluted 1:10 with water and serves as a good disinfectant for many articles. Besides being used for laundry, bleach can also be used to disinfect sponges and other linens. Do not use bleach to disinfect metal instruments. Chlorine is extremely corrosive to metals!

## DISPOSABLE MATERIALS

The best way to ensure aseptic procedure is to use disposable materials. These materials should be used once and discarded. There is no way to transfer microorganisms from one client to another if you are using disposable materials.

Popular disposable items include the following:

◆ cleansing pads made of sheet (roll) cotton
◆ disposable one-use lip brushes
◆ one-use mascara wands
◆ disposable eyeshadow sponges
◆ inexpensive cellulose sponges
◆ cotton swabs
◆ facial tissue
◆ wax strips
◆ disposable spatulas for wax or junior size tongue depressors
◆ paper towels and sheets

**Lancets should always be presterilized for one use and disposable. Never use a lancet more than once! Electrolysis needles and filaments are also available in disposable types.**

Disposables should be discarded in sealed plastic bags. Sharp items such as lancets and electrolysis needles should be disposed of in a "sharps box." A sharps box is a plastic box with a hole in the top in which you place used lancets and needles. The plastic box helps to prevent you or any other persons handling the refuse from accidentally injuring themselves with used lancets or needles. Even though blood is a rarity, it is best to protect everyone by using these precautions.

## NONDISPOSABLE ITEMS

Some items must be used more than once. Because of expense and practicality, items such as brush attachments, high-frequency electrodes, mask brushes, suction apparatuses, comedone extractors, and other items must be either sterilized or disinfected.

When cleaning utensils you must be careful not to cross-contaminate the utensils. Cross-contamination means that utensils are accidentally re-exposed to microorganisms during handling. Examples of cross-contamination are rinsing utensils in a non-disinfected bowl, handling clean brushes with dirty towels, and re-dipping used spatulas into the same jar of cream.

You must use extreme care not to ever contaminate any item used in treatment by touching it with something that is dirty or has been used on a client. The following are instructions for properly disinfecting implements, utensils, or equipment pieces.

Always wear disposable gloves when practicing disinfectant procedures.

## Disinfection of Brushes

Mask brushes should be autoclaved, if possible, but most brushes do not hold up well in the autoclave. The high temperature melts the glue that holds the brush together. In at least one state, the use of reusable mask brushes is against the sanitary code. Masks can also be applied with gloved hands or disposable spatulas. Soak brushes well in a disinfectant soap solution. The soak will help loosen mask materials from the brush. After soaking the brushes, put on a pair of gloves and rinse them well in a bowl. After they are thoroughly rinsed, place them in a solution of glutaraldehyde or other medical disinfectant. Let brushes soak for 20 minutes in the disinfectant. Remove them, rinsing well in a different rinsing bowl. It is best to label your rinsing bowls so that you don't rinse disinfected brushes in the soap-rinsing bowl. Remember to rinse very well so that you do not have disinfectant residue on the brushes. Store the disinfected brushes in a large jar until dry. After they are dry, they should be kept in a clean, closed container; a clean drawer; or a UV (ultraviolet) sanitizer.

UV sanitizers are good for storing clean, disinfected items. They kill some types of microorganisms with ultraviolet light. They do **not** sterilize. Utensils still must be disinfected before they are stored in a UV sanitizer.

Machine brushes should be washed well or soaked in a soap solution to remove all debris. They should then be soaked in a disinfectant solution, similar to mask brushes. Rinse machine brushes well and store in a clean, dry place.

High-frequency electrodes should be carefully cleaned with 70 percent isopropyl alcohol. After initial cleaning immerse the bulb part of the electrode (not the metal part) in a disinfectant solution for 20 minutes. Rinse the glass well with cool water, being very careful not to get the metal part of the electrode wet. Gently dry with a clean towel. Because high frequency treatment is performed after extraction, it is possible that small amounts of blood or bacteria may be present on a used electrode. You should have more than one electrode so that one may be used while another is being disinfected. Do not attempt to autoclave electrodes! Galvanic desincrustation attachments should be thoroughly cleaned with 70 percent isopropyl alcohol after each use. Using cotton covers over desincrustation attachments will also help to reduce contamination.

Iontophoresis rollers should be thoroughly cleaned with 70 percent isopropyl alcohol. The metal rollers can be detached and soaked in a disinfectant solution for 20 minutes. Follow manufacturer's directions for cleaning, because attachments may differ. Be careful not to immerse any electrical parts of the machine. Again, it is advisable to have additional machine attachments so that one can be used while another is being disinfected.

Suction attachments should be thoroughly cleaned with 70 percent isopropyl alcohol, then allowed to soak in a disinfectant solution for 20 minutes. Store in alcohol or in a clean, dry place.

Comedone extractors are very likely to contain small amounts of blood or debris after use. Clean them well with 70 percent alcohol. It is important to autoclave comedone extractors! If an autoclave is unavailable, soak the clean comedone extractor in a glutaraldehyde solution for 20 to 25 minutes. Rinse thoroughly. Never use an extractor on more than one person without sterilizing!

Tweezers should be cleaned well with 70 percent isopropyl alcohol after each use. Metal tweezers can be autoclaved or disinfected. Store tweezers in a bowl or jar with quaternary ammonia and rinse well before each use.

It cannot be stressed enough that it is important to have additional implements of all types available. It is also very important to be extremely systematic about cleansing and disinfecting all materials at all times. Your entire staff should be aware of salon sterilization procedures so that all staff members follow the same techniques and cross-contamination does not occur (Figure 2-3).

## Cleaning Sponges

Ideally, cleansing sponges should be used once and discarded. Many salons include the price of the sponges in the service and then give the used sponges to the client so that they may be used at home between salon treatments.

If disposable sponges are not a possibility, sponges should be washed in the washing machine with chlorine bleach. After washing they should be removed from

**COMMONLY USED DISINFECTANTS**

| Name | Form | Strength | How to Use |
|---|---|---|---|
| Quaternary Ammonium Compounds (Quats) | Liquid or tablet | 1:1000 solution | Immerse implements in solution for 20 or more minutes. |
| Formalin | Liquid | 25% solution | Immerse implements in solution for 10 or more minutes. |
| Formalin | Liquid | 10% solution | Immerse implements in solution for 20 or more minutes. |
| Alcohol | Liquid | 70% solution | Immerse implements or sanitize electrodes and sharp cutting edges 10 or more minutes. |

**COMMONLY USED ANTISEPTICS**

| Name | Form | Strength | Use |
|---|---|---|---|
| Boric Acid | White crystals | 2–5% solution | Cleanse the eyes. |
| Tincture of Iodine | Liquid | 2% solution | Cleanse cuts and wounds. |
| Hydrogen Peroxide | Liquid | 3–5% solution | Cleanse skin and minor cuts. |
| Ethyl or Grain Alcohol | Liquid | 60% solution | Cleanse hands, skin, and minute cuts. Not to be used if irritation is present. |
| Formalin | Liquid | 5% solution | Cleanse shampoo bowl, cabinet, etc. |
| Chloramine-T (Chlorazene; Chlorozol) | White crystals | ½% solution | Cleanse skin and hands, and for general use. |
| Sodium Hypochlorite (Javelle water; Zonite) | White crystals | ½% solution | Rinse the hands. |

Other approved disinfectants and antiseptics are being used in beauty salons. Consult your state board of cosmetology or your health department.

**Figure 2-3** Commonly used disinfectants and antiseptics

the washing machine and autoclaved. If an autoclave is not available, the following disinfecting procedure is recommended. Collect several dozen sponges after they have been washed in the washing machine. Place the sponges in a garment washing bag (the kind used for hosiery). Place the bag in the washing machine. Fill the washer with cold water and mix in about a gallon of household bleach. Allow the sponges to soak for 15 to 20 minutes in the bleach solution. Depending on the size of your washing machine, more or less bleach may be added. The bleach solution should be 1 part bleach to 10 parts cold water. After allowing sponges to soak for 15 to 20 minutes, put the washing machine on the rinse cycle. It may be necessary to run the sponges through two rinse cycles to remove all the bleach solution. The spin cycle will remove most of the water. Allow the sponges to dry in a clean place. It is best to store sponges in a UV sanitizer.

## GENERAL CLEANING

The facial room should be cleaned between clients. Utensils and equipment should be thoroughly disinfected. All towels and linens should be replaced between clients.

At the end of each day, the room should be very thoroughly cleaned.

The following are instructions for room "shut-down" procedures at the end of each day:

1. Put on a pair of latex gloves.
2. Remove all dirty laundry from the hamper. Spray the hamper with a disinfectant aerosol spray or wipe down with disinfectant. Mildew grows easily in hampers.
3. Remove all dirty spatulas, used brushes, and other utensils. Most of these should have been removed between clients during the day. Thoroughly disinfect all materials.
4. Wipe down all counters, the facial chair, machines, and other furniture with 70 percent isopropyl alcohol or other disinfectant. The magnifying lamp should be cleaned on both sides in the same manner.
5. Replenish the room with fresh linens, spatulas, utensils, and other supplies so it is ready for the next day.
6. Change disinfecting solution as necessary.
7. Maintain vaporizer as necessary.
8. Check the room for dirt or smudges on the walls, baseboards, or dust in corners or on air vents.
9. Vacuum and mop the room with a disinfectant.
10. Spray the air in the room with a disinfectant aerosol spray.
11. Replenish any empty jars. If you are reusing jars for dispensing creams from a bulk container, always use up the entire content of the small jar before replenishing. Never add cream to a partially used jar. Rinse the empty jar well with hot water and then disinfect with alcohol, rinsing thoroughly. Allow to dry before refilling the jar.

Following these procedures on a daily basis will serve three purposes:

◆ Your room will always be ready the next morning.
◆ Cleaning at night cuts down on the number of microorganisms that can breed overnight.
◆ Your room will always be spotless, making your clients confident and reassured that they are being treated in a hygienic environment.

## Laundry

Anyone handling dirty laundry should always wear thick rubber or latex gloves during the entire laundry procedure. Dirty lancets, sponges, and gauze may be contaminated and can accidentally get mixed in with the laundry. Sheets and towels should be washed well with chlorine bleach and immediately dried in the dryer. Headbands, turbans, smocks, and labcoats should also be washed in the same manner.

Linen service is an alternative to washing. Linen services are familiar with hospital sanitation procedures and are a good choice if you have little space in your salon.

## ABOUT OSHA

The **Occupational Safety and Health Administration (OSHA)** is a federal government agency, part of the Department of Labor, formed to help ensure that places of employment maintain a safe and healthy environment for employees.

Salons are expected to have a program in place to educate employees about possible hazards in the workplace. In the skin-care profession, we must educate employees about safe practices in sanitation and precautions to avoid possible exposure to chemicals, as well as precautions to avoid exposure to bodily fluids. Universal precautions for blood-borne pathogens include the use of protective equipment such as gloves, labcoats, and the proper disposal of used or contaminated tools such as lancets, waxing supplies, and other soiled or used implements.

Manufacturers of skin-care products are required to furnish **Material Safety Data Sheets (MSDS)**, which are special instruction sheets that describe safe concerns of products used in the skin-care practice. Data include how to safely clean up accidental spills and any special instructions regarding eye contact or accidental ingestion. Because skin-care products are designed to be applied to the skin, there are often very few, if any, precautions listed. Nevertheless, product manufacturers are required to furnish you with MSDS when requested.

MSDS are only necessary for professional products used in the salon. They are not necessary or required for retail products intended for home use.

In the skin-care salon, MSDS for antiseptics, germicides, disinfectants, and nail chemicals are probably the most important. Many of these types of chemicals are more dangerous if mishandled or accidentally spilled.

For more information on OSHA rules and precautions, contact the U.S. Department of Labor, Occupational Safety and Health Administration, 200 Constitution Ave. N.W., Washington, DC 20210. More information on this subject can also be found in *The Esthetician's Guide to Working with Physicians* by Susanne Warfield, available from Milady Publishing.

## PROTECTING YOU AND YOUR CLIENTS FROM DISEASE

Besides the many sanitation, disinfection, and sterilization procedures already discussed, it is important that you personally carry out personal sanitation procedures on a routine basis. You must be careful not to reuse disposable items or to contaminate your products by using a spatula more than once. To avoid cross-contamination while removing creams from jars, there are several good techniques to use:

1. Always remove creams from jars with a disinfected spatula. Use spatulas only once before discarding or disinfecting.

2. When removing creams from jars, remove enough for the entire service. It is better to remove too much product than to have to re-dip into a jar. If you need

**Occupational Safety and Health Administration (OSHA)** is a federal government agency, part of the Department of Labor, formed to help ensure that places of employment maintain a safe and healthy environment for employees.

**Material Safety Data Sheets (MSDS)** are special instruction sheets that describe safety concerns of products used in the skin-care practice.

more cream, use a fresh spatula. Place used spatulas in a soaking bowl for later cleaning and disinfecting. You should have at least six spatulas for each client you see per day.

3. It is a good idea to use small, disposable paper cups for dispensing creams. You may prepare measured portions of various products early in the day before clients arrive. Because you have measured the correct amount, this procedure eliminates all chances of contamination because you never touch a client's skin during preparation. Store cream portions wrapped in plastic wrap, or use small portion cups with plastic lids, like the kind used in restaurants for ketchup or sauces.

4. Pumps are another great idea, because they prevent contamination. Cleansers, fluids, and moisturizers can easily be dispensed from pumps. Squeeze bottles with flip-tops are another good type of dispenser. Using these types of dispensers also saves time in the treatment room.

5. Tubes or pumps are by far the most sanitary method for retail client use products. Your clients should also be instructed to use spatulas for jars at home. Using tubes or pumps eliminates this problem.

6. Wax should also be dispensed using one spatula per dip. Again, a larger amount of wax may be removed and placed in a paper cup for application.

## Use of Antiseptic Washes

Always wash your hands between clients with a good antiseptic soap or wash. Dispensers are the most sanitary method of accomplishing this. Bar soap is not appropriate because you touch and retouch the bar each time you wash your hands.

## Gloves

You absolutely must use latex gloves when performing waxing, or any service that might involve exposure to blood or body fluids. It is strongly suggested to use gloves from start to finish of all facial treatments, electrolysis, and waxing (Figure 2-4).

Gloves will protect your hands from exposure to many microorganisms. If you don't use gloves for the entire facial treatment, at least wear them during and after extraction, through the remainder of the treatment. If you have any cuts, abrasions, or irritations on your hands, you must use gloves at all times!

The best type of glove to use is latex examination gloves. They conform much better to the hands than vinyl or plastic gloves and are much more comfortable for both the esthetician and the client. Many estheticians think that gloves take away the "personal touch" from the client. The truth is that most clients think that gloves feel smoother than hands for massage, and they appreciate your efforts to use sanitary procedures.

Some people, however, are allergic to latex. It is important to have vinyl gloves on hand in case you have a client who is allergic to latex. The problem with vinyl gloves is that they generally are not as formfitting as latex gloves. Neoprene® gloves are made of a special synthetic polymer. These gloves fit like latex, but they are not latex. Latex gloves can also break down when used with many oils. If you use oils for massage, it is best to use vinyl or Neoprene® gloves.

Some gloves are powdered with talc or cornstarch for ease in putting on the gloves. Unfortunately, health care workers, including estheticians, often become allergic or develop contact dermatitis from glove powders. There are gloves available now that are completely powderless. Also be sure to purchase gloves that are the right size. Gloves that are too tight can rub and irritate the skin.

Gloves need not be sterile. Nonsterile, disposable, latex gloves usually are available in small, medium, and large sizes from a medical, dental, or esthetic supply house.

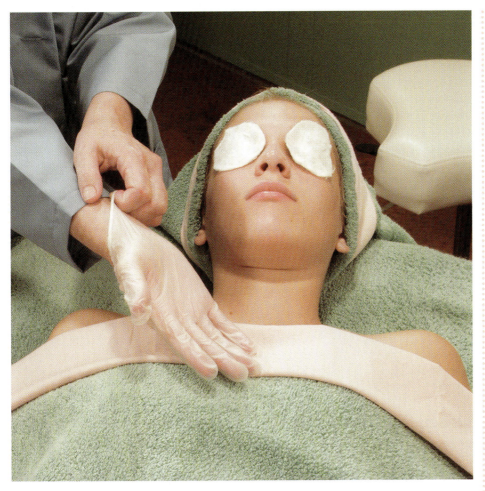

**Figure 2-4** It is important for estheticians to wear gloves during many procedures including facial treatments, extraction, waxing, and electrolysis

## Avoiding Cross-Contamination

**Contamination** means that a surface or substance has been exposed to microorganisms. **Cross-contamination** occurs when you touch a contaminated surface or substance and then touch a noncontaminated item. For example, if you touch the client's skin with your fingers and then get makeup out of a bottle by dumping it on your forefinger, you have cross-contaminated the makeup in the bottle. If you went to a party and someone took a potato chip, dipped it in dip, ate part of it, and then re-dipped it, that person cross-contaminated the dip. Don't be a "double-dipper"!

The solution would be to use a sanitized or disposable spatula to remove the makeup from the bottle and then place the makeup in a disposable plastic cup. You can re-dip into the disposable cup because it is going to be thrown away.

Another common source of cross-contamination in the salon is the use of bowls that have not been disinfected properly between clients. If you have a bowl of clean water and dip your hands in it after you touched the client, the bowl has been contaminated. You *must* disinfect all bowls between clients using a hospital-grade disinfectant, or you should autoclave the bowls. The best solution is to have a lot of wet sponges, so that you *never* have to rinse sponges, and use the same rinsed sponges on the same client. Also, *never* rinse sponges by placing them in a sink. Sinks are loaded with bacteria!

**Contamination** means that a surface or substance has been exposed to microorganisms.

**Cross-contamination** occurs when you touch a contaminated surface or substance and then touch a noncontaminated item.

## Techniques for Avoiding Blood Exposure during Treatment

Always begin extractions from the chin and work upward on the face. If you should encounter blood, gravity will pull the blood down the face and away from areas you will be extracting from next. While wearing gloves, try to avoid touching anything but the client's skin. Prepackaged, portioned products discussed earlier will help to prevent you from touching any bottles, jars, or other utensils while extracting.

Using a magnifying lamp during extraction helps protect your eyes from exposure to debris. Although masks and eye goggles are necessary for many health care workers, they are not necessary for estheticians. If you work with an assistant, the person should also wear gloves. Blood may accumulate under a mask in an acne treatment, for example. Wear gloves when removing masks or finishing the treatment. It is generally not necessary to wear gloves during makeup application unless you are working with a patient with acne or performing paramedical makeup on a client with open abrasions or incisions. Makeup brushes should also be washed and disinfected between uses. Makeup brushes are damaged much more easily during disinfection than are mask brushes. Be careful to use a mild disinfectant for makeup brushes.

When applying gloves, carefully slip your hand into the glove and then check the glove for any small tears or holes. Gloves with holes should be immediately discarded. To remove soiled gloves, grab a section of the cuff (the wrist part of the glove) and remove the glove, turning the glove inside out. Repeat with the other glove. Turning the gloves inside out will prevent accidental contact with the soiled part of the glove. Discard used gloves immediately.

## Other Diseases

Most states have cosmetology laws that prevent cosmetology professionals from working on clients with infectious diseases or on clients who have open sores suggestive of infectious disease. Taking a good client history on all new clients will help inform you of diseases that the client may have. Clients with infectious diseases such as conjunctivitis (pinkeye), impetigo, herpes infection, or other infectious diseases should not be worked on until a doctor certifies that they are well.

## IN CONCLUSION

The esthetician is at relatively little risk of infection with most microorganisms. However, it is important to take precautions to always avoid contact with blood or other body fluids. Always wear gloves and use the disinfection and sterilization procedures outlined in this chapter. Laws vary slightly from state to state. Make sure you are thoroughly acquainted with your state sanitation rules and laws regarding the practice of esthetics. Most important, use common sense. Always be aware of your professional hygiene techniques. Constantly practicing good techniques will become a habit.

## TOPICS FOR DISCUSSION

1. What is the difference between disinfection and sterilization?
2. What is an invasive procedure?
3. What is aseptic procedure?
4. Discuss various methods for disinfecting equipment and materials.
5. Discuss general cleaning procedures.

6. Why are gloves important?
7. Discuss the correct ways to put on and take off latex gloves.
8. Why is it important to have both latex and vinyl gloves?
9. What is OSHA and why is it important?
10. What is an MSDS?

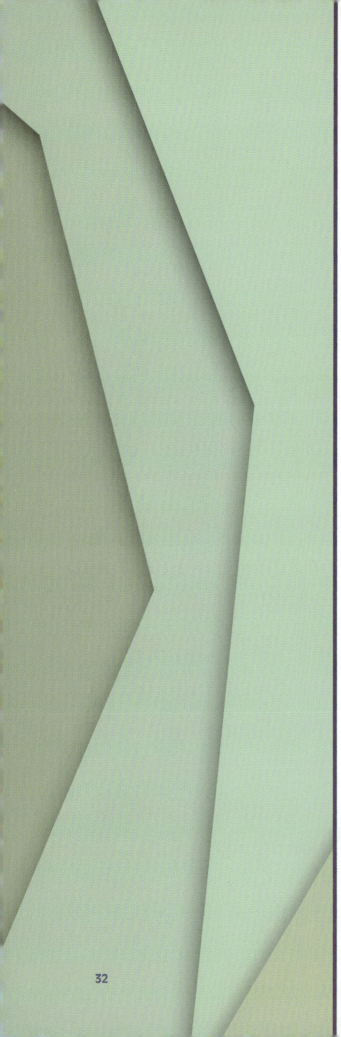

# CHAPTER 3

# The Immune System

## OBJECTIVES. . .

The body's immune system is a very complex system. It is the body's defense mechanism against disease and other invaders. This chapter describes how the immune system functions and some of the many reactions that take place in the body's fight against disease. You will learn the many immune functions of the skin and why the skin is one of the most important parts of the immune system.

The **immune system** is the body's mechanism for fighting disease. The immune system involves a complex series of specialized cells, the blood, the nervous system, organs, hormones, and many complex chemical reactions. When a person possesses the necessary substances and characteristics to avoid getting a disease, that person is said to be **immune** to that disease.

Let's suppose that your body is invaded by a pathogenic organism. A **pathogenic organism** is a type of bacteria, virus, or other one-celled organism that causes disease. This kind of bacteria is, of course, foreign material to the body. An **antigen** is a foreign substance that the body recognizes as foreign and therefore attempts to defend against. The body will produce a special kind of protein called an **antibody** that helps to neutralize foreign organisms entering the body. When you have already had chickenpox, you cannot get chickenpox again. This is because your body produced antibodies the first time you had the illness. When your body builds antibodies to diseases when you are sick, the process is called **acquired immunity**. In other words, you acquired immunity to a future illness of the same type that you did not have before you were ill.

**Natural immunity** is immunity to certain diseases that you have had since you were born. You obtain the antibodies for natural immunity from your mother's blood and your parents' genes before you are born. In Chapter 1, we mentioned white blood cells. White blood cells are largely responsible for fighting disease in the immune system. White blood cells are produced by the bone marrow, but also by the spleen, liver, and lymph nodes. There are 8,000 white blood cells per milliliter of blood. When the body has an infection, there may be up to 50,000 white blood cells per milliliter!

## COMPONENTS OF THE IMMUNE SYSTEM

There are two kinds of white blood cells. **Polymorphonuclear leukocytes** are referred to as **polymorphs**. Polymorphs are divided into three types: esoinophils, basophils, and neutrophils. Polymorphs attack bacteria and other pathogenic organisms in a process called **phagocytosis**. They surround foreign bodies and destroy them. They also help in disposing of **necrotic** (dead) tissue. Pus is largely comprised of defeated, dead polymorphs. You can understand this better if you think about a pimple. When acne bacteria take over a pore, polymorphs rush to the rescue. Some are killed by the bacteria and some die during the struggle. Their bodies are the main component of pus in the pustule.

A very large variety of white blood cells is called a **macrophage**. Macrophage means "large phagocyte." It acts as a guard, constantly patrolling the body looking for foreign invaders. Its cell membrane will surround and "swallow" bacteria. It is large enough to swallow and destroy even a hundred bacteria at a time. Macrophages can identify foreign bodies and determine that they are invaders and not part of the body's cells. In other words, they can tell the difference between the body's own cells and foreign invading organisms.

The other type of white blood cell is called the **lymphocyte**. Lymphocytes are produced by the lymph nodes, the spleen, and the thymus gland. The thymus gland is located under the breastbone in the chest. It secretes hormones and helps to trigger synthesis of more lymph tissue.

There are two types of lymphocytes. They are called B lymphocytes and T lymphocytes, also known as **B cells** and **T cells**. T cells are of three types. T-helper cells help alert the immune system. Think of T-helper cells as messengers. When a macrophage identifies a foreign organism, the T-helper cell runs to the lymph nodes, where another type of T cell, the T-killer cell, is waiting. T-killer cells are activated and rush to the invasion site of the foreign organism. The T-killer cells work to kill the organisms. After the battle is won, another type of T cell called T-suppressor cells stop the T-killer cells from fighting and signal them that the battle is over.

The T-helper cell also plays another role in the immune system. It signals the B cells, which are in the lymph nodes. The B cells make antibodies that are, as we discussed previously, proteins that help to prevent further infection or reoccurrence. Antibodies are also called **immunoglobulins**, called Igs by scientists. Igs float through the bloodstream and help protect against invasion by organisms they recognize.

Let's put all this information in perspective. Think of the body as a community. The immune system is the "fire department" (Figure 3-1). The macrophage is the fire

**Immune system** is the body's mechanism for fighting diseases.

**Immune** describes the body's defense against disease and inability to contract an illness due to excellent function of the immune system.

**Pathogenic organism** is a type of bacteria, virus, or other one-celled organism that causes disease.

**Antigen** refers to a foreign substance recognized by the immune system as an invader.

**Antibody** is a protein that helps to neutralize foreign organisms entering the body.

**Acquired immunity** is the process of building antibodies to disease when you are sick.

**Natural immunity** is immunity to certain diseases that you have had since you were born.

**Polymorphonuclear leukocytes** are white blood cells that attack bacteria and other pathogenic organisms.

**Polymorphs** are white blood cells that attack bacteria and other pathogenic organisms.

**Phagocytosis** is the process in which polymorphs attack bacteria and other pathogenic organisms.

**Necrotic** tissue is dead tissue.

**Macrophage** is a large type of white blood cells that act as a guard, constantly patrolling the body looking for foreign invaders.

**Lymphocyte** is produced in the lymph nodes, the spleen, and the thymus gland.

**B cells,** also called B lymphocytes, make antibodies that are proteins that help to prevent further infection or reoccurrence.

**T cells,** also called T lymphocytes, help alert the immune system.

**Immunoglobulins,** or Igs, are antibodies that protect against specific invaders.

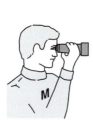
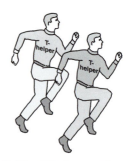

**1.** The macrophage spots a "fire" and signals the T-helper cells.

**2.** The T-helper cells run to the "fire department."

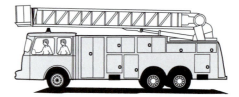

**3.** The T-killer cells rush to the scene of the "fire."

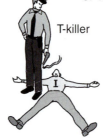
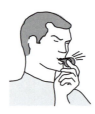
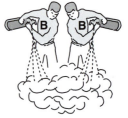

T-killer

**4.** The T-killer cells kill invading organisms.

**5.** T-suppressor cell "blows whistle" to let T-killer cells know that everything is under control.

**6.** B cells manufacture antibodies ("fireproofing"), helping to prevent another invasion.

**Figure 3-1** The Immune Fire Department

patrol unit, constantly looking for "fires" (foreign organisms). If it spots a "fire," it holds it and checks it out, making sure it is not a "false alarm." Once the macrophage has established that the organism is real, it signals the T-helper cells, who rush to the "fire station" to alert the T-killer cells, who are waiting to "slide down the pole." The T-killer cells rush to the scene, fiercely battling the "blaze" of foreign organisms, killing all the organisms. Watching the battle is the T-suppressor cell—sort of a lookout. When the "fire is out," the T-suppressor cells blow the whistle to let the T-killer cells know that the fire is under control. The T-helper cells have also alerted the B cells in the lymph nodes. The B cells start producing "fireproofing materials" (antibodies, Igs). The Igs serve as safety officers to make sure that this type of "fire" never starts again.

## HOW THE IMMUNE SYSTEM COMMUNICATES WITH ITSELF

In Chapter 1 we discussed how DNA replicates itself in cell division and how each cell is a self-contained life system connected to other cells, specialized into the different tissues.

The information contained in the DNA of each cell allows the cell to duplicate an exact copy of itself, passing on the instructions from one cell generation to the next. This is a unique code in each individual person.

Just as the DNA is coded, so is the surface of the cell membrane. Each cell membrane has on its surface special codes called **receptors**. Receptors are basically how cells communicate. Receptors can receive messages from other cells or other tissues. Hormones often communicate to cells via their receptors. Receptors inform T cells of what type of cell it is and that it is an "official" cell of the body and not an antigen (foreign body). The receptors on the cell membranes are made of special proteins. These proteins specifically fit similar protein structures on the surface of immune system cells, such as macrophages. It works like a lock and key (Figure 3-2). As long as the macrophage's "key" fits a cell's "lock," the macrophage recognizes the cell as part of the body's tissue. When the key does not fit, the macrophage starts the process of investigating the unidentified body.

The T cells communicate with each other by releasing a hormone-type substance called **interleukin**. Interleukin is present in the cytoplasm of T cells and is released as an alarm system when the T cell is alerted to a foreign body. It is sort of like a skunk spraying when it is disturbed. The other T cells receive a similar alarming message from the interleukin.

## ABOUT CANCER

Cancer is one of the most intriguing and destructive diseases. Cancer starts in one cell. The cell becomes deformed and then duplicates through mitosis, but the process of mitosis does not stop. The abnormal cell keeps dividing, creating more and more cancerous cells.

With the thousands of cell duplications happening constantly in our bodies, some cells become **mutated**, or changed, from time to time. They become deformed and are recognized as deformed by the immune system. The immune system will kill these cells. So it is theoretically probable that cancerous cells develop periodically but that these cells are usually killed by the immune system. However, when the immune system does not function properly, or when the cancerous cells divide too fast to be killed by the immune system, cancer, as we know it, develops.

Cancer cells can also "disguise" themselves. The T cells are trained to react to receptors on the cell membrane that help them distinguish body cells from foreign bodies. In a cancerous cell, the cell membrane is actually the same as the membrane of a normal body cell. The T cells cannot tell that the cell is cancerous. The T cell treats the cell as a normal cell, ignores it, and does not attack. Cancerous cells that have abnormalities in their cell membrane may be recognized as unusual, but normal cell membranes will indicate no problem to the immune system. Cancer is abnormal cells duplicating out of control. This is how cancer can spread so quickly. Spreading of cancer is called **metastasis**; the cancer is said to be metastasizing.

> **Receptors** inform T cells of what type of cell it is and that it is an "official" cell of the body and not an antigen.

> **Interleukin** is present in the cytoplasm of T cells and is released as an alarm system when the T cell is alerted to a foreign body.

> **Mutated** means changed.

> **Metastasis** is the spreading of cancer.

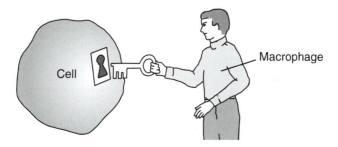

**Figure 3-2** Lock and key of the membrane

T cells, as we have already discussed, are produced by the thymus gland in the chest. The thymus gland is very productive early in life and then significantly reduces production. T cells, unlike other body cells, live for about 60 years, then start to die. This may explain why older people are more likely to get cancer and illnesses of any kind.

*Onco-* means "tumor," and *-ology* means "the study of." **Oncology** is the study of cancer. Physicians who specialize in the treatment of cancer are called **oncologists**.

**Oncology** is the study of cancer.

**Oncologists** are physicians who specialize in the treatment of cancer.

Let's review for a moment some things we learned in Chapter 1. In the nucleus of cells in our body lies the DNA. DNA contains instructions for running the cell. In the DNA are the genes, which determine our hereditary traits.

Among the genes are the **oncogenes**. Oncogenes play an important part in cell duplication. They help trigger the replication process. Everything is fine unless they get out of control. Scientists believe that oncogenes out of control may initiate the beginning of that one cancerous cell.

**Oncogenes** are specialized genes that regulate and trigger cell duplication.

## Cancer Causes

What specifically causes oncogenes to go out of control is not known. However, some substances are **carcinogenic**. Carcinogenic means "cancer-causing." Substances that are carcinogenic are called **carcinogens**. There are many well-known carcinogens. Let's start with the one discussed the most—smoking!

**Carcinogenic** means cancer-causing.

**Carcinogens** are substances that cause cancer.

Smoke insults the body like almost no other substance. Smoke is, of course, foreign to the body. So the body tries to get rid of it like any other foreign substance. The chemicals within smoke kill cells and contain more free radicals (defined later in this chapter) and poisons than almost any other substance. Exposure of the cells to these substances severely damages cells. The cells have to work hard to repair the tissue damaged by the chemicals. This hurried process to repair the cells in the tissues, along with possible aggravation of the oncogenes by the chemicals, may cause abnormal cell replication and therefore cancerous cells. Because the body is stressed by the repair process, the immune system is overworked during this rebuilding process. The "tired" immune system is less likely to react well to invaders. So one effect of smoking is that it decreases immune functions in the body.

Many other substances can contribute to "slowing" of the immune system. Excessive alcohol intake, illegal drug use, stress, improper diet, too much fat, lack of exercise, and many other factors can contribute to malfunctions of the immune system. Let's think about these factors individually.

Alcohol in excessive amounts can cause tremendous stress on all body systems. It is, in fact, a poison in significant quantities. Continual, repetitive damage is done day after day to the body of an alcoholic. Alcoholics also tend not to eat correctly, not to get enough sleep, and to cause themselves stress by creating problems for those around them.

Illegal drug use also damages the body. The effects are similar to that of alcohol. High stress levels, poor diet, and irritation to the tissues are all effects of drug use. Drug users also risk the danger of overdose, which often kills.

Stress insults every function of the body. Scientists and physicians are learning more and more about stress and its influence on disease. It is generally accepted that stress can be a factor in almost every disease. When the body is under stress, the immune system is overworked. **Immunosuppression** refers to the slowing of the immune system by any of the factors mentioned in this section.

**Immunosuppression** refers to the slowing of the immune system.

Improper diet robs the body of its fuel—the fuel it needs to carry out all the chemical reactions that take place in every single cell in the body. Imagine how you would feel if you were not able to eat for several days. The cells cannot function properly without proper nutrition. And the immune system is made of cells!

Too much fat in the diet causes a buildup of cholesterol and triglycerides in the blood vessels. This **plaque** obstructs blood flow. How do cells receive their food and oxygen? From the blood! If the "road" is blocked, the supplies cannot get through. And the cells of the immune system are on the delivery route.

Regular aerobic exercise such as walking, biking, aerobics, or swimming improve the oxygen transport system of the body. This means that the body gets more oxygen. Exercising regularly also can lower blood pressure, reduce cholesterol and triglycerides, and reduce stress. All of these factors we have just discussed involve one thing—common sense! Treat your body with respect and it will treat you with respect.

## FREE RADICALS

Anyone who reads health magazines has heard of free radicals. **Free radicals** are wild, unstable atoms or molecules. Often they are unstable oxygen atoms. Oxygen occurs in the atmosphere as $O_2$, or two oxygen atoms linked together. They are stable because they have a stable number of electrons in their outer orbit. (See Chapter 8, Essential Knowledge of Chemistry.) When a cell or a chemical reaction within the body needs an atom of oxygen, it takes one of the two atoms, leaving one unstable atom that no longer has the right number of electrons to be stable. This is a free radical, which, in this case, is also referred to as **singlet oxygen**.

It is the sole mission of every atom to become stable by obtaining enough electrons in their outer energy levels. (See Chapter 8.) So the unstable oxygen atom desperately looks for electrons to fill its outer energy orbital. One great source for electrons is fat. Fatty materials tend to have electrons that are easy to steal. Lipids and, more specifically, lipids within a cell membrane are easy targets. Singlet oxygen steals electrons from these fats to stabilize itself, but creates another free radical called **lipid peroxide**. Lipid peroxide can create yet another free radical called **hydroxyl radical**, one of the most aggressive and destructive free radicals. Different kinds of free radicals are known as **reactive oxygen species (ROS)**.

So what's the big deal about losing an electron or forming a new substance? Chemical reactions are very dependent on electron transfer, or trading electrons to form new compounds and reactions. So, if a substance or atom has the wrong number of electrons, this can easily interfere with proper chemical reactions and, therefore, proper body and cellular functioning.

Let's pretend there are three estheticians who work in the same salon: Deborah, Joanne, and Lisa. Each has her own room and her own equipment.

Deborah arrives at work at 8:45 and discovers that her steamer is broken. She looks into Joanne's room and sees that she is not there yet. So Deborah borrows Joanne's steamer for her 9:00 client.

Joanne arrives around 9:00 for her 9:20 appointment and discovers that her steamer has been taken. She looks into Lisa's room and sees that Lisa is not there yet, so she borrows Lisa's steamer.

Lisa arrives at 9:15 for her 9:30 appointment and discovers her steamer is missing. She looks into Deborah's room, whose client is now under a mask, and sneaks Deborah's (really Joanne's!) steamer out of the room.

And so goes the day! We have all known days like this, whether it is a broken steamer, or a series of clients late for their appointments. The point of this story is that the estheticians taking the steamers from each other's rooms work like free radicals stealing electrons from various other atoms. What would that day be like in the salon? Chaotic? Irritating? Free radicals do create havoc and chaos, and often real irritation, even it is not clearly visible. Irritation that does not have physical objective symptoms is called **subclinical inflammation**.

---

**Plaque** is a buildup of cholesterol and triglycerides in the blood vessels.

**Free radicals** are oxygen atoms that are unstable because they have lost an electron in their outer orbit. They are attracted to fats and lipids, which have extra electrons available to stabilize these oxygen atoms.

**Singlet oxygen** describes a very reactive single oxygenation, lacking the proper electrons for stability.

**Lipid peroxide** is a fat that has been attacked by singlet oxygen.

**Hydroxyl radical** is a very destructive form of free radical.

**Reactive oxygen species (ROS)** defines any type of molecule that is a free radical and contains a form of oxygen.

**Subclinical inflammation** is an irritation with no obvious physical symptoms.

DNA damage from free radicals can occur and is possibly a factor in skin cancer. It has also been suggested that hyperpigmentation is linked to free radicals. One of the biggest causes of free radicals is sun exposure.

Although free radical oxygen atoms are a by-product of many normal chemical reactions within the body, free radicals are also formed readily from smoking, alcohol, stress, and pollution. Whereas free radicals can affect all the body cells and are probably significantly responsible for the aging of the entire body, free radicals have a particularly strong effect on the skin. We will discuss treating and preventing free radical formation in future chapters.

## HOW MEDICINE HELPS THE IMMUNE SYSTEM

### Vaccines

**Vaccines** are an artificial way of tricking the immune system into making antibodies, or Igs. Vaccines introduce very small amounts of antigen (foreign organisms) into the body. Not enough of the organism is introduced to cause the body to become ill, but enough that it triggers the B cells to make immunoglobulins (Igs) to protect against whatever organism is being used in the vaccination process.

Sometimes the vaccination process will produce minor symptoms of the illness. You have probably heard of people getting slightly ill after receiving a flu vaccine. In cases where small amounts of the organisms are enough to trigger disease, doctors sometimes use dead viruses or irradiated organisms in vaccines. Irradiated organisms used in vaccines have been treated with some form of radiation before being used. They are still alive, but the radiation treatment renders the organisms unable to reproduce. These are sometimes called **modified live vaccines**.

Vaccines are available against a large variety of diseases, including polio, smallpox, measles, mumps, certain types of influenza (flu), and many other diseases.

### Antibiotics

**Antibiotics** are drugs that are made from extracts obtained from living organisms. Penicillin is probably the best known form of antibiotic. It is derived from a type of mold. Antibiotics do not produce long-term, or active, immunity. They simply kill the bacteria.

Science has yet to develop much effective treatment for viruses. Viruses are different from bacteria in that they do not have the same characteristics as one-celled organisms. Viruses are particles instead of cells. They do not have the same structure as a cell. They invade the body by "injecting" themselves into healthy cells. They reproduce in great numbers inside the body cell, eventually killing the cell. When the cell dies, the many viruses are released to invade other cells.

The immune system is our best protection against viruses. Scientists have developed immune system stimulants and synthetic immunoglobulins that may help the body's own immune system fight viruses. However, no drugs to kill viruses are yet available that are as effective as antibiotics against bacterial infections.

Sometimes antibiotics kill the wrong bacteria as well as the ones they were intended to kill. It is not unusual for someone taking antibiotics to have gastrointestinal disturbances while they are taking antibiotics. This is because the antibiotics also kill "good guy" bacteria while they are attacking the pathogenic organisms. Many bacteria present in our bodies help with necessary chemical reactions that happen within the body constantly. These "good guy" bacteria are referred to as flora. When these bacteria are killed by an antibiotic, normal body functioning may be affected.

**Vaccines** are an artificial way of tricking the immune system into making antibodies, or Igs.

**Modified live vaccines** are still alive, but radiation treatment renders the organisms unable to reproduce.

**Antibiotics** are drugs that are made from extracts obtained from living organisms that fight bacterial infections.

# THE IMMUNITY ROLE OF THE SKIN

The fact that the skin is the outer shield of the body makes it an immune barrier. Keratin in the corneocytes helps to protect the body against invasion by foreign bodies and organisms. The fact that the skin will resist being punctured by a needle illustrates this point. If you press your finger against the point of a needle, the skin will not be pierced unless pressure is applied to the needle.

Microorganisms are found all over the surface of the skin at all times. These organisms generally do not penetrate the skin because of the layers of corneocytes preventing absorption. The **acid mantle**, or the layer of lipids and sweat secretions on top of the skin, help kill many bacteria. What if we tear the skin or puncture it with that needle? When we puncture the skin, we break the barrier of the corneocytes and expose the broken skin and blood to the many microorganisms that are on the needle, as well as those on the surface of the skin.

**Acid mantle** is the layer of lipids and sweat secretions on top of the skin that help kill bacteria.

Diseases that cause breaks in the skin surface, such as eczema, acne, and dermatitis, make the skin more susceptible to invasion by microorganisms. Dermatitis is often accompanied by a secondary infection such as a fungus or bacteria.

The second possibility for passing the barrier of the corneum is through the routes of skin penetration we discussed earlier. It is physically possible for a microorganism to penetrate the skin through the intercellular fluids or cement that we discussed in Chapter 1. But this organism would have to penetrate the corneum, its layers of keratinized cells, the acid mantle, and the intercellular cement.

Let's suppose that a microorganism gets through the outer layer. The microorganism is first noticed by the **Langerhans cell**. Langerhans cells are "guard" cells that constantly patrol the epidermis. Langerhans cells look like spiders, because one end has many tentacle-like structures called **dendrites**. On the other end of the Langerhans cell is a pseudopod. **Pseudopod** means "false foot." The Langerhans cell is able to extend this oval-shaped foot to help it move.

**Langerhans cells** are "guard" cells that constantly patrol the epidermis.

**Dendrites** are tentacle-like structures on the end of some cells including nerves, melanocytes, and Langerhans cells.

**Pseudopod** means false foot.

When the Langerhans cell is stimulated by a foreign body, it breaks off a sample piece of the antigen. The Langerhans cell then presents the sample piece to the macrophage, which is present in the epidermis just under the Langerhans cell. The macrophage then identifies the antigen, and if it is indeed a pathogenic organism, it signals the T cells to the rescue.

The Langerhans cells are particularly sensitive to sun exposure. A moderate amount of sun exposure will knock them out of commission for a few days. Repeated sun exposure may knock them out of commission long enough for skin cancer cells to get a good start. With the Langerhans cells "on sick leave" from the sun exposure, the skin is left vulnerable to other microorganisms. This explains why many people get flares of herpes simplex (fever blisters) when they are exposed to the sun. This lack of immune protection may also have a domino effect on other parts of the immune system within other parts of the body.

For many years scientists thought that the epidermis was dead and had no chemical processes. Whereas keratinocytes are technically dead or dying, we now know that there are numerous functions and vital chemical reactions that are carried out in the epidermis.

The keratinocytes in the epidermis also help to secrete a number of important immune substances. The keratinocytes secrete a protein substance called apolipoprotein-E, apo-E for short. Apo-E helps transport cholesterol, which makes up a part of the intercellular cement. Keratinocytes also help to neutralize potential carcinogens and produce two different forms of interleukin, the hormone-like substance that helps immune cells communicate. The keratinocytes also produce another substance called granulocyte-macrophage colony-stimulating factor (GM-CSF), which helps promote replication of the macrophages in the granular layer of the epidermis. Last but not least, the keratinocytes produce a substance very similar to that produced by the thymus gland. These hormones help cause T cells to mature.

Also present in the epidermis are the Granstein cells, which are believed to play a part in suppressing immune function. It is theorized that the Granstein cells act similarly to T-suppressor cells in discontinuing actions of the immune system.

Cosmetic and medical scientists are now learning more and more about the function of the epidermal cells and how they may be manipulated by topical agents. It is now possible to stimulate lipid synthesis, speed up epidermal cell turnover, and send signals to the cells to perform other functions. Research of this type may be important to both the cosmetic and medical worlds because this type of treatment might help a number of problems ranging from wrinkles to wound healing.

## AUTOIMMUNE DISEASES

**Autoimmunity** is a condition in which the immune system cannot distinguish the difference between antigens and its own body cells. The immune system essentially starts attacking the body cells. A good example of an autoimmune response is what happens sometimes after an organ transplant. We have all heard about a kidney transplant patient who "rejected" the new kidney. The immune system sees the new kidney as a foreign body and works to attack and reject the new kidney.

Autoimmune diseases also cause rejection, but the person's own body cells are being rejected. In autoimmune diseases, it is theorized that the B cells produce antibodies in an out-of-control way. It has been theorized that the suppressor cells, for some reason, do not stop the B cells from producing antibodies. The antibodies produced that are responsible for attacking the body's cells are called **autoantibodies**.

There are many autoimmune diseases including **rheumatoid arthritis** and some forms of **psoriasis**, a disorder in which skin cells turn over too quickly. **Scleroderma** is another autoimmune skin disease that causes a thickening of skin tissue. Schleroderma actually means "hardening of the skin." The skin becomes thick and tight. Schleroderma severity varies with individual cases, but it can affect connective tissues throughout the body as well as internal organs.

**Lupus** is a disease that affects more than a half a million Americans, predominantly women. The word lupus means "wolf" in Latin because one of the major symptoms of lupus is a butterfly-shaped rash across the cheeks and nose that resembles the bite of a wolf across the face.

In patients with lupus, the immune system is producing too many antibodies, including antibodies to the body's own cells.

There are two main forms of lupus: systemic lupus erythematosus and discoid lupus. **Systemic lupus erythematosus**, also referred to as **SLE**, is the most severe form of lupus. SLE can affect the skin, joints, nervous system, and kidneys, and it may affect virtually any body tissue or organ. The severity of SLE varies greatly. Some patients with lupus have very mild symptoms, whereas others have almost chronic problems. Lupus symptoms, in many patients, can come and go. When someone is having a problem caused by lupus, they are said to be having a **lupus flare**. When the disease is not flared, the patient is said to be in **remission**.

The body is constantly cleaning itself of dead body cells. In SLE, the lymphocytes also produce antibodies to these dead cells. When the lymphatic and blood systems are still trying to rid the body of these dead cells, the antibodies produced by the malfunctioning immune system bind themselves to the dead cells, creating "traffic jams" in the blood vessels. Damage to the blood vessels results.

**Discoid lupus erythematosus (DLE)** is a form of lupus that primarily affects the skin. **Discoids** are hard, red round lesions that form around hair follicles and that appear mainly on the face, neck, scalp, and inside the ears (Figure 3-3). DLE, fortunately, generally does not affect internal organs, but about 10% of patients with DLE eventually develop a mild form of SLE.

---

**Autoimmunity** is a condition in which the immune system cannot distinguish the difference between antigens and its own body cells.

**Autoantibodies** are antibodies that attack the body's own cells.

**Rheumatoid arthritis** is an autoimmune disease that affects the joints in the body.

**Psoriasis** is an autoimmune disease that causes rapid desquamation of the skin, resulting in severe inflammation of the skin.

**Scleroderma** is an autoimmune disease that causes thickening of the skin.

**Systemic lupus erythematosus (SLE)**, commonly known as **lupus**, is an autoimmune disease that primarily affects the skin, the joints, the nervous system, and the kidneys.

**A lupus flare** occurs when someone is having a problem caused by his or her lupus.

**Remission** is a period of time when a disease stops being active.

**Discoid lupus erythematosus (DLE)** is a form of lupus that affects the skin, producing hard, round lesions.

**Discoids** are the hard, round lesions that form around hair follicles when a person has DLE.

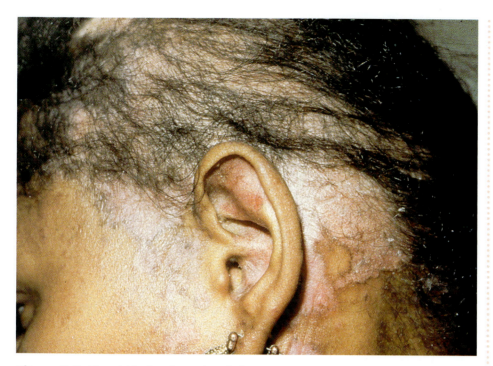

**Figure 3-3** Discoid lesion in systemic lupus (Courtesy Rube J. Pardo, M.D., Ph.D.)

## Causes of Lupus

There is no known cause or cure for lupus. However, lupus varies greatly in severity and can be managed with drug therapy, symptom relievers, and steroids. There also are new drugs available that help to calm the immune system. Doctors who manage patients with lupus are **rheumatologists**.

## Skin Problems Associated with Lupus

Sun exposure is a major problem for patients with lupus. Sun exposure, especially prolonged sun exposure, can cause flares. In fact, many patients with SLE are first diagnosed with lupus when experiencing a flare after a sunburn or prolonged sun exposure. It seems that the immune system in patients with lupus reacts violently to sun exposure.

Daily sunscreen protection is important for everyone, but it is even more important for patients with lupus. Daily use of an SPF-15 or higher broad-spectrum sunscreen is essential. Because patients with lupus tend to have more sensitive skin, choose a product that has been thoroughly irritancy tested. A sunscreen containing zinc oxide or titanium dioxide is generally a better choice because these agents reflect rather than absorb sunlight.

Generally speaking, treat the skin of the patient with lupus as you would sensitive skin, avoiding fragrances, stimulating ingredients, and common allergens.

Treating the skin during a flare may be risky. There have been incidences of skin reactions from procedures such as electrolysis, extraction, and waxing. Lupus is often treated with **corticosteroids**, drugs such as prednisone, to suppress the excessive immune responses. Patients using steroid drugs are more likely to react to these procedures, but there is no real rule, and some patients tolerate the procedures with no problem.

It is a good idea to check with the client's rheumatologist and have the doctor tell you what might need to be avoided in esthetic care of the patient with lupus. Many patients with lupus can really benefit from esthetic care because they require help in choosing products appropriate for their skin.

**Rheumatologists** are physicians that specialize in treating autoimmune diseases.

**Corticosteroids** are drugs used to suppress symptoms and the overactive immune system.

# TOPICS FOR DISCUSSION

1. What is the function of the immune system?
2. What is the difference between acquired and natural immunity?
3. Describe the process of the immune system functioning on a foreign body.
4. What are some factors that suppress the immune system?
5. Discuss the skin's immune function.
6. What is an autoimmune disease? What is one of the most prevalent autoimmune diseases the esthetician sees?
7. Explain why free radicals are bad for cells.

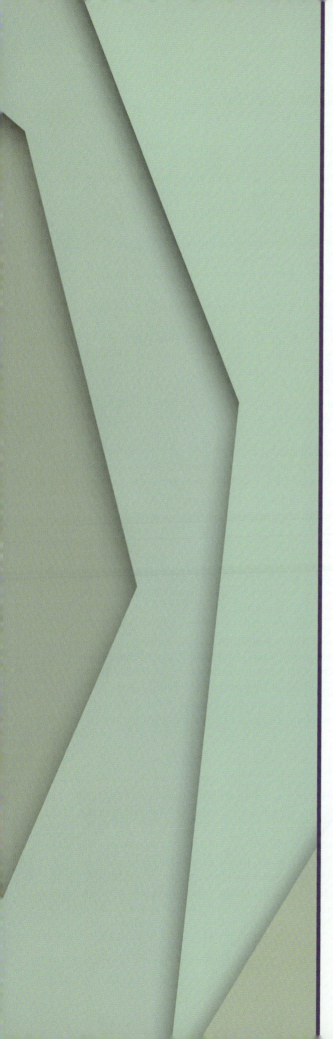

# AIDS and Communicable Diseases

## OBJECTIVES. . .

Because estheticians work with the public, they must be familiar with common diseases that are **communicable diseases**. Communicable diseases are diseases that can be transferred from one person to another. In this chapter, we will discuss common communicable diseases and ways you can prevent these diseases from affecting you or your clients.

Some of these diseases are not devastating and are easily curable. Others, such as AIDS (acquired immune deficiency syndrome) and hepatitis, can severely threaten the health and lives of persons they affect.

This chapter is intended to make you knowledgeable about these diseases, including how they are spread and how to prevent spreading them. Precautions you can take in the salon or clinic to help prevent the spread of these diseases are explained. It is also intended to enable you to talk to clients intelligently about these diseases, particularly when you have a client who has one of these diseases.

**Communicable diseases** are diseases that can be transferred from one person to another.

# COMMON DISEASES THAT AFFECT THE SKIN-CARE PRACTICE

The following are common diseases that are frequently seen in the salon. These diseases are communicable, and precautions must be taken by the skin-care professional. The skin-care professional is not a medical doctor and should never attempt to diagnose, treat, or give advice to clients about these diseases. However, the esthetician should be able to recognize these diseases so that they may refer the client to a doctor for treatment.

Further, the estheticians must not expose themselves or other clients to these diseases by performing services on clients who have **infectious diseases**, which are highly contagious diseases that can easily be transferred by contaminating hands or skin-care implements.

**Conjunctivitis** is a bacterial disease of the eye, commonly known as pinkeye. The eye or eyes appear red or pink and have a yellowish discharge that easily forms a crust. Clients may comment that their eyelids are stuck together when they awake. Conjunctivitis is extremely contagious and spread by touching the eye and spreading the bacteria to skin-care or makeup implements either at home or in the salon or clinic. Mascara wands, eye creams in which the client has dipped her finger, eye shadows and eye shadow brushes, and essentially anything that the client has touched may be contaminated with bacteria. Clients must discard any eye product or implement that they have touched.

Estheticians must *never* work on a client with conjunctivitis. The client must be referred to a doctor and wait until the doctor approves of further esthetic treatment. Normally, it only takes a few days using antibiotic eye drops to cure conjunctivitis. Should you accidentally treat a client with conjunctivitis, you must discard or sterilize any item that may have been touched or contaminated during the service.

> **Infectious diseases** are highly contagious diseases that can easily be transferred to another person.
>
> **Conjunctivitis** is a bacterial eye infection; commonly called "pinkeye."

## Herpes Simplex

**Herpes simplex** is a virus that causes outbreaks of blisters on and around the lips and mouth, commonly known as fever blisters or cold sores (Figure 4-1). Herpes can flare easily when the immune system of the body is suppressed, which can be caused by illness, stress, or sun exposure. Many people experience severe flares with prolonged sun exposure. Herpes simplex is managed with antiviral drugs such as **acyclovir**.

Estheticians should *never* treat clients with open herpes blisters because this is when the virus is most contagious. Clients should be referred to a doctor for treatment. Occasionally, herpes will flare after a facial treatment, especially chemical exfoliation treatments. If you have a client who has herpes, he or she should be referred to a doctor for pretreatment with acyclovir before using chemical exfoliation products in the salon.

> **Herpes simplex** is the virus that causes fever blisters or cold sores.
>
> **Acyclovir** is a prescription antiviral drug used to treat and prevent herpes viruses.

## Impetigo

**Impetigo** is a bacterial infection of the skin often seen in children, but it can be spread to adults. Crusty lesions that ooze or weep are symptoms of impetigo. They often occur on the face but can occur anywhere on the skin.

Clients with impetigo must be referred to a doctor for antibiotic treatment. They should not be treated in the salon until cleared by the physician.

**Methicillin-resistant *Staphylococcus aureus*** (**MRSA**, pronounced MERSA) is a type of staphylococcus (staph) bacteria that is antibiotic resistant. In other words, antibiotics commonly used to treat staph infections do not work on these bacteria. Most often, MRSA is present in hospitals. However, in the last few years, **community-acquired MRSA** has shown up outside the hospital environment.

> **Impetigo** is a bacterial skin infection resulting in weeping sores; commonly seen in children.
>
> **Methicillin-resistant *Staphylococcus aureus* (MRSA)** is a dangerous type of antibiotic-resistant bacteria.
>
> **Community-acquired MRSA** is a type of MRSA that can result in boil-like skin lesions. It must be referred to a physician.

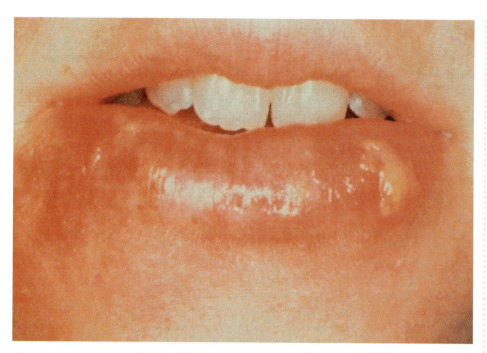

**Figure 4-1** Herpes simplex

Skin-related community-acquired MRSA infections appear as large, boil-like eruptions that do not respond to normal treatments. MRSA lesions can weep and be spread from person to person by body contact. Athletes who participate in contact sports such as wrestling can be more susceptible to MRSA infections. All clients who have obvious skin infections should never be treated in the salon and should be immediately referred to a doctor.

## ABOUT AIDS

AIDS is a devastating disease that has already affected millions of people and continues to affect millions more. In this chapter you will learn how the AIDS virus affects the immune system and the body. We will discuss how AIDS is transmitted and what can be done to prevent further spread of AIDS. We will discuss AIDS symptoms in the body, including many symptoms that may appear in the skin. Management of the patient with AIDS will be reviewed so that you will be knowledgeable about the medical treatment of AIDS and AIDS-related conditions.

AIDS is a syndrome caused by a virus known as the human immunodeficiency virus (HIV), which is capable of destroying the immune system in persons infected with it. The immune system is the vital natural defense system against diseases. Without a properly functioning immune system, the body is unable to fight off infections that threaten it.

As we have already learned, viruses work by "injecting" themselves into healthy cells. Once they are inside the healthy cells, they reproduce in great numbers, eventually killing the cell. The cell ruptures, releasing millions of new viruses. Each of these new viruses can "inject" other cells, repeating the process and duplicating even more viruses.

When the body is infected with HIV, the virus invades certain types of white blood cells known as T cells or CD4 cells, and the genetic material of the virus becomes a part of the blood cell. The virus tricks the blood cell into duplicating its genetic material, eventually overtaking the cell while breeding new virus capsules. It essentially uses the cell to duplicate itself, and the new viruses attack other T cells. Eventually, the number of T cells dwindles to the point where there are not enough to defend the body against invasion by disease-causing organisms. These organisms, normally kept in check by a properly functioning immune system, begin attacking the body. Such diseases are called **opportunistic infections**, which means they are diseases that rarely affect a normal, healthy body and cannot be eradicated as they normally would by a properly functioning immune system.

**Opportunistic infections** are sicknesses that the immune system normally has no trouble fighting off.

When persons die of AIDS, it is because the body simply can no longer defend itself against disease. No one actually dies of AIDS; they die of infections or diseases that infest the body owing to failure of the immune function.

## HOW PEOPLE GET INFECTED WITH AIDS

HIV has been linked to a similar virus in African green monkeys. The monkeys carry this similar virus but are not always affected by it. When viruses or other organisms duplicate many times, the DNA in the organism sometimes changes slightly. This change is called a **mutation**. Many scientists believe that the AIDS virus mutated in a human after the human was bitten by a monkey in Africa. The virus was then probably spread sexually. There are many, many cases of AIDS in Africa, mostly in heterosexuals. Because HIV attacks white blood cells, it can spread very rapidly in the body. Blood, as you know, flows through the body. There are some blood cells in every body fluid. Body fluids are blood, semen, urine, vaginal secretions, spinal fluid, tears, saliva, and amniotic fluids in pregnant women. Semen and blood appear to be the only real sources of infections. No infection from tears or saliva has ever been documented.

**Mutation** means change.

Intravenous drug users are infected by the AIDS virus by using dirty hypodermic needles that contain small amounts of blood from another person. When they inject their illegal drugs, they also inject the other person's HIV-infected blood.

Many patients who received blood transfusions before blood was being checked for HIV contamination became infected. Organ donors infected with HIV donated organs that were also contaminated, causing AIDS to develop in some people. However, now that there are tests to screen blood and tissue donations, infection through blood transfusions or organ transplants is highly unlikely.

The number one risk source for HIV infection is sexual intercourse. Sexual intercourse involves direct transmission of body fluids from one individual to another. The vagina, the penis, and the rectum all have many small blood vessels that can break during intercourse, causing direct exposure. When HIV-infected blood enters the body, infection can occur. Once the virus enters the body, it can spread very quickly. However, symptoms caused by the breakdown of the immune system may not be noticed for months or years.

Anyone who has been infected by HIV can transmit the virus to others through sexual contact, whether or not that person has symptoms. During the early stages of the disease, it is virtually impossible to tell if an individual is infected by simply looking at that individual.

## TESTING FOR THE AIDS VIRUS

When the body is infected with HIV, the B cells produce antibodies to the virus. These antibodies can be identified by blood tests, which are able to isolate the antibody.

The first test done for the HIV antibody is called the ELISA (enzyme-linked immunosorbent assay) test. This test is a screening test for the HIV antibody. If the test is positive, this indicates that the patient has antibodies to the virus. Confirmation of a positive ELISA test is completed by a second blood test called a Western blot test. If the second test is also positive, the patient definitely has HIV antibodies. Doctors refer to these patients as HIV positive. Persons who do not have the virus or antibodies are called HIV negative. Individuals who are HIV positive, as we said before, may not show symptoms of AIDS for months or for as long as ten years or more. Medical scientists believe, however, that without antiviral treatment, all individuals who are HIV positive will eventually develop AIDS symptoms.

Sometimes a person with HIV infection will not test positive for the virus immediately. Let's suppose an individual was exposed through sexual contact but did not test positive when he was tested for HIV two months later. However, several months later he tested positive for the virus. This delayed reaction occurs because the B cells have not yet produced antibodies to the virus. The B cells eventually produced antibodies, and they were identified during the later test. The period of time between exposure to HIV and the time antibodies are made is called a **window phase**. Individuals will not test positive if there are no antibodies, because the test identifies the antibodies, not the virus. For high-risk individuals, several tests should be performed at intervals over a period of a year to eighteen months. During that time the individual must abstain from contact to prevent the possibility of another window phase from occurring.

There have been more than 500,000 cases of AIDS diagnosed in the United States. More than a million individuals are HIV positive, a few of whom have not shown symptoms in 15 years and most of whom developed AIDS in the first ten years. That is about 1 in 250 Americans. Persons who are HIV positive may infect an uninfected person through sexual contact or exchange of blood, semen, or other body fluids. The test for HIV is now available through private physicians, state and local health departments, and other health care facilities. There is currently an at-home mail-in test available that can be purchased at pharmacies.

> **Window phase** is the period of time between exposure to HIV and the time antibodies are made.

## THE SYMPTOMS OF HIV INFECTION

Many small infections can occur in a person who is HIV positive before strong symptoms develop. Strange skin rashes and lesions, repeated infections such as frequent flu-like symptoms, chronic tiredness, and other symptoms may be caused by HIV infection. Of course, many other diseases can have these same symptoms. Because a person has symptoms like these does not necessarily mean the person is infected with HIV. The beginning of immune system breakdown, however, may result in multiple minor infections.

In order to call HIV infection AIDS, a person must both be HIV positive and show signs of advanced immune system breakdown, identified by the presence of a definite opportunistic disease or extremely low T cell counts. We will discuss these diseases shortly. Doctors often refer to patients with these symptoms as having "full-blown" AIDS.

## Common AIDS Symptoms

*Pneumocystis jiroveci* pneumonia (PCP), formerly known as *Pneumocystis carinii*, affects AIDS patients. This form of pneumonia produces high fever and a horrible hacking cough owing to fluid in the lungs, and almost always results in hospitalization.

Other forms of lung infection are also prevalent in patients with AIDS. Fungal and yeast infections of the lungs are common, as well as fungal and yeast infections of the esophagus. Other forms of bacterial infection may also occur in the lungs. Some of these infections may occur simultaneously.

Swollen lymph nodes are also common in individuals with HIV. The immune system is trying to fight off infection but is losing the battle. Swollen lymph nodes may indicate the presence of a large number of dead T cells killed by HIV.

**Dementia** is an infection of the brain or cerebrospinal tissues resulting in abnormal thought processes.

**Chronic wasting syndrome** refers to rapid, unexplained weight loss.

**Dementia** is an infection of the brain or cerebrospinal tissues. This may result in personality disorders or mental illnesses. Various forms of cancer are much more likely to occur in patients with AIDS. Again, the immune system no longer can protect the body. **Chronic wasting syndrome** refers to rapid, unexplained weight loss. Any sort of recurrent infection may be a symptom. A simple infection may be treated with antibiotics but reoccurs in a short period of time. These are only a very few general symptomatic diseases of AIDS. Again, it must be stressed that all of these diseases may occur in healthy persons. But, they are most likely to occur when the immune system is not functioning well, as is the case with HIV infection. These diseases are sometimes called AIDS-indicator diseases. Doctors know that if a person with HIV has these diseases, AIDS is often indicated.

## TREATMENT OF AIDS AND HIV INFECTION

Although there is still no cure for AIDS, there has been much progress made in understanding the biochemistry and physical aspects of the virus and its physiology in relation to the immune system.

Great strides have been made in the management of the patient with HIV. It is important that patients with HIV receive testing regularly to monitor their immune systems. Constant monitoring can help doctors slow the progress of the disease. New tests have been developed that measure **viral load**, which is an indication of how many viral particles are actually in the infected patient's blood. Other tests can now monitor CD4 cells, a specific type of T cell severely affected by HIV. A low CD4 is an indication of low resistance to diseases.

**Viral load** is a measurement of how many viral particles are in a patient's blood.

The immune system must be in good shape to fight off disease and infections. To help restore or partially restore the immune system in patients with HIV, scientists have developed drugs known as **enzyme inhibitors**, which interfere with the normal activity of the HIV virus. AZT is an example of this type of drug. This drug therapy results in reduction of the virus replicating process and therefore reduces the amount of HIV in the body, allowing the body to restore immune function or at least partially restore it. Combinations of drugs, known as **"drug cocktails,"** interfere with various biochemical reactions the virus needs to complete its replication.

**Enzyme** inhibitors are chemicals that interfere with enzyme activity. In the case of HIV infection, they interfere with enzymes that cause viral replication.

**Drug cocktails** are mixtures of several different drugs that work well together.

By combining antiviral drugs, doctors can now lower and keep viral loads in check, thus keeping CD4 counts higher. These drug groups are already keeping patients with HIV healthy, enabling them to live much longer, productive lives as well as have a higher quality of life. There are some indications, although it is very early to tell, that patients with HIV will be able to live out normal lifespans, if they are properly monitored.

Some of these drugs have side effects in some people, and not all patients are able to take them. Side effects include intestinal symptoms, such as diarrhea, and tiredness. Many of these drugs are also very expensive, placing financial burdens on the patient, on the patient's family, and society.

Unfortunately, in some cases, the drugs stop working or stop working as effectively. This may mean that the virus has adapted to the drugs. At this point the virus could spread again and immune suppression could take place, leaving the patient susceptible to many infections. Fortunately, there are several types of drug cocktails, and doctors can sometimes adjust the combination of drugs to try a new approach.

There also has been progress in the preparation of a vaccine against AIDS. Although tests are not complete as of this writing, scientists have prepared a vaccine that has proved successful in monkeys for a period of one year. This, however, does not mean that the vaccine will necessarily work in humans, nor does it mean that it will work for longer periods of time. It is significant progress, however, and it does mean that there is hope for more long-term treatment. Even if a cure is not found, perhaps someday it can be managed, like diabetes or thyroid disease.

One of the problems with the virus is that it mutates frequently, and there are several types or **strains** of HIV. This means that the virus can change and adapt itself to the drug therapy. In fact, 20 percent of persons with AIDS today have now been infected with viruses mutated from the cocktails, indicating that they probably had sexual intercourse with persons being treated with the enzyme inhibitors.

## PREVENTION OF AIDS

Prevention is still the best treatment for AIDS. Prevention means taking steps to stop people from getting a disease. In this case, it means stopping people from becoming infected with HIV. The best way to prevent the spread of the virus is through education. This is where the esthetician can play a very important part. If you are knowledgeable about AIDS you can help your clients understand the syndrome as well as answer questions about preventing the spread of AIDS. It is, therefore, very important that all estheticians, and in fact all health and personal care professionals, be aware of prevention techniques.

### Prevention Techniques

There are basically only two ways to get HIV infection or AIDS through contact with infected individuals. Both ways involve the exchange of blood, blood products, or body fluids contaminated with HIV between individuals.

Because sexual contact is the number one cause of the spread of AIDS, "safe sex" practices must be implemented. Any exchange of blood, semen, or vaginal fluids during sexual contact may cause HIV infection if one person is infected. Precautions must be carefully carried out to prevent exchange of these fluids. The absolute safest prevention technique is abstinence. **Abstinence** means that the persons do not engage in sexual intercourse at all. If sexual partners choose to have sexual intercourse, using a condom (rubber) is important. A latex condom is the only type that is safe to use. Some condoms are made of skin taken from lambs. Skin, as we discussed in Chapter 1, can be permeable. It is possible that a condom made of lambskin will leak semen and cause infection. Condoms must be worn throughout sexual relations, from start to finish.

Avoiding body penetration is also helpful in preventing AIDS. When the penis enters any body orifice, such as the vagina, rectum, or mouth, the disease transmission possibility is greatly increased.

Monogamy means that two persons who engage in sex are faithful to one another and never have sex with any person other than their spouse or partner. Persons who are in a monogamous relationship where both persons have tested negative for HIV and have received medical counseling regarding proper HIV testing need not worry about HIV infection, as long as there are no other risk factors. Other risk factors include use of intravenous drugs.

The use of intravenous drugs (illegal drugs that are injected by a hypodermic needle into the body) is terrible for the health of any individual. Besides the many health risks that illegal drug use causes, HIV infection is also very possible. People who are addicted to intravenous drugs are often careless about health and hygiene. They use other addicts' needles or share needles that are dirty and contaminated with HIV or many other diseases. Direct injection of HIV-infected blood almost certainly leads to HIV infection.

One of the newest concerns is complacency due to the news of successful drug therapy. Some people are being careless about safe sex and needles, thinking AIDS is controllable. It isn't.

HIV infection among homosexual males has declined, but the infection rate has increased among women and teenagers and is increasing among African-Americans and Hispanics.

**Strains** are slightly genetically different forms of the same virus.

**Abstinence** means that the persons do not engage in sexual intercourse at all.

# PERSONAL PRECAUTIONS

HIV infection and AIDS are preventable. Following are some general tips for prevention:

1. Do not have unprotected sex. Use a latex condom from start to finish.
2. Sex with multiple partners is extremely risky. Anal and oral sex are also very risky. Any sexually active persons with multiple sexual partners, regardless of sexual preference, expose themselves to blood or semen.
3. Do not use intravenous drugs or have sex with anyone who does. AIDS is rampant among IV drug users, many of whom are also prostitutes.
4. HIV infection is on the rise in teenagers, heterosexuals, and females.
5. Never assume that anyone is not HIV positive. Persons may have HIV and appear perfectly healthy.
6. Even if a potential sexual partner tells you that he or she has tested negative for HIV, there is a "window phase" in which a person being tested may not have developed antibodies to the virus yet. All HIV tests detect antibodies in the blood. Someone who is in a window phase may test negative, yet still have the virus. Always use a condom.

# DISPELLING MYTHS ABOUT AIDS

When people do not fully understand something that is life threatening like AIDS, they tend to be afraid. Because they are afraid, rumors often get started about how the disease spreads. Let's stop some of those rumors. These are the facts about AIDS.

1. The only way to get AIDS is to exchange blood or body fluids contaminated with blood from a person with HIV.
2. You cannot get AIDS from casual contact. Sitting next to someone who is infected cannot transmit HIV.
3. You cannot get AIDS by drinking after someone or sharing eating utensils.
4. You cannot get AIDS by hugging, touching, social kissing (on the cheek), or eating food prepared by someone who is infected.
5. You cannot get AIDS from mosquito or insect bites.
6. No cases of AIDS have ever been associated with French kissing.
7. AIDS is not a "gay disease." Anyone can become infected if they engage in unsafe sex or share needles with an infected person.

# AIDS AND THE ESTHETICIAN

Exposure to HIV in the cosmetology workplace has not been documented, but it is extremely important to use the hygiene and sterile techniques listed later in this chapter.

There have been some incidences where a health care worker became infected with HIV due to needle-stick injuries. This means that the health care worker was accidentally stuck with a used, dirty needle from a patient with HIV.

This, of course, can cause infection in the same way as it does in intravenous drug users. It is very important that all health care workers and personal care workers take precautions to avoid such accidents.

We, of course, do not work with body fluids as health care workers do. However, certain procedures performed by estheticians may sometimes result in very small amounts of blood surfacing on the skin. Extraction, waxing, tweezing, and electrolysis are examples of such procedures. Clients may express concern about your salon's techniques for sterilizing equipment to prevent HIV infection. Because we work in a field that sometimes involves contact with small amounts of body fluids and blood, we must take special precautions when handling clients. We must make sure to follow strict sanitation guidelines and make sure that all our utensils and equipment are thoroughly disinfected at all times. We discussed techniques to prevent transmission of AIDS and many other diseases in Chapter 2, Hygiene and Sterilization Techniques.

## SKIN SYMPTOMS ASSOCIATED WITH AIDS

Fortunately, early detection of HIV now allows medical management of the HIV-positive patient. Skin problems as well as other problems that occur due to immune system dysfunction are therefore less likely to occur. Nevertheless, we should discuss the skin symptoms and problems that may be associated with HIV and AIDS.

There are many HIV-related symptoms that may occur in the skin. These include unusual or severe cases of common diseases such as shingles (herpes zoster), herpes simplex, genital herpes, genital warts, seborrheic dermatitis, unexplained rashes, warts, impetigo, fungal infections, folliculitis, athlete's foot, and other infections of the mouth and throat. Although these infections can occur in people who are HIV negative and in people with HIV, they are often recurrent or extremely severe. They may also prove resistant to normal treatment. All of the preceding symptoms are medical conditions, regardless of patient type, and should be referred to a physician immediately.

The skin is a major organ of the immune system, where some of the first symptoms of HIV infection or AIDS show up. HIV and AIDS are often first diagnosed in a dermatologist's office. Although estheticians are not in the business of diagnosing or treating disease, it is important to be aware of these possible symptoms and encourage clients who show signs of these illnesses to see a physician, regardless of HIV status.

Again, it is important to remember that these symptoms may all be present in normal, healthy, HIV-negative individuals. The esthetician should never mention the AIDS relationship of these symptoms to the client. The esthetician should only refer these problems to a doctor, as you should for any medical condition.

The symptoms, which affect many people anyway, tend to be much more severe and chronic in those with HIV. The treatments for these symptoms administered by physicians are often more intensive to treat skin problems associated with patients with AIDS. Many of these symptoms may also affect mucous membranes, such as the inside of the mouth, rectum, vagina, and eye.

### Herpes

Herpes is a virus that comes in many different forms. Most people think of genital herpes when they hear the word **herpes**. But, as explained later in this chapter, there are many different herpes viruses and not all are transmitted by sexual contact (Figure 4-2).

Cold sores, for example, result from one form of the herpes virus. Genital herpes is another form. In patients with HIV, herpes flareups tend to be much more severe and happen more often. Physicians may give these patients antiviral medications to help the depressed immune system heal the lesions associated with a herpes infection.

Another form of herpes is called **herpes zoster**, better known as **shingles**. Shingles is actually an adult manifestation of chickenpox. It can be very painful. Shingles in patients with HIV is often much worse and widespread than in normal healthy individuals (Figure 4-3).

### Warts

**Warts** are often recurrent and more widespread in HIV-positive patients. They may occur in unusual places such as the beard area, mouth, and tongue. Plantar warts on the feet or hands may also be present. The physician may find that these warts are resistant to normal treatment. Warts on the genitals, anus, and vagina are also often seen.

**Herpes** refers to a group of viruses.

**Herpes zoster** is the virus that causes both shingles and chickenpox.

**Shingles**, known also as herpes zoster, is caused by the same virus that causes chickenpox. The lesions of herpes zoster look like multiple red blisters.

**Warts** are caused by a variety of viruses known as papovaviruses or verrucae.

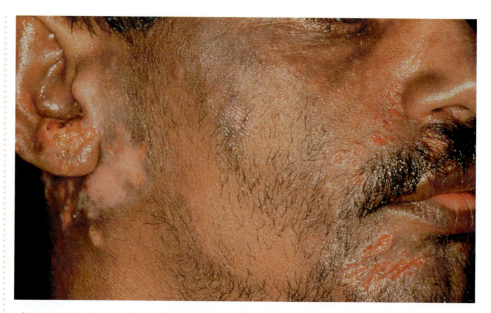

**Figure 4-2** Herpes Type II in patient with HIV (Courtesy Rube J. Pardo, M.D., Ph.D.)

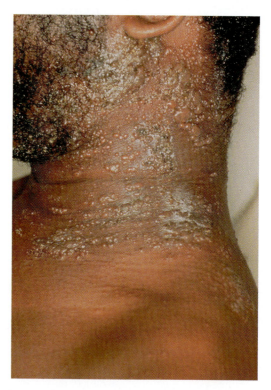

**Figure 4-3** Shingles on the neck and face of a patient with HIV (Courtesy Rube J. Pardo, M.D., Ph.D.)

**Molluscum contagiosum** is a viral infection frequently seen on the faces of children, which appear as groups of small, flesh-colored papules.

**Impetigo** is a skin infection that is characterized by large, open, weeping lesions.

**Molluscum contagiosum** is often seen in normal children. It often looks like a large group of warts and is frequently seen on the face.

## Infections

**Impetigo** is a bacterial infection, again often seen in small, normal children. In patients with AIDS, the lesions can be much worse. Impetigo is characterized by multiple lesions, often in the mouth and chin area. They have a crusty top but ooze transparent fluid. Impetigo is extremely contagious. Refer the patient to a physician immediately.

**Mycosis** infections are fungal infections. Many fungal infections can affect both the skin and the internal organs of the patient with AIDS. Skin infections from fungi may be indicative of internal fungal infections in patients with AIDS. Fungal infections may show many different forms of symptomatic lesions.

**Folliculitis** is an irritation of the hair follicle and is caused by a bacterial infection. The follicles appear inflamed, are in groups or patches, and often may appear as patches of very tiny pustules.

Severe **seborrheic dermatitis**, or seborrhea, may be seen in patients with HIV. Many clients may have a small area of seborrheic dermatitis, but in patients with AIDS the seborrhea may be much worse. Red, scaly patches in all areas of the face, but especially the hairline and ears, are apparent. Severe seborrhea may cause cracks in the skin and bleeding. Oozing lesions may also be present. The scalp can be severely affected as well. Again, seborrhea affects many healthy individuals, but in patients with AIDS it is much more widespread, inflamed, and chronic. Normal treatment may prove to be unresponsive. More potent topical steroids are often needed to control the disorder (Figure 4-4). Psoriasis may develop or worsen in patients with AIDS.

## Mouth Symptoms

One of the earliest symptoms of AIDS may be a yeast infection of the mouth called **oral thrush**. *Candida albicans* is the name of the yeast that causes thrush. Thrush symptoms include an abnormally thick, white paste covering mouth tissues. It often occurs in patients with HIV. It looks like cotton stuck to patches in the mouth. Thrush is often a problem for small children who do not have AIDS. It is not seen as often in normal, healthy adults.

**Hairy leukoplakia** is a tumor-like eruption that can occur on the tongue or the insides of the cheeks. It is hard and scaly looking. Herpes lesions, or "fever blisters," may also affect the inside of the mouth of patients with AIDS.

**Mycosis** are fungal infections.

**Folliculitis** is a bacterial infection of the hair follicle.

**Seborrheic dermatitis**, or seborrhea, is an inflammation of the sebaceous glands and follicles resulting in redness, flaking, and itching in oily areas of the face.

**Oral thrush** is an infection of the mouth and throat caused by the yeast known as *Candida albicans*.

**Hairy leukoplakia** is a tumor-like eruption that can occur on the tongue or the insides of the cheeks.

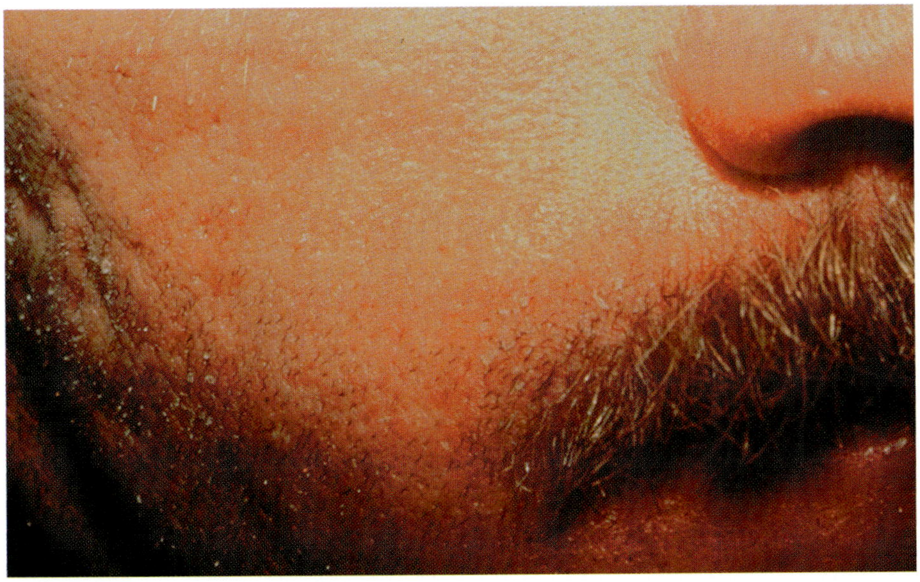

**Figure 4-4** Seborrheic dermatitis in a patient with HIV (Courtesy Rube J. Pardo, M.D., Ph.D.)

## Other Skin Symptoms

Many unusual skin lesions plague patients with HIV. Strange skin bumps and lesions may be apparent. Because patients with AIDS have lowered resistance to infection, physicians constantly see new and strange lesions on the skin of patients.

## SKIN CANCERS ASSOCIATED WITH AIDS

**Kaposi's sarcoma** is a rare form of skin cancer characterized by purple–brown lesions.

**Kaposi's sarcoma** (KS) was, at one time, a frequent skin symptom of AIDS. It appears as purple–brown lesions. It is a rare form of skin cancer, but it can affect patients with AIDS because this patient's body is immunosuppressed. Because progress has been made in antiviral treatment, patients with HIV are now much less likely to develop Kaposi's sarcoma (Figure 4-5).

Other skin cancers are also seen in AIDS patients. Although not as prevalent as Kaposi's sarcoma, basal and squamous cell carcinomas have been detected in patients with AIDS and seem to spread much faster in these patients. Malignant melanoma may also be seen and also has a tendency to spread faster in patients who are immunosuppressed.

## THE MENTAL AND EMOTIONAL STATE OF PATIENTS WITH AIDS

It is possible for a patient with AIDS to experience many different emotions concerning the illness. Because it is a relatively new disease, much is still to be learned about AIDS. Although we basically understand its transmission and its effect on the immune system and the body, we are still learning about management of the individual

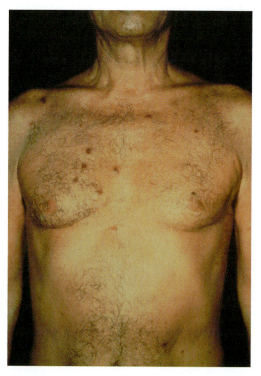

**Figure 4-5** Kaposi's sarcoma in an AIDS (HIV-positive) patient (Courtesy Rube J. Pardo, M.D., Ph.D.)

with HIV. Because of these uncertainties, patients with AIDS may have great difficulty coping with their situations. There is no permanent cure for AIDS.

Patients with AIDS or who are HIV positive may feel anger toward others or themselves about the disease. They may also deny having the disease. They experience many of the same emotional conflicts felt by patients with cancer. The stigma originally attached to AIDS, a so-called "gay disease," is decreasing, but many people are still not educated about its transmission. This, again, is where the esthetician can play a part in helping to educate the public. If a client says something incorrect about AIDS, tactfully correct the client. Only by getting the right word out can the many misunderstandings about this illness be clarified.

## HANDLING CLIENT QUESTIONS ABOUT AIDS

Clients may have questions regarding AIDS and the salon, specifically questions about sanitation and sterilization. It is acceptable for clients to ask these questions and for you to answer. It is very important that you are knowledgeable about the salon's sterilization procedures and that you are familiar with the requirements of your state regarding proper sanitation in the salon.

The client may be completely misinformed about AIDS and HIV. Cosmetology professionals are in a unique position to educate the consumer about issues such as AIDS. Rumors about AIDS are rampant, and it is important for you to always remain well informed to help dispel these rumors.

Following are some tips about handling questions:

1. Answer the questions factually and briefly, but do not dwell on the subject.

2. Reassure the client that everything you use is sterile or disposable and that you have taken all the precautions possible. (Make sure that you do!) A poster or plaque listing your sterilization and sanitation practices is a good idea. There is one available from EMDA—the Esthetics Manufacturers and Distributors Alliance, 401 North Michigan Avenue, Chicago IL 60601.

3. Make sure that your salon is always spotless. Let your client observe you washing your hands and following aseptic procedures. The impact of an immaculately clean salon or clinic will squelch most doubts the client may have.

4. Make sure that all coworkers are equally informed with the facts about AIDS and aseptic and sterile procedures.

5. A client may confide in you or come to you for advice concerning his or her exposure or sickness. Refer the client to a physician immediately. Use the same caring attitude you would with any client.

## AIDS AND THE FUTURE

At the time of this writing, 1 in 250 people in the United States is HIV positive. In your lifetime it is likely that you will know someone who is HIV positive or who has AIDS. Although great progress in treatment has been made, we all hope that a cure or a vaccine is on the horizon.

## ABOUT HEPATITIS

**Hepatitis** is an inflammation of the liver that is caused by a viral infection. There are five known viruses that cause hepatitis: hepatitis A, B, C, D, and E.

The liver is an extremely important organ in the body. It helps break down fats and helps store energy. It helps with food digestion and also acts as a disposal

**Hepatitis** is an inflammation of the liver.

system for toxins and blood wastes. A person cannot survive without a functioning liver.

Hepatitis interferes with the liver's ability to function properly. Severe viral infection can cause liver failure, which is often fatal. Hepatitis viruses are extremely infectious, and the odds of becoming infected with a hepatitis virus are much higher than with HIV. This is a result of the virus being present in much higher numbers. Symptoms of hepatitis include **jaundice**, which is a yellowing of the skin and eyes, abdominal pain, fever, and constant fatigue. Hepatitis can result in permanent damage to the liver. The hepatitis virus can also live quietly in the liver after symptoms have gone away. If the virus lives after the initial disease, the person can still infect other people and is known as a **carrier**.

**Jaundice** is a yellowing of the skin and eyes.

**Carrier** refers to a person who is infected with an illness and able to transmit it to another person. A carrier may or may not show symptoms of the disease.

## Types of Hepatitis

Hepatitis A is caused by eating food contaminated with the virus, usually through fecal material and poor sanitation. This is the type of hepatitis associated with eating raw oysters and other raw shellfish. Oysters eat by filtering water, and bay water can be contaminated with human waste from sewage. Hepatitis A is the least dangerous of the hepatitis viruses, and most people recover completely.

Hepatitis B is a much more serious type of infection and is most often spread by sexual contact or body fluids, similar to HIV. Unlike HIV, however, hepatitis B can be contracted by kissing. Hepatitis B symptoms may last for months. Although most people recover fully from it, a few develop permanent liver damage, and about 10 percent become carriers. Liver cancer is known to often occur in long-term carriers after 30 or more years.

Hepatitis C was identified only a few years ago. The symptoms are similar to hepatitis B, and it is sometimes associated with HIV infection.

Hepatitis D affects those already infected with hepatitis B. This is a serious infection and permanent damage is much more likely to occur.

Hepatitis E, which is similar to hepatitis A, occurs mainly in underdeveloped countries.

## Vaccines and Prevention of Hepatitis

Hepatitis B and C can be prevented or avoided by the same precautionary measures as for HIV. Hepatitis A can be prevented by proper sanitation, by proper hand washing, and by following general cleanliness guidelines.

There are now vaccinations available for hepatitis A and B. They are administered in a series of injections, which slowly builds the body's immunity to the virus. Hepatitis vaccinations are highly advisable for estheticians, because they are periodically exposed to blood and body fluids.

## Hepatitis and the Salon

Proper sterilization of implements, proper disposal of contaminated materials, the use of one-use implements, and the use of hospital-grade disinfectants as discussed in Chapter 2, Hygiene and Sterilization Techniques, are the best methods for preventing accidental exposure to hepatitis viruses in the salon.

Technically, hepatitis viruses are harder to kill than HIV and are much more numerous in body fluids. It is much more likely for someone to contract hepatitis rather than HIV from an improperly sanitized or contaminated implement. Risk can be reduced greatly by use of proper sanitation and sterilization procedures.

For much more information on these subjects, read *HIV/AIDS and Hepatitis* by Doug Schoon, available from Milady Publishing.

# AIDS/HIV KNOWLEDGE QUIZ

## True or False

____ **1.** Any person can get AIDS.

____ **2.** To become infected with HIV, infected blood or body fluids must enter the body.

____ **3.** One in 250 Americans is now infected with HIV.

____ **4.** Prevention is still the best treatment for HIV and AIDS.

____ **5.** AIDS can be spread by mosquitoes.

____ **6.** Anyone who gets AIDS is a promiscuous individual.

____ **7.** There are other diseases more transmissible than AIDS.

____ **8.** You can easily spot a person with HIV.

____ **9.** It is against the law to discriminate against patients with AIDS or HIV.

____ **10.** If a person has a negative HIV test, the person absolutely does not carry the virus.

____ **11.** The best way to prevent diseases of any type in the salon is to assume that all your clients are HIV positive.

____ **12.** Persons with HIV may not show symptoms for years.

____ **13.** The biggest increase in AIDS is currently seen in teenagers, women, African-Americans, and Hispanics.

## Answers

1. True.
2. True.
3. True.
4. True.
5. False. No cases of AIDS or HIV infection have ever been traced to mosquito bites, casual contact, kissing, swimming pools, toilet seats, contact through cosmetology, pets, drinking fountains, food handling, or donating blood. You can only get AIDS from exchange of blood, blood products, or body fluids.
6. False. Although promiscuous sex is risky, anyone can get HIV from unprotected sex with an infected person.
7. True. Hepatitis and many other diseases are much easier to catch than AIDS/HIV.
8. False. Symptoms of AIDS may not show up for years. It is often impossible to tell by sight if a person has HIV or AIDS.
9. True.
10. False. HIV tests may be false-negative if the person has yet to develop antibodies to the virus, which is what HIV tests detect. Persons should be tested several times, several months apart, without participating in any risky activity during that time.
11. True. The very best way to ensure proper hygiene is to assume that all clients are HIV positive.
12. True.
13. True.

# TOPICS FOR DISCUSSION

1. Why is it possible for an HIV-infected person to show no symptoms?
2. Discuss the medical management of the person with HIV.
3. What can be done to prevent the spread of AIDS?

4. Why is it important to know that AIDS often affects the skin?

5. Why are skin infections in patients with AIDS so much more severe than in healthy individuals?

6. Discuss the future of the AIDS epidemic.

7. What progress has been made in the management of individuals with HIV?

CHAPTER **5**

# Hormones

## OBJECTIVES. . .

Every esthetician needs to be familiar with the endocrine system and hormones. Hormones have very definite effects on the skin, and their functioning is directly related to many skin problems. This chapter will familiarize the esthetician with the major glands of the endocrine system and their function. You will also learn about the menstrual cycle, pregnancy, menopause, and diseases and disorders of the endocrine system. How hormones affect the skin will be discussed in depth.

**Hormones** are basically chemical messengers that are manufactured or **secreted** by glands within the body. As you have previously learned, many glands are present in the body. **Exocrine glands** such as the sebaceous glands and the sudoriferous glands have ducts through which chemicals move. **Apocrine glands** are present in the groin and armpit. **Endocrine glands** secrete hormones. The endocrine glands empty hormones directly into the bloodstream. Although most people think of hormones in terms of sex hormones, sex hormones are only a few of the hormones that the endocrine system produces.

Hormones work by transmitting chemical messages to the various body cells. The hormones have special "keys" that fit the "locks" on the cell membranes that they are intended to affect. The key fitting the lock causes the cell membrane to produce enzymes that stimulate other chemical reactions within the cell. The "locks" on the cells are called **receptors** or receptor sites. Each hormone affects specific cells in different ways, and each endocrine gland produces different hormones.

**Hormones** are special chemicals that are manufactured or secreted by glands within the body.

**Secreted** means synthesized or released by various cells or organs.

**Exocrine glands**, such as the sebaceous glands and the sudoriferous glands, have ducts through which chemicals move.

**Apocrine glands** are present in the groin area and armpits. They produce a thicker form of sweat and are responsible for producing the substance that, when in contact with bacteria, produces body odor.

**Endocrine glands** secrete hormones directly into the bloodstream.

**Receptors** inform T cells of what type of cell it is and that it is an "official" cell of the body and not an antigen.

**Pituitary gland** is found in the center of the head. It serves as the "brain" of the endocrine system.

**Hypothalamus gland** controls some involuntary muscles, such as the muscles of the intestines that help move food through the gastrointestinal system.

**Trophic hormones** are chemicals that cause other glands to make hormones.

**Hypothalamus** manufactures hormones that stimulate the pituitary gland to make other hormones. It is also able to detect needs of various parts of the body by chemically monitoring the blood.

# THE ENDOCRINE GLANDS

There are eight major endocrine glands in the human body (Figure 5-1).

The **pituitary gland** is found in the center of the head. It serves as the "brain" of the endocrine system. It is connected to the brain by another endocrine gland called the **hypothalamus gland**.

The pituitary gland secretes many hormones called **trophic hormones**. Trophic hormones are chemicals that cause other glands to make other hormones. Trophic hormones are "signal hormones." Trophic hormones secreted by the pituitary gland include follicle-stimulating hormone (FSH), which is the pituitary hormone that causes production of sex hormones in the glands present in the sex organs. The pituitary gland also produces special hormones that cause regulation of the amount of fluid retained by the body, hormones that control growth, and special hormones that cause the female breast to produce milk.

The **hypothalamus** controls some involuntary muscles, such as the muscles in the intestines that help move food through the gastrointestinal system. The hypothalamus also manufactures a variety of hormones that cause stimulation of the pituitary gland to make other hormones. You might say that the hypothalamus is the

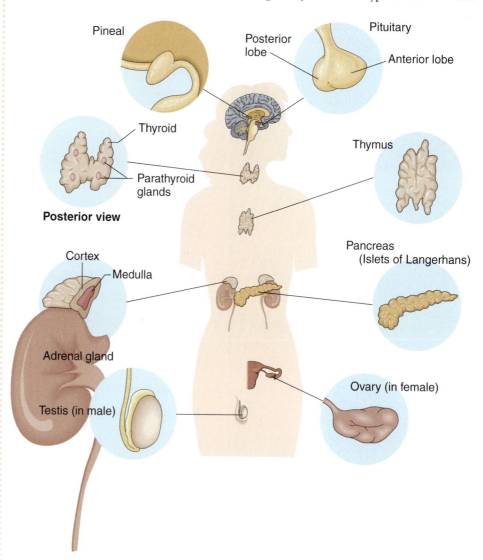

**Figure 5-1** The endocrine system

"interpreter" between the brain and the pituitary gland. The hypothalamus is able to detect needs of various parts of the body by chemically monitoring the blood that flows through it.

The **thyroid gland** is located in the neck. It regulates both cellular and body metabolism and produces hormones that stimulate growth. One of the hormones secreted by the thyroid gland is called **thyroxine**. Without thyroxine dwarfism occurs in children.

The thyroid gland uses a lot of iodine in its manufacture of hormones. This is why it is important to have some iodine in the diet. Iodine is present in fish, meat, and some vegetables.

Behind the thyroid gland lies a related glandular structure called the **parathyroid gland**. The parathyroids are responsible for regulating calcium and phosphates in the bloodstream, which are necessary for proper bone growth. Vitamin D is an important element in the regulation of calcium also.

The **adrenal glands** are located just above the kidneys. Like hair, they have an inner part called the medulla and an outer core called the cortex. The medulla makes the two main hormones called adrenaline and noradrenaline. These two hormones are needed by the nervous system to transport nerve impulses.

**Adrenaline** is also secreted when the body is under stress. Many of us have experienced an "almost accident" when a car pulls out right in front of us. That feeling immediately after an "almost accident" is caused by adrenaline. You could call adrenaline the "emergency hormone." No doubt you have heard stories of people having almost super-human strength during emergencies. This is also caused by the adrenal hormones. When a large amount of adrenaline is secreted suddenly into the bloodstream, the body responds by preparing for an emergency. The heartbeat increases, pupils of the eyes dilate, the bronchi in the lungs expand, and the body generally focuses all its attention on the impending emergency. The cortex of the adrenal glands manufactures steroids, which are very small hormone molecules that are able to penetrate cell membranes and enter cells for specific reasons. The steroid hormones produced by the adrenal cortex are called corticoids. The corticoids help regulate the metabolism and the body's use of carbohydrates, proteins, and fats. They also help to maintain water balance in the body and regulate sodium and potassium levels.

The **pineal gland** is located in the brain, like the pituitary gland. It is very small and is funnel shaped. Its function is not well understood, but it is theorized that it is related to the sex hormones.

The **pancreas** is located in the abdomen. It has several functions. It secretes pancreatic enzymes that are delivered into the intestine. These enzymes help digest foods taken into the body.

Within the pancreas are a group of specialized cells called the islets of Langerhans. These cells manufacture a hormone called insulin, which regulates blood sugar or glucose levels. **Diabetes** is a disease that results from the pancreas not secreting enough insulin. Diabetics must take synthetically produced insulin.

The **thymus gland** has already been discussed in Chapter 3, The Immune System. As you know, it produces specialized lymphocytes to help the body fight disease. The thymus gland grows during childhood and begins shrinking in later years.

The last, but not least, of the major endocrine glands are the sex glands. These are the **ovaries** in females and the **testes** in males. The ovaries are located above the uterus and are connected to the uterus by two hollow tubes called the fallopian tubes (Figure 5-2). The ovaries contain eggs that will eventually be released into the fallopian tubes for possible fertilization by sperm. The testes are present within the scrotum. The testes are connected to another tube called the vas deferens. The vas deferens leads to a holding sac called the seminal vesicle, which holds sperm manufactured by the testes. This series of tubules continues and eventually joins the urethra, which is the tube that leads to the outside of the penis (Figure 5-3).

**Thyroid gland** is located in the neck. It regulates both cellular and body metabolism and produces hormones that stimulate growth.

**Thyroxine** is one of the hormones secreted by the thyroid gland.

**Parathyroid gland** is responsible for regulating calcium and phosphates in the bloodstream.

**Adrenal glands** are located just above the kidneys and produce hormones needed by the nervous system to transport nerve impulses.

**Adrenaline** is secreted when the body is under stress.

**Pineal gland** is located in the brain. Its function is not well understood, but it is theorized that it is related to the sex hormones.

**Pancreas** is located in the abdomen. It secretes pancreatic enzymes that are delivered into the intestine.

**Diabetes** is a disease that results from the pancreas not secreting enough insulin.

**Thymus gland** is located under the breastbone in the chest. It secretes hormones and helps to trigger synthesis of more lymph tissue.

**Ovaries** are located just above the uterus and are connected to the uterus by two hollow tubes called fallopian tubes.

**Testes** are present within the scrotum and produce sperm.

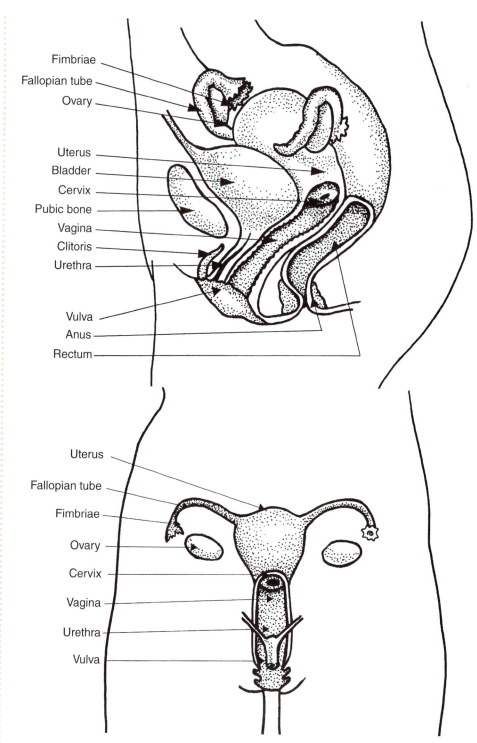

**Figure 5-2** Female reproductive organs

# HORMONES PRODUCED BY THE OVARIES AND TESTES

The sex glands of both men and women produce hormones. The testes secrete testosterone. **Testosterone** is the male hormone responsible for development of typical male characteristics such as a deep voice, broad shoulders, body hair, and other male characteristics. Male hormones are called **androgens**.

**Testosterone** is the male hormone responsible for development of typical male characteristics.

**Androgens** are male hormones.

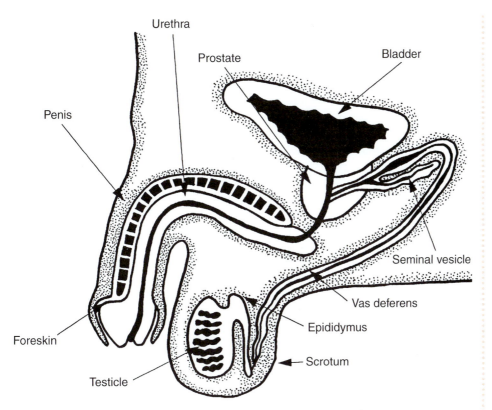

**Figure 5-3** Male reproductive organs

The ovaries produce three hormones. **Estradiol** is one of the female hormones, better known as estrogen. **Estrogen** is the hormone that gives a woman female characteristics, such as breasts, and also helps with the development of the menstrual cycle. Another hormone secreted by the ovaries is **progesterone**, which is a steroid hormone that helps prepare the uterus for pregnancy and is an important hormone in the menstrual cycle. A third hormone manufactured by the ovaries is **relaxin**, which helps enlarge the pelvic opening during childbirth.

Both male and female sex glands receive many of their "cues" for hormone production from the pituitary and the hypothalamus. The pituitary makes a hormone called **follicle-stimulating hormone**, referred to as **FSH**. FSH from the pituitary gland causes the testes to produce sperm. Another pituitary hormone called **luteinizing hormone**, or LH, causes the testes to manufacture testosterone.

The same types of pituitary hormones cause production of female hormones in the ovaries. The FSH produced by the pituitary causes the development of the ovum, or egg. Luteinizing hormone (LH) causes the actual process of ovulation or the release of the egg (ovum) from the ovary.

## HORMONAL PHASES OF LIFE

There are several phases of life in humans that are dramatically influenced and caused by the presence or lack of hormones. Although we produce hormones to some extent throughout life, there are several stages during which pronounced changes occur.

## Puberty

**Puberty** is the stage of life when physical changes occur in both sexes and when sexual function of the sex glands begins to take place. Sexual reproduction is physically possible at puberty.

**Estradiol** is a steroid made from the hormone estrogen that gives women female characteristics.

**Estrogen** is the hormone that gives women female characteristics.

**Progesterone** helps prepare the uterus for pregnancy and is an important hormone in the menstrual cycle.

**Relaxin** is a hormone manufactured by the ovaries that helps enlarge the pelvic opening during childbirth.

**Follicle-stimulating hormone (FSH)** is a hormone secreted by the pituitary gland that causes the development of the egg, or ovum.

**Luteinizing hormone** causes the actual process of ovulation or the release of the egg from the ovary. It also causes the testes to manufacture testosterone.

**Puberty** is the stage of life when physical changes occur in both sexes and when sexual function of the sex glands begins to take place.

At the beginning of puberty, which is usually about 12 to 14 years of age (females may be earlier than males), the hypothalamus begins producing a hormone called luteinizing hormone releasing hormone, which in turn stimulates the pituitary gland to manufacture much larger amounts of FSH and LH.

The FSH and LH are trophic hormones. They cause the ovaries and testes to secrete more hormones, specifically estrogens and androgens. The sudden production of these hormones starts a number of drastic changes in physical appearance. Girls begin developing breasts, fat deposits form around the hips to provide feminine curvature, and the sweat glands begin producing body odor. Androgen production in females gives rise to pubic, leg, and underarm hair. In males, these changes in appearance include muscle development, development of the masculine form, broader shoulders, deeper voice, body and facial hair, and general physical growth. Puberty, of course, also triggers sexual attraction to the opposite sex.

It is interesting to note that just when sexual attraction begins, the maintenance of attractiveness gets more difficult! Many changes happen within the skin at puberty. As hormone production of the sex organs begins at puberty, many hormone changes occur that affect the skin. Probably the biggest change is related to the production of androgen, the male hormone, which is produced by both males and females. As the production of androgen begins, the sebaceous glands produce more and more sebum. Androgen is a sebaceous gland stimulant. As androgen enters the bloodstream, it carries its hormonal messages, resulting in appearance changes such as body hair growth and the development of body odor. At the same time androgen also affects the sebaceous glands.

The increase in sebaceous gland activity and production causes dilation of the follicles. This is when "pores" are first easily visible. You may notice that small children have no easily visible pore structure on the skin's surface. The pores become dilated due to increased sebum production. As the sebum fills the follicle, it begins pushing against the follicle walls, stretching them and making the pores on the surface appear larger. The nose is usually the first to develop visible pores. This development of the pore structure will continue into the bridge of the nose, then the forehead, and then the chin. You may notice that a 12-year-old client has visible follicles only in these areas. The scalp also becomes oilier due to androgen production. This is the beginning of what many refer to as the "T-zone," so named because of its pattern (Figure 5-4).

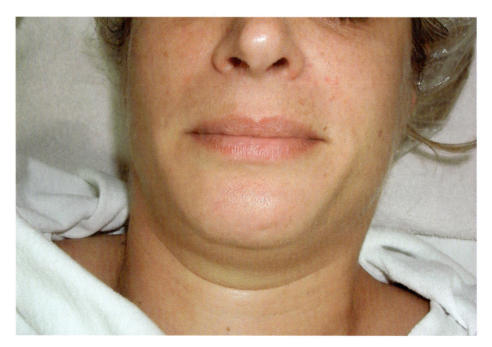

**Figure 5-4** Combination skin can be recognized by an oilier T-zone, down the middle of the face, and smaller pores, indicating drier skin in the perimeter of the face (Courtesy Mark Lees Skin Care, Inc.)

Puberty is also for many teenagers the beginning of acne and break-out tendencies. You may see a young client with large comedones in the nose, chin, and forehead areas or occasionally only very small comedones in the nose only. The smallness of the comedones at this age is because the follicle walls have yet to stretch out much. The androgens have not yet had their full effect on the sebaceous glands.

Mothers often bring in their young teenagers with all of these problems. The young client should be advised of proper home care, but it is extremely important to keep it simple! Children of this age are often not used to daily skin care. Please be very thorough in your explanation of home care procedures. Although it is important to instruct them in proper care, they cannot be expected to perform a seven-step regimen twice a day! They should be instructed to use a washable, foaming cleanser twice a day, followed by a gentle, low pH toner. A mild antiacne product should be used at night if necessary. A 2 percent salicylic or a 2.5 percent benzoyl peroxide gel is recommended.

Sunscreen should be used daily. It is important to convince young clients to start using sunblocks on a daily basis. This is the best way to prevent future sun damage. Teaching good health habits at a young age will help the client maintain good skin for a lifetime. Emphasize the dangers of excess sun and give helpful hints about using sunscreens at the beach. Moisturizers are rarely needed by pubescent teenagers, except in very cold climates. Make sure you always recommend products that are noncomedogenic (see Chapters 15 and 16, Acne and the Esthetician and Comedogenicity, respectively).

Treatment in the salon should follow these steps:

1. Cleanse the face well with a cleansing milk for oily or combination skin. Do not use toner or astringent at this point in treatment—the follicles are usually already tight and small. Using toner on this skin at the beginning of treatment will only make extractions more difficult.

2. Presoften the clogged areas by using a desincrustant solution or pre-mask. Steam with this solution on the face for about eight minutes. It is very important that the skin is hydrated for this type of treatment.

3. Remove the pre-mask or desincrustant solution. Gently pat the skin dry.

4. Begin extraction, being careful to explain to the young client what you are doing. Explain to the client that extraction should always be performed by a professional. You may have difficulty extracting these tightly packed comedones. Be gentle, and take your time. Remember, this is the young client's first experience with extraction! Slow, gentle pressure applied in small areas is most effective.

5. After extraction is complete, apply a toner or antiseptic astringent.

6. Apply a light hydrating fluid and use high frequency.

7. Apply a clay-based drying mask for oily skin.

The first facial treatment for a teenage client should be an educational experience, rather than a "feel-good" treatment. You should help the young client understand (in simple terms) what is happening to the skin and the need for consistent hygiene. Explain the use of noncomedogenic cosmetics and the need for professional advice in choosing the right products.

Acne development should also be explained to the teenage client so that the client is aware of possible future occurrences and their prevention.

If the young client already experiences acne flareups, you should make the proper treatment recommendations. (See Chapter 15, Acne and the Esthetician.) Treatment for most pubescent teens is only necessary bimonthly until further development of the pore structure or the beginning of acne flareups occurs.

Another problem associated with puberty is the development of a condition called **keratosis pilaris**. Keratosis pilaris appears as small pinpoint bumps, usually on the cheeks, accompanied by generalized redness. This condition is often seen in

**Keratosis pilaris** is a condition in which the skin exhibits redness and irritation in patches, accompanied by a rough texture, and small pinpoint white papules that look like very small milia.

"rosy-cheeked" children. In this condition, the androgens have affected the growth of either terminal or lanugo hairs, which have started growing but are not strong enough to push through the follicle opening. The hairs remain trapped inside the follicle and as a result irritate the follicle and the surrounding skin. Although this condition is usually treated by a dermatologist who uses mild retinoids or other exfoliating agents, it is sometimes seen in the salon. You should treat this condition very gently by using mildly abrasive scrubs and light extraction. The routine use of a mild abrasive, such as granular scrubs that are not excessively drying, will help open the follicle and allow the hair to come out, cutting down on irritation. A 10 percent glycolic gel, with a pH 3.5 or higher, should be used in the area once or twice a day.

## Appearance Changes in Adolescence

As the teenager gets older and further into the teenage years, the client will usually experience more problems with acne. Salon treatments should then be administered on at least a monthly basis, except in cases of more severe acne, when they should be more frequent.

## The Menstrual Cycle

**Menarche** is a girl's first period.

**Menstruation** is the body getting rid of an unused ovum and accompanying endometrium.

With puberty and adolescence comes **menarche**, the beginning of the menstrual cycle in females. Menarche is the girl's first "period." **Menstruation** is the correct name for the "period." Menstruation is actually the body getting rid of an unused ovum and accompanying endometrium, which is the lining of the uterine wall, that occurs each month in females. The endometrium is formed by the uterus in response to the hormone progesterone. The menstrual cycle is a 27- to 30-day cycle in which the female's ovaries manufacture an ovum and hormonal changes take place that prepare the uterus for pregnancy in case the ovum is fertilized by sperm. When the ovum is not fertilized, the uterus sheds the lining (endometrium), which is menstruation (Figure 5-5).

**Figure 5-5** The menstrual cycle

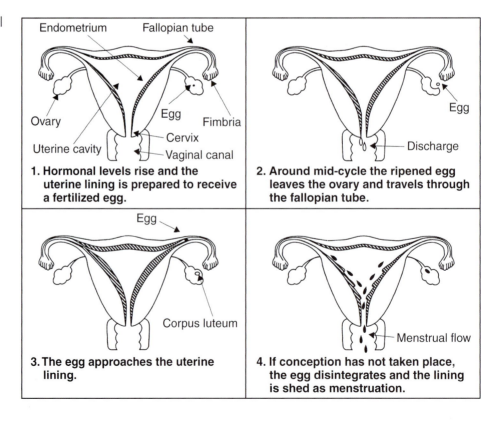

1. Hormonal levels rise and the uterine lining is prepared to receive a fertilized egg.

2. Around mid-cycle the ripened egg leaves the ovary and travels through the fallopian tube.

3. The egg approaches the uterine lining.

4. If conception has not taken place, the egg disintegrates and the lining is shed as menstruation.

There are actually six phases to the cycle:

Phase 1 occurs during the first five days of the cycle. The hypothalamus senses low levels of estrogen and progesterone and signals the pituitary gland to secrete FSH and LH. The ovaries then begin producing larger amounts of estrogen and progesterone, which prepare and release the ovum, or egg.

In Phase 2, the hypothalamus detects that the ovaries are secreting the right amount of estrogen necessary for ovulation, shuts down the pituitary gland's large production of FSH, and begins producing more LH. This occurs during days 6 to 12 of the cycle.

In Phase 3, the hormone levels of estrogen and progesterone are adjusted again. The estrogen level reaches a high point, which signals the pituitary gland to release a very large amount of LH, which then causes the release of the egg from the ovary. The surge in LH occurs in the 12th and 13th days of the cycle.

Phase 4 is on the 14th day, when the egg (ovum) is released from the ovaries and begins its journey down the fallopian tube to the uterus. What is left of the follicle from which the egg was released turns into a hormone-producing structure called the corpus luteum, which produces large amounts of progesterone. The progesterone produces the uterine lining, or endometrium, which is the "nest" that the uterus builds for a fetus. This 14th day is when a sperm can fertilize an egg and the woman becomes pregnant.

Phase 5 is essentially the last two weeks of the 28-day cycle. If fertilization of the egg has not occurred, the pituitary hormones FSH and LH drop substantially. The corpus luteum shrinks, substantially lowering its production of progesterone. This decrease in progesterone causes the breakdown of the endometrium.

Phase 6 begins menstruation, or the "period." The whole cycle begins again on the 28th day.

Many women experience differences in the actual days on which different phases of the menstrual cycle take place. Stress, obesity, anorexia, and other endocrine system disorders can all affect the cycle.

# PREGNANCY

If the ovum is fertilized by a sperm on the 14th day of the cycle, the female becomes pregnant. The corpus luteum continues to produce progesterone, and the endometrium becomes much thicker. The fertilized egg goes through a series of transformations, begins mitotic division, and forms a mass of cells. The embryo begins to form, surrounded by a capsule-like structure called a trophoblast. The trophoblast, in simple terms, provides nutrition for the embryo. The membrane of the trophoblast eventually evolves into the placenta, which is a thick layer of hormone-producing cells that serves as the nutrient, oxygen, and waste exchange system between the growing embryo and the blood system of the mother.

The placenta manufactures many hormones, including those that affect the corpus luteum, the growth of the embryo, and the production of milk in the mother's breasts.

## Skin and Appearance Changes during Pregnancy

A vast number of obvious changes take place in the human body during pregnancy. Many of these changes affect the skin. Hyperpigmentation is often seen in pregnant women. The skin often tans much more easily than normal. Pregnancy mask, or **melasma**, is a condition in which the face develops significant hyperpigmentation, resembling a dark facial mask (Figures 5-6 and 5-7). Light areas surround the eye

**Melasma** are splotchy, pigmented complexions that may be present after use of birth control pills.

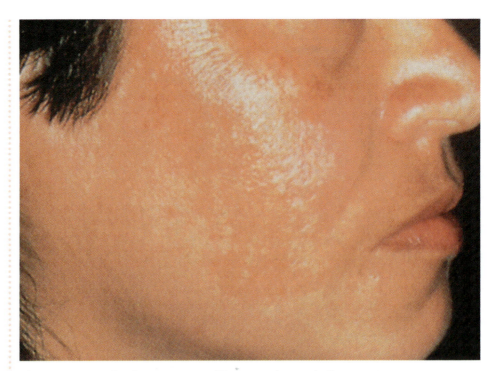

**Figure 5-6** Mask of pregnancy with hyperpigmentation (Courtesy Timothy G. Berger, M.D.)

areas, and the rest of the face is dark with pigment. Pregnancy masks and pregnancy-related hyperpigmentation are caused by a hormone secreted by the placenta that stimulates the melanocytes in the skin. Normally, hyperpigmentation subsides after the birth of the child, but sometimes the condition will need to be treated in the salon after childbirth. Treating hyperpigmentation during pregnancy is not advisable. Even if there is a bleaching effect achieved by the use of skin bleaches such as hydroquinone, the placenta continues production of the melanin-producing hormone, only to result in more hyperpigmentation. It is best to wait until the pregnancy is over. Observe whether the hyperpigmentation decreases significantly with the shutdown of placental hormones. If the hyperpigmentation does not fade within several months, it can then be treated. Avoiding exposure to the sun will help cut down on the amount of pigment produced during pregnancy.

Stretch marks, or striae, are marks that occur in pregnant women. These strip-like lines may be red or brown–tan in appearance and are the result of rapid weight gain during pregnancy. The skin simply stretches quickly, and the marks occur in the areas of the abdomen, breasts, buttocks, and legs. Unfortunately, little can be done for stretch marks. Many stretch marks fade after childbirth. The use of good, hydrating body creams and lubricants during the pregnancy seems to keep some women from developing stretch marks or at least reduces the severity. The creams must be applied on a daily, consistent basis for best results. In some women creams seem to have no effect. Some theories indicate that the development of stretch marks may be hereditarily or genetically connected. Research is currently being conducted using retinoids, electrical stimulation, and other methods to treat post-pregnancy stretch marks.

An increase in blood flow and blood pressure during pregnancy may lead to the development of **telangiectasias**, or small, red, enlarged capillaries on the face and other areas of the body. Avoiding sun and hot temperatures will help reduce the possibility of telangiectatic development. Telangiectasias are sometimes called **couperose** by European estheticians.

**Telangiectasias** are small, red, enlarged capillaries of the face and other areas of the body.

**Couperose** refers to diffuse redness, including telangiectasis of the face and other areas of the body.

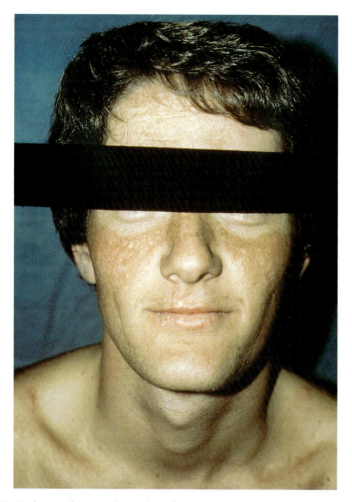

**Figure 5-7** Melasma in a male patient is very unusual (Courtesy George Fisher, M.D.)

Telangiectasias usually fade rapidly after childbirth. If there are still obvious red lines after several months, they may be treated by a dermatologist or plastic surgeon using a special type of current called **diathermy**, or they can be treated by injecting saline or using a laser.

Varicose veins may also develop on the legs during pregnancy, due to weight and pressure on the legs. Resting with the legs elevated helps to prevent their occurrence. Use of support hose is also helpful in preventing varicose veins. Most varicose veins, again, fade after pregnancy, but those that do not can be treated by a dermatologist, plastic surgeon, or vascular surgeon.

Waterproof leg makeup may be used to conceal varicose veins or telangiectasias. Pregnant women may also have problems with their facial skin. Fluctuations in hormones may make problem skin worse, or significantly better. In many cases, acne-prone skin will become worse in the beginning of pregnancy, then become much better in the third or fourth month, resulting in clear skin for the rest of the pregnancy. This is the result of the abundant female hormones present in the bloodstream during pregnancy. Acne will often flare up again after the baby is born, or just after the mother stops nursing. This, of course, results from a dramatic drop in female hormones in the bloodstream.

Acne in the pregnant woman should be treated as you would any case of acne (see Chapter 15, Acne and the Esthetician), except that therapy with galvanic and

**Diathermy** is a special type of current used in the treatment of telangiectasias.

high-frequency current should be eliminated. Check with the client's physician if you have any doubts about treatment or products.

## Precautions for Treating the Pregnant Woman

No type of electrical therapy, specifically galvanic or high-frequency therapies, should be administered to a pregnant woman, except with written permission from her physician. Physicians will often approve of electrolysis treatment, but it is important to get a written note from her doctor and keep it on file with the client's record for legal reasons.

Many topical preparations, including alphahydroxy acids, have never been extensively evaluated as to their safety when used in pregnant women. Although there is no currently available cosmetic agent known to affect the fetus, it is best to be conservative when using topical treatments and products, particularly newer functional agents. If you are in doubt about recommending a particular treatment to a pregnant client, check with her physician before administering that treatment or any questionable product for home use.

Most routine procedures may be performed on pregnant women. Special courses in body massage therapy for pregnant women are available from certified massage therapy schools. Make sure you have taken such a course before performing body massage on a pregnant woman.

Pregnant women may sometimes develop strange reactions to otherwise well-accepted treatments. Waxing, for example, may suddenly be very irritating to the skin. The only way to predict these types of reactions is to start slowly and patch-test areas for treatment. The woman's physician should supervise any internal or external drugs she takes during pregnancy. Pregnant women need lots of esthetic help during pregnancy. Pedicures may become a necessity, rather than a luxury service. Changes in the nails, skin, and hair may occur. It is also very important to be sensitive to a pregnant client's needs, because pregnancy is a wonderful, but sometimes emotional, time for some women.

## PREMENSTRUAL SYNDROME

**Premenstrual syndrome** is a condition in which some women experience uncomfortable physical changes before menstruation. These changes are caused by the fluctuating levels of hormone in the bloodstream. Increased estrogen levels may lead to water retention that can cause bloating, swelling of the breasts, swelling of the hands and feet, and general heaviness. The increase in hormones can also cause mood swings and may make the woman more susceptible to stress.

Controlling stress is one of the best ways to deal with premenstrual syndrome, frequently referred to as PMS. Stress-reducing techniques such as deep breathing exercises, aerobic workouts, massage, or general relaxation techniques may help reduce the symptoms. Esthetic care plays an important role in helping women with PMS feel better, both physically and psychologically. Wearing looser clothes may help constricted feelings associated with water retention.

In severe cases, hormones and other therapy administered by a physician may be warranted. Physicians may use drugs for high blood pressure or hormone-suppressing drugs to treat women with severe PMS.

## PMS and Acne Flareups

Women frequently experience acne flareups seven to ten days before menstruation. The specific days in the cycle associated with acne flareups may vary in some women. The cause of premenstrual acne is not completely understood. It is theorized that large levels of progesterone, present in the bloodstream during the cycle days

**Premenstrual syndrome** is a condition in which some women experience uncomfortable physical changes before menstruation.

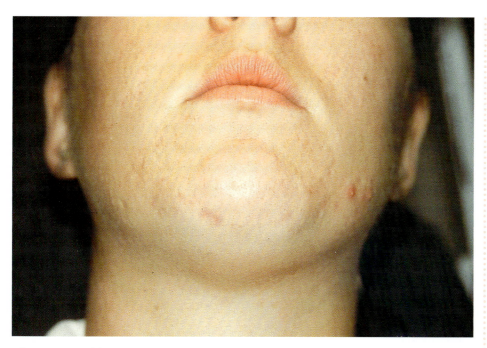

**Figure 5-8** Chin acne

normally associated with premenstrual acne, switch on the sebaceous glands, which quickly fill the follicles with sebum. This sudden surge of sebum inflames the follicle walls, causing acne papules to erupt.

Often, these flares occur in the chin and jawline area. This is referred to as chin acne (Figure 5-8). The flares present as large, sore papules. Many times they do not develop into pustules but clear up after a few days. Treatment at home with 2.5% benzoyl peroxide gel or a sulfur-resorcinol drying lotion may dry them up faster.

Women who experience constant, recurrent breakouts during premenstrual times should be referred to a dermatologist, gynecologist, or endocrinologist (hormone specialist) for treatment. Ortho Tri-Cyclen® is a birth control pill that has been developed that can help clients who have chin acne during premenstrual periods.

Premenstrual acne should be treated in the same manner as any acne flareup. Administering a good deep-cleansing facial treatment one week before the normal monthly breakout seems to help many women reduce or eliminate the flareups. Use of noncomedogenic products also can help control the breakouts, as can other therapies recommended in Chapter 15, Acne and the Esthetician. Increased stress during PMS can also cause breakouts or sudden acne flareups. Help your client choose some stress-reducing techniques or suggest that she treat herself to a body massage or other special pampering salon service to reduce stress and make herself feel better.

## BIRTH CONTROL PILLS

Birth control pills work by regulating hormones normally associated with the menstrual cycle. They interfere with the normal development of the ovum by preventing or obstructing ovulation.

There are two basic types of birth control pills. One type contains both estrogen and progesterone and works by preventing the egg from maturing, therefore preventing ovulation. The other type is mainly progesterone. These are often called "mini-pills." The mini-pills work by exposing the bloodstream to extra amounts of progesterone, which causes thickening of the uterine fluids, keeping the egg from becoming fertile.

## Skin Problems Associated with Birth Control Pills

A skin problem often associated with the use of birth control pills is the tendency to have acne flares. This does not occur in all women using birth control pills, but it does occur in a substantial number. It is common that estheticians see clients with acne flares who have just started using a new type of birth control pill. The hormones in the pills change normal hormone levels, affecting sebum production.

Birth control pills that contain little or no estrogen tend to be more aggravating to acne conditions. Estrogen-dominant pills tend to improve acne-prone skin.

In the past, birth control pills with high levels of hormones often caused very frequent acne flares. More modern birth control pills contain smaller amounts of hormones and do not cause as many problems with acne flares.

Starting and stopping birth control pills may have a dramatic effect on acne. Starting an androgen-dominant or progesterone-dominant pill may make acne immediately worse, whereas starting an estrogen-dominant pill may make acne-prone skin immediately better.

Stopping the pill may have like effects. Because the pill has a tendency to suppress natural hormone levels, discontinuing the pill may throw off natural hormone levels, making acne worse. It may take some time for the body to adjust to not having the hormone "supplement" present in the birth control pills. Some women take much longer to adjust.

## Hyperpigmentation and the Birth Control Pill

The other appearance problem related to birth control pills is that of hyperpigmentation, or melasma. Splotchy, pigmented complexions may be present after use of birth control pills. This hyperpigmentation usually is located in the forehead and cheeks. The upper lip is also often affected by melasma. Some women can develop a full-scale pregnancy mask associated with birth control pills.

Sunlight, especially deliberate exposure such as sunbathing, can make melasma much worse. Advise a client with melasma to stay out of the sun, and if she must go in the sun to use a strong sunblock. Sometimes the doctor can adjust the dosage or the type of the client's pill to reduce the possibility of melasma resulting from its use.

You should treat hyperpigmentation with hydroquinone and glycolic acid. See Chapter 20, The New Science of Aging Skin Treatment, for more information on treating melasma. Paramedical camouflage cosmetics can also be used.

## MENOPAUSE

**Menopause** is the time in a woman's life when the ovaries stop producing ova.

**Perimenopause** is the time before and around menopause.

**Osteoporosis** is a weakening of the bone associated with aging that is predominant in women.

**Menopause** is the time in a woman's life when the ovaries stop releasing ova. Menopause normally occurs when a woman is in her late forties or early fifties. The time before and around menopause is called **perimenopause**. What actually happens during menopause is that the ovaries have run out of follicles containing eggs. A female is born with 700,000 to 2 million eggs, which are contained in the follicles within the ovaries. Many die or atrophy, but at puberty about 400,000 remain. The pituitary gland secretes FSH and LH, but the ovaries stop responding. When no follicles are left to respond to follicle-stimulating hormone, no estrogen is produced in the ovary, and the preparation of the uterus does not occur.

The drop in hormone levels in the bloodstream causes a variety of physical symptoms. Hot flashes, rapid heartbeat, decreases in vaginal secretions, emotional irritability, bloating, and other signs may occur.

The same symptoms may be produced after a hysterectomy. If a woman has a hysterectomy early in life, the gynecologist will often leave the ovaries and remove only the uterus. The presence of the ovaries helps secure hormone levels in the bloodstream, at least until true menopause takes place. Medical science has discovered that women who lose their ovaries early in life are more likely to develop **osteoporosis**, a weakening of the bones associated with aging that is predominant in women. Many women have **hormone replacement therapy (HRT)** after menopause or after a hysterectomy. Use of synthetic estrogen and progesterone, taken in the sequence of the normal menstrual cycle hormone secretions, helps prevent many of the symptoms associated with menopause. It, of course, will not make women ovulate again. Estrogen is believed to have a positive effect on reducing the chances of osteoporosis development, offers a decreased chance of cardiac problems, and may help prevent rheumatoid arthritis.

Some recent studies indicate that there may be an increased risk of breast cancer in women who use HRT longer than five years. If there is a family history of breast cancer in the immediate family (sister, mother), there may be a greater risk. The use of HRT should be an individual and personal decision based on personal and family history; menopausal symptoms and their severity; and, most importantly, a thorough consultation with a doctor.

## SKIN CONDITIONS ASSOCIATED WITH MENOPAUSE

In the next two decades 40 million women will go through menopause. Esthetically, a woman may have any number of symptoms associated with perimenopause. This may include thinning hair, excess hair growth on the face or other body areas, or even increased oiliness or dryness of the skin.

Recent research indicates that the presence of estrogen has a strong influence on collagen formation. As menopause occurs, estrogen levels drop dramatically and may have an obvious effect on the appearance of wrinkles and lack of elasticity. Use of HRT may improve and reduce the loss of collagen, therefore causing skin to regain more of its previous elasticity and suppleness.

Lack of estrogen may significantly affect barrier function, increasing sensitivity of the skin, dehydration, possible hyperpigmentation, and fluctuations in blood flow. Estrogen is responsible for sending many hormonal messages to the skin, and a decrease can affect many functions of the skin and, therefore, its appearance.

Many aging problems associated with menopause may actually be the result of cumulative sun exposure earlier in life. It is coincidental that the damage of years of sun exposure happen to surface about the same time as menopause in some women. Having both sun damage and menopausal effects on the skin can cause real esthetic problems and is even more reason why your client needs lots of care at this important time.

### Hot Flashes and Flushing

Hot flashes are caused by a fluctuation in blood flow resulting from decreased estrogen, which normally helps with smooth blood flow. Without estrogen, there are sudden "spurts" in blood flow, resulting in redness and the feeling of heat in the skin. Flushing and hot flashes can be reduced or eliminated with hormone replacement therapy.

Rarely, women experience a condition called **formication**, which feels like continuous tingling and itching. Some women have described it as feeling like "bugs crawling on the skin." Again, this can be treated with HRT.

Use of nonfragranced creams with lipid replacement ingredients such as sphingolipids or ceramides may help with dryness and itching. The skin may be more sensitive to any stimulating product, so be careful with these, especially stimulating aromatherapy products.

### Moodiness

Women may experience moodiness during menopause. Although some of this may be caused by hormonal fluctuations, it may also be stress related or may be complicated by depression. It is important that you are understanding of the needs of your

**Hormone replacement therapy (HRT)** uses oral or injectable female hormones to control or prevent symptoms of menopause. HRT may also help prevent skin changes or osteoporosis in women.

**Formication** is an itching and tingling feeling of the skin experienced by some women during menopause.

client who is menopausal and offer stress-reducing services such as massages or aromatherapy.

## Perimenopausal Acne

Clients may experience a sudden flare of acne during or just after menopause. This is again caused by a decrease of estrogen in the bloodstream, which, in turn, increases the percentage of the male hormone androgen that turns on the sebaceous glands. This results in increased oiliness, hirsutism, and acne lesions. You should treat this as you would any other acne case, but remember that the client may more readily experience dehydration and be concerned about aging skin. Be careful not to overdry the skin.

## Esthetic Management of Menopausal Skin

The esthetician can play a significant role in helping the client going through menopause with skin problems. The esthetician may actually notice small symptoms in the skin before the client is even fully aware that she is beginning menopause.

Keep a client's age in mind when noticing some of the symptoms we have discussed here. Adjusting a client's home care and treatment schedule may help a great deal.

For clients experiencing aging symptoms, recommend lipid-based creams, which can help improve barrier function. Soothing antioxidants can help reduce redness and discomfort. Alphahydroxy acids may also relieve various symptoms. More frequent salon treatments may help esthetic symptoms as well as help with stress management.

## Menopausal Skin Symptoms

1. Dryness and itchy skin on the face and body
2. Increased sensitivity
3. Sudden flares of acne
4. Sudden hair growth on the face
5. Mood swings
6. Client complains of "suddenly aging" skin
7. Hot flashes and flushing
8. A "tired" look to the skin, with increased elastosis

## ABOUT HIRSUTISM

**Hirsutism** refers to excessive hair growth.

**Hirsutism** refers to excessive hair growth. Women who have hormonal fluctuations may experience hirsutism. Excess hair growth, primarily on the face, may happen at any time in a woman's life, but especially after menopause. The dominance of the androgenic hormones after menopause is the main cause.

Hirsutism may be treated by waxing or electrolysis in the salon. Excessive facial hair growth is often best treated by electrolysis because the electrolysis is eventually permanent. Waxing may provide temporary relief in minor cases. Stiffer hairs in the chin and lip areas are best treated by electrolysis. Estheticians and electrologists should be aware of other symptoms that may require referral to a physician. Although most excessive hair is mainly a cosmetic nuisance, accompanying symptoms such as thinning of the hair, deepening of the voice, and loss of menstruation should be referred to a gynecologist.

# OBESITY, ANOREXIA, AND HORMONES

Women who are extremely obese may experience a loss of hormone activity, resulting in menstrual irregularity, hirsutism, and acne. Women who are anorexic may have hormonal fluctuations and irregular menstrual cycles.

Women athletes who have a very low body fat percentage may also experience similar hormonal problems. Many estheticians have observed a correlation between avid female athletes and low body fat, hirsutism, and acne.

# OTHER HORMONAL DISORDERS THAT AFFECT THE SKIN

Although it is not the esthetician's job to diagnose illness, you should be aware of some symptoms that you may connect with certain skin problems or be able to discuss a client's skin symptoms related to an endocrine illness. You should always refer suspicious skin problems to a physician. If you have a client who has multiple symptoms of any kind of illness, always refer the client to a doctor.

**Hyperthyroidism** is a condition in which the thyroid gland secretes too much thyroid hormone. Physical symptoms may include heart palpitations, weight loss, and fatigue. Esthetic symptoms include thinning of the skin, hair loss, and rapidly growing nails. **Hypothyroidism** is just the opposite of hyperthyroidism. The thyroid gland does not produce enough hormone. Puffy eyelids, facial swelling, and coarse skin that is very dehydrated are esthetic symptoms of hypothyroidism, if they are also associated with weight gain, poor balance, or hearing problems.

Adrenal gland disorders can also result in skin symptoms. Cushing's syndrome is a disease of the adrenal glands. Persons with Cushing's syndrome secrete too much hydrocortisone. Too much medicinal hydrocortisone can also cause the disease. Symptoms are thinning of the skin and bruises that occur easily. Addison's disease is the exact opposite of Cushing's syndrome. The adrenal glands do not produce adrenal hormones. Skin symptoms include severe hyperpigmentation on the face, dark freckles on the torso, as well as hyperpigmentation on the palms of the hands. Addison's disease is easily treated with hormone therapy.

**Hyperthyroidism** is a condition in which the thyroid gland secretes too much thyroid hormone.

**Hypothyroidism** is a condition in which the thyroid gland secretes too little thyroid hormone.

# TOPICS FOR DISCUSSION

1. What are the major endocrine glands?
2. What is puberty, and what hormonal changes take place with puberty?
3. What precautions should the esthetician take when treating a pregnant woman?
4. What are some esthetic side effects of birth control pills?
5. What are some esthetic problems associated with menopause?
6. Name several endocrine disorders and discuss their effects on the skin.

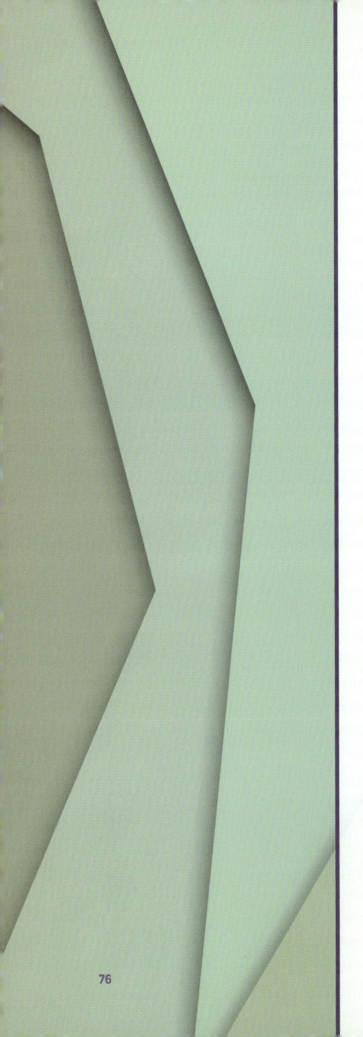

# CHAPTER 6

# Skin Analysis

## OBJECTIVES. . .

**Skin analysis** is the process of determining the client's skin type and conditions that require esthetic care. It is a very important skill for all estheticians. Skin analysis is the key to determining correct skin treatment programs.

In this chapter, we will discuss differences in esthetic and dermatological skin typing, proper health screening, and techniques used in professional skin analysis. You will learn about properly recording your analysis and how to use charts for the client.

You will learn how to recognize very basic skin conditions and lesions. This chapter is not intended to provide extensive information on particular skin conditions. For more information on any of the conditions discussed within, please refer to other chapters on the specific skin conditions.

# FITZPATRICK SKIN TYPING

When a dermatologist speaks about the skin type of a patient, he or she will probably use a term such as "type 1" or "type 2." Dermatologists do not generally refer to clients' skin types as oily, normal, or dry, as estheticians do. They assess skin in terms of genetic pigment coloration. This type of skin typing was originated by Dr. Thomas Fitzpatrick, a famous research dermatologist.

**Fitzpatrick Skin Typing** is a system of classifying the client's individual skin by hereditary pigmentation, indicating their resistance to sun-related damage and sunburn. The lower the number, the lighter the skin coloration and the more the client is susceptible to sun-related damage or disease (Figure 6-1).

The system describes skin coloration, eye color, and hair color of each skin type and states the typical scenario regarding the tendency of skin to burn or tan when exposed to the sun (Table 6-1).

# ESTHETIC SKIN TYPING

## Client Health History

The first treatment for every client should begin by taking a health history for the client. This will give you important information about the client, including his or her habits, medical conditions, and other information that can affect your treatment of the client's skin.

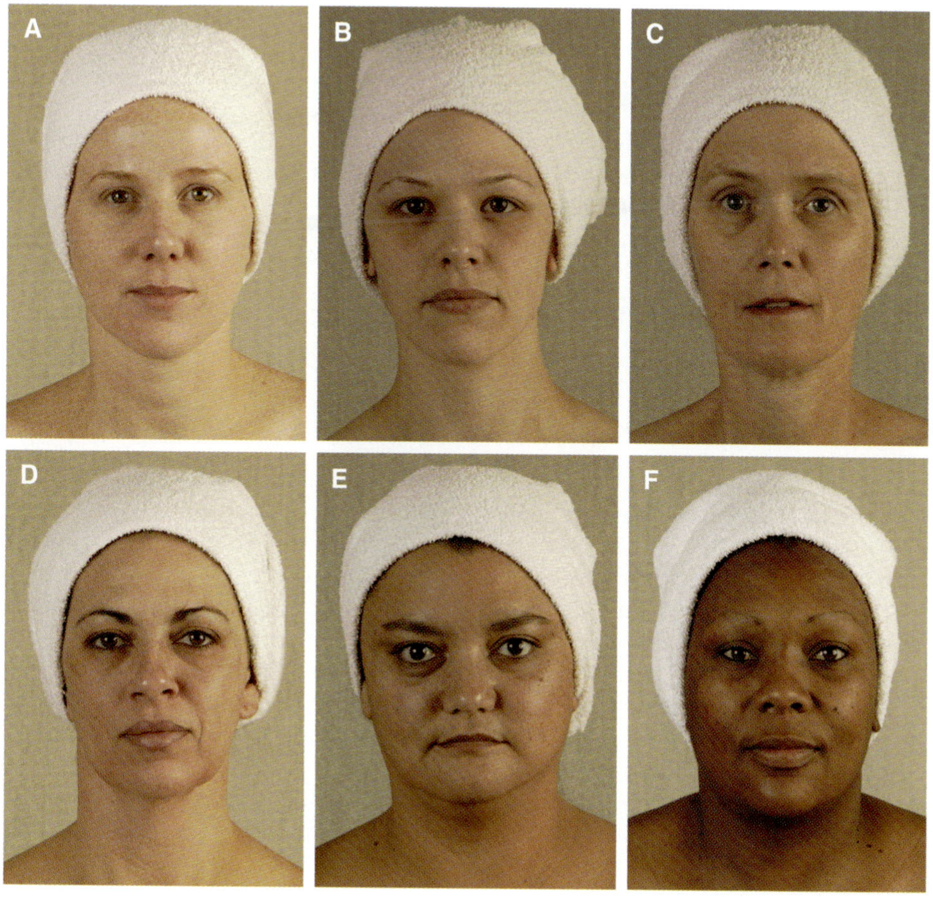

**Skin analysis** is the process of determining a client's skin type and conditions.

**Fitzpatrick Skin Typing** is a system that classifies skin by hereditary pigmentation and resistance to sun damage and sunburn.

**Figure 6-1** *A*, Fitzpatrick I; *B*, Fitzpatrick II; *C*, Fitzpatrick III; *D*, Fitzpatrick IV; *E*, Fitzpatrick V; and *F*, Fitzpatrick VI

**Table 6-1**

| Fitzpatrick Skin Types | | |
|---|---|---|
| **Skin Type** | **Burns or Tans** | **Characteristics** |
| Type I | Always burns, never tans | Very fair skin, red or blonde hair, blue eyes, likely freckled skin |
| Type II | Burns easily, tans minimally | Fair skin; blue, green, or hazel eyes; blonde or red hair |
| Type III | Sometimes burns, gradually tans | Very common coloring; still fair, but with any color hair and eyes |
| Type IV | Rarely burns, always tans | Typical Mediterranean Caucasian skin; medium to heavy pigmentation |
| Type V | Very rarely burns, always tans | Middle-Eastern skin types, not sun sensitive |
| Type VI | Almost never burns | Black skin; generally never sun sensitive |

**Contraindications** are treatment techniques, products, or ingredients that must be avoided because of individual client conditions that may cause side effects or possibly endanger the client's health.

The client should fill out the client health form (Figure 6-2). After the client completes the form, you should discuss any questions you have with the client, and when in doubt, postpone treatment until the client has approval for the treatment from her doctor.

**Contraindications** are treatment techniques, products, or ingredients that must be avoided because of individual client conditions that may cause side effects or somehow endanger the client's health. For example, when a client tells you she is allergic to all forms of nuts, you must avoid using any products containing nuts or nut by-products. In this case, the use of nuts is contraindicated.

Using, for example, a honey and almond scrub on this client will likely cause an allergic reaction. If a client has a pacemaker or is pregnant, the use of electrical current is contraindicated. If a client is already using prescription peeling agents prescribed by her dermatologist, the further use of more peeling agents is contraindicated.

## What to Ask About

Here we will review some of the more common contraindications. This is intended only as an overview of common contraindications. For much more information on health screening and contraindications, see *Milady's Standard Comprehensive Training for Estheticians.*

**Allergies.** Does the client have any known allergies to any cosmetics, foods, or drugs? You must avoid using any chemical or ingredient to which the client is allergic. Common allergies include fragrances, nuts, iodide allergies (avoid seaweed products), specific sunscreen ingredients, and hydroquinone (melanin suppressant for hyperpigmentation). There may be many other ingredients to which the client is allergic. You need to discuss this thoroughly with the client before treatment begins to make sure you are clear about the client's specific allergies. Carefully check labels on products to determine if the product contains the allergic ingredient. If there is any doubt, always check with the client's doctor or dermatologist.

Clients sometimes mix up irritant and allergic reactions, so it is important that you try to establish if the client is actually allergic or simply overused a product and had an irritant reaction.

Patients with rosacea also must avoid many ingredients and treatments to avoid flares. For more information on allergic and irritant reactions, see the chapters on sensitive skin and rosacea.

**Confidential Skin Health Survey**

**PLEASE PRINT**

Today's Date _____
First Name _____ Last Name _____ Date of Birth ___/___/___
Street _____ Apt. # _____ City _____ State _____ Zip _____
Phone—Home ( )_____ Work ( )_____ Mobile ( )_____ Dermatologist/
Physician _____ Phone ( )_____
Emergency Contact _____ Phone ( )_____
Your Occupation _____
Referred By  ❏ Friend  ❏ Mailer  ❏ Walk-by  ❏ Yellow Pages  ❏ Gift Certificate  ❏ Other _____
Esthetician Name _____

1. Is this your first facial?  ❏ Yes  ❏ No
2. What is the reason for your visit today? _____
   _____
3. What special areas of concern do you have? _____
   _____
   _____
4. Are you presently under a physician's care for any current skin condition or other problem?  ❏ Yes  ❏ No
   What? _____
5. Are you pregnant?  ❏ Yes  ❏ No
6. Are you taking birth control pills?  ❏ Yes  ❏ No
   If so, what type? _____
7. Hormone replacement?  ❏ Yes  ❏ No
   If so, what? _____
8. Do you wear contact lenses?  ❏ Yes  ❏ No
9. Do you smoke?  ❏ Yes  ❏ No
10. Do you often experience stress?  ❏ Yes  ❏ No
11. Have you had skin cancer?  ❏ Yes  ❏ No

12. Are you now using (or used in the past):  ❏ Azelex
    ❏ Differin  ❏ Renova  ❏ Retin-A
    ❏ Tazarac  ❏ Glycolic or alphahydroxy acids
    If so, when and for how long? _____
13. Are you now using or have you ever used Accutane?
    ❏ Yes  ❏ No
    If so, when and for how long? _____
14. Do you have acne?  ❏ Yes  ❏ No
    Experience frequent blemishes?  ❏ Yes  ❏ No
    If so, how frequently? _____
15. Do you have any allergies to cosmetics, foods, or drugs?
    ❏ Yes  ❏ No
    Please list _____
16. Are you presently taking medications—oral or topical?
    ❏ Yes  ❏ No  If so, please list
    _____
    _____
17. What products do you use presently?  ❏ Soap
    ❏ Cleansing milk  ❏ Toner  ❏ Scrub  ❏ Mask
    ❏ Creams  ❏ Sunscreen  ❏ Other

Please circle if you are affected by or have any of the following:

| | | |
|---|---|---|
| Asthma | Hepatitis | Metal bone, pins, or plates |
| Cardiac problems | Herpes | Pacemaker |
| Eczema | High blood pressure | Psychological problems |
| Epilepsy | Hysterectomy | Sinus problems |
| Fever blisters | Immune disorders | Skin diseases—other |
| Headaches—chronic | Lupus | Urinary or kidney problems |

Please explain above problems or list any significant others: _____

I understand that the services offered are not a substitute for medical care, and any information provided by the therapist is for educational purposes only and not diagnostically prescriptive in nature. I understand that the information herein is to aid the therapist in giving better service and is completely confidential.

**SALON POLICIES**
1. Professional consultation is required before initial dispensing of products.
2. Our active discount rate is only effective for clients visiting every 4 weeks.
3. We do not give cash refunds.
4. We require a 24-hour cancellation notice.

I fully understand and agree to the above salon policies.

_____     _____
Client's signature                                       Date

**Figure 6-2** Confidential skin health survey

# Drugs and Medications

There are many drugs that can cause skin treatment side effects. Many of these are topical drugs such as tretinoin (Retin-A®, Renova®, etc.), tazarotene (Tazorac®), azelaic acid (Azelex®), adapalene (Differin®), and others. Ask specifically if the client is using *any* topical drug. The main contraindications for these drugs are the use of other exfoliants or peeling agents, fragrances, and any stimulating product that increases blood circulation. Accutane® (isotretinoin) is an oral drug used primarily for treating grade IV acne that has *many* cosmetic side effects. Clients using Accutane *must avoid other peeling agents and waxing on any part of the body.* For more information on Accutane, see the chapter on acne. Clients using the oral drug Prednisone® usually have an autoimmune disease such as lupus. Clients using Prednisone should avoid waxing, peeling, and other stimulating treatments. Again, when in doubt, check with the client's physician.

**Medical Conditions.** There are many medical conditions that can affect skin treatment. Specifically, you need to know if the client has heart (cardiac) problems, epilepsy or seizure disorders, cancer, lupus, hepatitis, or fever blisters (herpes simplex) or if she is pregnant.

As a general rule, if you have any doubt about treating a client with medical conditions, check with the client's doctor before treating the client.

Any treatment involving the application of electrical current should be avoided on patients with heart problems, clients who are pregnant, patients with a seizure disorder, and clients with implanted metal bone pins or plates.

Clients with lupus sometimes react unusually to any stimulating treatment. Be careful with extraction, stimulant treatments, and waxing on these clients.

Clients who have had problems with fever blisters, especially chronically, should have any skin treatment cleared by the doctor. Peeling treatments, specifically, have been known to aggravate herpes simplex outbreaks.

## SKIN TYPES VERSUS SKIN CONDITIONS

We need to distinguish the difference between skin types and skin conditions. **Skin types** are related to the amount of sebum being produced by the sebaceous glands. Skin types are hereditary and generally cannot be changed through esthetic treatment. **Skin conditions** are treatable disorders of the skin. Skin conditions are often changeable through esthetic treatment.

Certain skin types have typical conditions associated with them. For example, oily skin often has skin conditions such as comedones, clogged pores, and frequent acne breakouts. Dry skin often has a condition of dehydration because there is not enough sebum to prevent the skin from dehydrating.

Estheticians can treat comedones through extraction and exfoliating products and can improve dehydration through the use of moisturizers and hydrating treatments and products. They cannot, however, change the hereditary skin type.

Some conditions can affect any skin type. Sun damage conditions, such as wrinkles, elastosis (sagging skin), or hyperpigmentation can affect oily, combination, or dry skin.

The importance of establishing skin type is to determine the type of product to be used on the skin. For example, sunscreens are available in a variety of **vehicles**, the carrying base and spreading agent of the product. A sunscreen in a vehicle that contains oils and emollient ingredients is more appropriate for dry skin types, whereas a sunscreen in a lightweight vehicle with lesser amounts of emollients is more appropriate for oilier skin that does not need as much oil and lubrication.

Consumers as well as estheticians often choose a product or treatment to help a skin condition that is in the wrong vehicle for the client's skin type. They are focused only on the skin condition and are not paying attention to the skin type. They may choose a product to help symptoms of sun damage, but the product is not in the correct vehicle for their skin type. An anti-aging product that is in the wrong vehicle can create other unwanted conditions.

It is essential that skin type be firmly understood for success in any skin-care program.

## THE ANALYSIS PROCEDURE

1. Begin by cleansing the skin with a gentle cleansing milk or lotion. Thoroughly remove all makeup. Do NOT tone the skin after cleansing when performing an

---

**Skin type** is the determination of the hereditary oiliness or dryness level of an individual's skin.

**Skin conditions** are generally treatable disorders of the skin that are often related to environmental damage or the client's skin type.

**Vehicles** are the spreading agents in skin-care or cosmetic products.

analysis because this can make pores look smaller than they actually are and interfere with an accurate analysis.

2. Look at the client's skin carefully through a magnifying lamp (mag lamp). Most magnifying lamps enlarge the appearance of the skin 3–5 times. Carefully observe the entire skin from top to bottom (Figure 6-3).

3. To determine the skin type, look for the presence or absence of visible pores. **Pore** is a lay term for the follicles, but specifically we are looking at the top view of the follicle, commonly referred to as a pore. Where you can see clearly visible pores, the sebum flow from the follicle is either normal or oily. The larger the pore, the oilier the skin area. The smaller the pore, the less oil is reaching the surface to lubricate and help prevent surface dehydration. The pore size is, in general, a good indication of how much sebum is being produced and reaching the skin surface. Some clients appear to have no pores. The follicles *are* actually present, but they are simply not dilated because there is little sebum passing through the follicle. Follicles stretch to accommodate the amount of sebum being produced by the sebaceous glands. **Oily skin** areas are characterized by larger pores (Figure 6-4), **normal skin** by average size pores, and **dry (alipidic) skin** by very small, sometimes barely visible pores (Figure 6-5). We refer to dry skin as alipidic, meaning there is a lack of lipids being produced by the sebaceous gland. Clients often call their *dehydrated* skin "dry," and we want to distinguish between a lack of sebum flow and a lack of moisture in the skin surface, which is dehydration. **Combination skin** is characterized by oily, normal, and dry skin in different areas. Combination skin is the most common type of skin, usually with oilier areas in the center of the face and pores becoming visibly smaller as you look across the face toward the perimeter (toward the ears), indicating alipidic skin. The **perimeter** of the face is the outside edges, bordered by the ears, lower chin and neck, and top edge of the forehead. The **T-zone** is the area of the forehead, nose, and chin. This area is often oily and may often have larger pores (Figure 6-6). Estheticians frequently refer to combination skin as **combination-dry** or **combination-oily.** This means that the client has combination skin, but it tends to be more dry or oily.

**Pore** is the lay term for follicle, most often used for the appearance of the top view of the follicle.

**Oily skin** is a skin type characterized by enlarged pores, indicating active sebaceous production.

**Normal skin** is a skin type characterized by evenly distributed average-sized pores.

**Dry (alipidic) skin** is a skin type characterized by very small or barely visible pores, indicating below-average sebaceous production.

**Combination skin** is facial skin characterized by a mix of oily and dry skin areas.

**Perimeter** is the outside edge of the face, bordered by the ears, lower chin and neck, and top of the forehead.

**T-zone** is the middle area of the face, including the forehead, nose, and chin.

**Combination-dry** is a skin type that has both oily and dry areas but is predominantly dry. It is indicated by larger pores through the middle of the T-zone only.

**Combination-oily** is a skin type that has both oily and dry areas but is predominantly oily. It is indicated by larger pores through the T-zone, expanding into the outer cheeks, with smaller pores in the facial perimeter only.

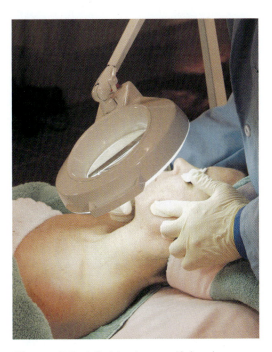

**Figure 6-3** A lighted magnifying lamp

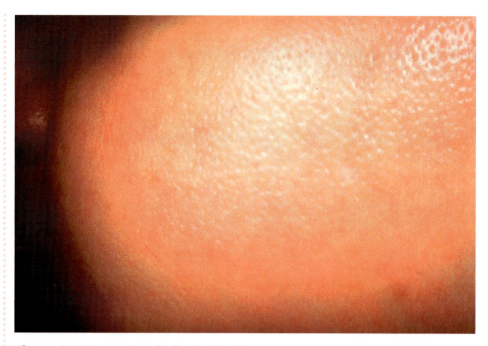

**Figure 6-4** Large pores indicate oily skin areas (Courtesy Mark Lees Skin Care, Inc.)

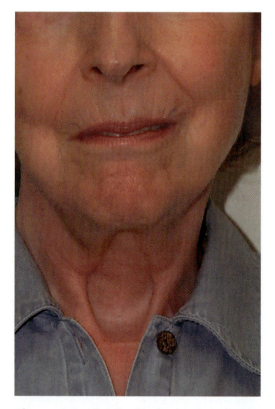

**Figure 6-5** Alipidic skin is characterized by a lack of visible pore openings (Courtesy of Mark Lees Skin Care, Inc.)

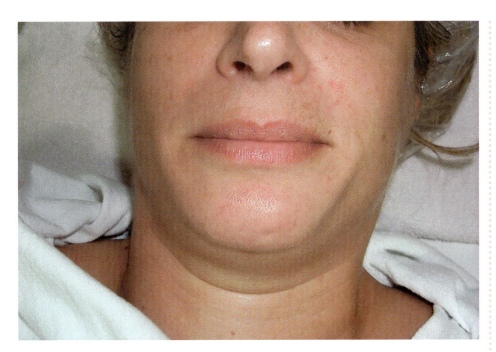

**Figure 6-6** Combination skin (Courtesy Mark Lees Skin Care, Inc.)

Because acne is hereditary, acne is considered by many to be a skin type. There are four different grades of acne. For information about this skin type, please read the chapter on acne.

4. After you have established the skin type, you must observe any conditions of the skin. The following is a basic guide for different conditions frequently seen during skin analysis. For much more information on any of these conditions, consult the specific chapters on aging, sun damage, acne, sensitive skin, and "recognize and refer" medical conditions. Some of these terms are not medical or scientific, but they are included because they are commonly used among estheticians.

**Table 6-2**

| Skin Type | Characteristics | Comments |
|---|---|---|
| Normal | Perfectly even pore distribution | Very unusual |
| Oily | Enlarged pores throughout the face. May be very shiny with obvious oiliness. | Usually also has many clogged pores, open or closed comedones. |
| Dry/Alipidic | Very small or invisible pores | May also be very dehydrated. Typical in older skin. |
| Combination-Oily | Larger pores through the "T-zone" (nose, chin and forehead), with smaller or less visible pore structure in the perimeter areas of the face. | Very typical skin type, especially in clients who are younger than 40–50 years of age. |
| Combination-Dry | Pore structure visible only through the very center of the face, especially in the nose area. Fine or invisible pore structure on the cheeks and outer areas of the face. | Typical in older skin, especially older female clients. |

# PORE OR FOLLICLE-RELATED CONDITIONS

Follicle-related conditions are generally symptoms of oily skin or oily areas.

**Open comedones**—Enlarged clogged follicles, commonly known as blackheads, generally associated with oily areas.

**Closed comedones**—small, white bumps just under the skin surface. Careful observation will indicate a very small pore opening. Associated with oily and acne conditions (Figure 6-7).

**Sebaceous filaments**—small clogged pores with black tops often seen in the nose and center areas of the face (Figure 6-8).

**"Orange peel" texture**—refers to large areas of enlarged pores, indicative of oily skin.

**Sebaceous hyperplasias**—often said to look like a "daisy" or "donut," these lesions are indicative of oily and sun-damaged areas. They are caused by overgrowth of sebaceous glands (Figure 6-9).

**Papule**—a red bump, usually acne-related.

**Pustule**—a red bump with a white head, usually an acne lesion.

**Ingrown hairs**—these may look like papules or pustules but are caused by hairs that have broken off in the follicle and irritated the follicle walls, usually as a result of improper shaving or tweezing. Look for these in areas of the face such as the chin, where clients may be tweezing unwanted hair. These also may be frequently seen on the neck of male clients.

**Milia**—perfectly round white bumps that resemble sesame seeds. Milia contain impactions of keratinized cells and sebum (Figure 6-10).

**Cyst**—large bump under the skin surface; must be referred to a dermatologist.

**Scarred ostia**—often called "open pores" or ice pick scars, these are small scarred follicles that always appear enlarged.

**Figure 6-7** Open and closed comedones
(Courtesy Michael J. Bond, M.D.)

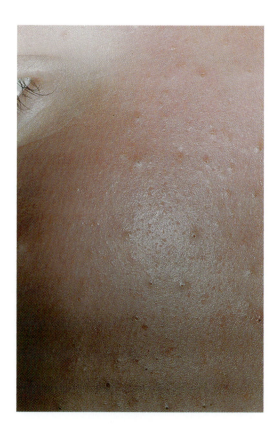

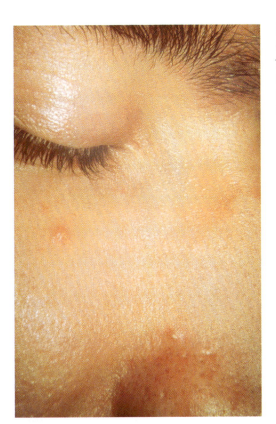

**Figure 6-8** Sebaceous filaments, often called clogged pores, are follicles filled with solidified sebum. The black tip is oxidized sebum in the top of the follicle
(Courtesy Mark Lees Skin Care, Inc.)

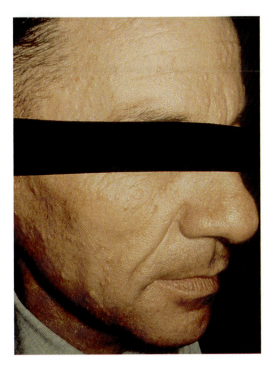

**Figure 6-9** Multiple sebaceous hyperplasia in an adult male with oily skin and sun damage. Sebaceous hyperplasias usually are found on the forehead, temple, and upper cheeks, but they can appear anywhere on the face
(Courtesy George Fisher, M.D.)

**"Pseudopores"**—a European esthetic term referring to enlarged pore structure in older, sun-damaged skin. Usually appear in groups on the cheeks immediately on the sides of the nose; these open pores are not clogged and always appear enlarged. This is a symptom of sun damage. The skin be typed as dry but still show these obvious pores, but the client generally has dry or combination-dry skin (Figure 6-11).

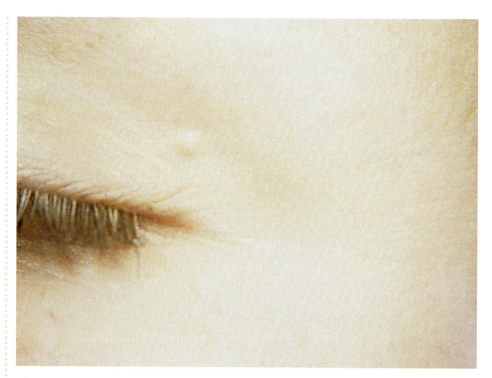

**Figure 6-10** Milia are often seen around the eye area, as seen on this client's upper lid (Courtesy Mark Lees Skin Care, Inc.)

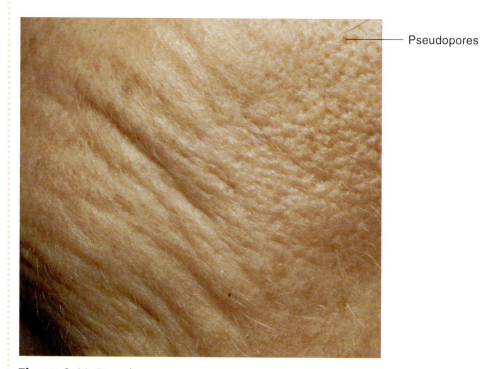

Pseudopores

**Figure 6-11** Pseudopores

# AGING AND SUN-DAMAGE CONDITIONS

Sun damage and aging symptoms can appear on any skin type. Although skin tends to become drier as it ages, aging skin can be dry, oily, or combination.

**Rhytides** are wrinkles. Intrinsic wrinkles, also known as expression lines, may be caused by constant facial expressions. Sun damage–related wrinkles are often not in the facial expression areas. Expression lines in sun-damaged skin are deeper and more pronounced.

**Elastosis** is lack of skin firmness and lack of elasticity. Sagging skin is a symptom of elastosis. Skin that does not "snap back" when lightly pinched lacks elasticity. Elastosis is caused by gravity, sun exposure, and other factors.

**Tactile roughness**—refers to a rough texture to the touch.

**Chloasma**—refers to sun-related freckles, splotches, or hyperpigmentation.

# REDNESS CONDITIONS

Redness conditions can appear on any skin type. Skin that is red with oily skin symptoms is often classified as **sensitive-oily** skin. Skin that has redness without obvious pore structure is classified as **sensitive-dry** skin. Redness, of course, can be a sign of inflammation, which can affect any skin type.

**Telangiectasias**—dilated red capillaries (Figure 6-12).

**Couperose**—the European term for areas of telangiectasias

**Diffuse redness**—areas of mild constant redness.

**Pinkness**—usually indicative of sensitive skin.

**Erythema**—the medical term for redness. There are numerous medical conditions that are erythemic and need medical referral.

**Rosacea**—medical condition characterized by nose redness, other diffuse redness, and telangiectasias.

> **Sensitive-oily** is a skin type that is both oily and tends to be red and reactive.
>
> **Sensitive-dry** is a skin type that is both dry (alipidic) and tends to be red and reactive.

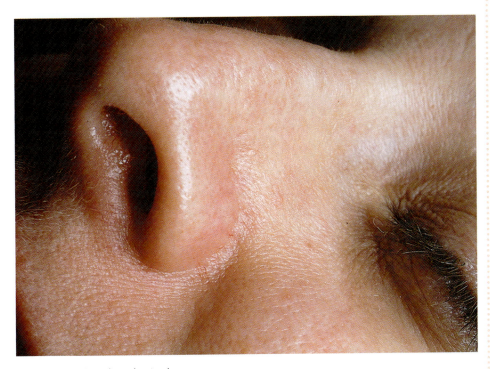

**Figure 6-12** Telangiectasias

## PIGMENTATION CONDITIONS

Pigmentation conditions are variations in skin coloration. Most pigmentation conditions are caused by abnormalities in pigment production in the melanocytes. Pigmentation problems can affect any skin type.

**Hyperpigmentation**—over-production of melanin, resulting in dark splotches, and **hypopigmentation**—is lack of melanin production, resulting in light-colored areas.

**Solar lentigenes**—freckles caused by sun exposure (Figure 6-13).

**Mottling**—speckled hyperpigmentation, also usually caused from cumulative sun exposure (Figure 6-14).

**Vitiligo**—a medical condition resulting in absence of pigment in splotches (Figure 6-15).

**Post-inflammatory hyperpigmentation**—dark splotches or spots related to skin trauma. Dark spots of pigmentation left from acne blemishes are the result of pigmentation produced from inflammation of the acne lesion. They can also result from scratching or chronic picking at acne lesions. These are particularly common in darker skin types.

**Melasma**—commonly referred to as "pregnancy mask." This presents as mask-patterned splotches of hyperpigmentation. Sometimes this only affects part of the face, but it still has a pattern to it and is most often symmetrical, equally affecting both sides of the face (Figure 6-16).

## SKIN ABNORMALITIES

While analyzing the skin, you should also make note of any unusual skin problems or abnormalities, even if you will not be treating these conditions.

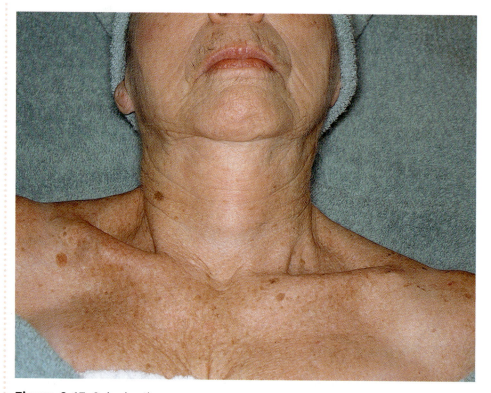

**Figure 6-13** Solar lentigenes

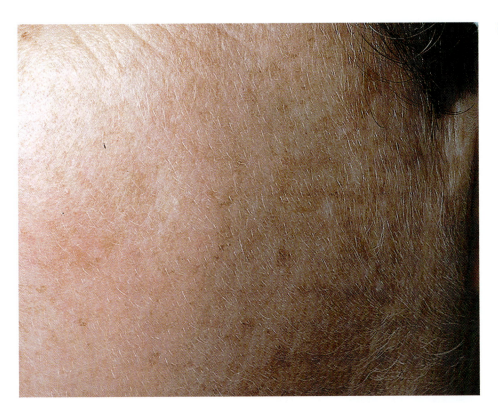

**Figure 6-14** Mottling

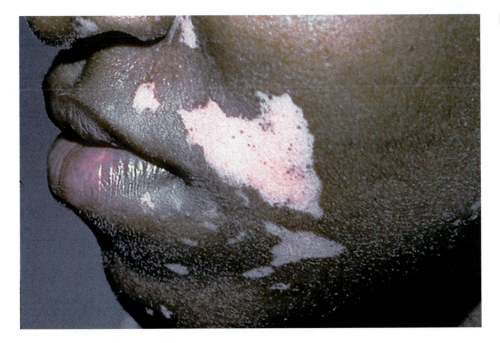

**Figure 6-15** Vitiligo

**Birthmarks**—often splotches of hyperpigmentation that are **congenital** (have been present since birth.) Some birthmarks may be treated by dermatologists.

**Port-wine stains**—large red-to-purple splotches that are vascular (involving blood vessels). They are congenital and can be treated with lasers by dermatologists or plastic surgeons.

**Scars**—should be noted in the client's chart. Location of the scar should also be noted. **Hypertrophic** scars are above the skin. **Hypotrophic** scars are depressions in the skin such as **pockmarks**.

**Congenital** refers to conditions present since birth.

**Hypertrophic** describes a raised scar above the skin's surface.

**Hypotrophic** describes a depressed scar.

**Pockmark** is a hypotrophic scar often caused by chickenpox or acne.

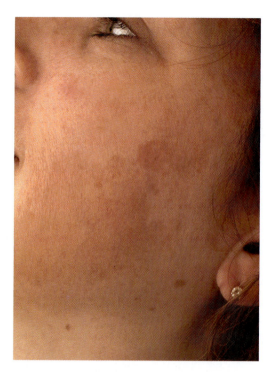

**Figure 6-16** Melasma

## MEDICAL CONDITIONS OF THE SKIN

Although estheticians do not diagnose medical conditions or administer medical procedures, notes should be made during the analysis of any diagnosed medical condition that affects the client. Notes should also be made of any areas that currently exhibit symptoms of the medical condition. This would include areas affected by rosacea, seborrheic dermatitis, skin cancer or scars from skin cancer treatment, and so on.

During analysis, you may notice signs of probable medical conditions that require referral to a dermatologist or other doctor. Although you should never tell a client she has a disease or medical condition, you must refer the client to a doctor any time that you suspect a client has a medical condition. Medical referrals to doctors to diagnosis and treat your client's medical conditions should also be recorded. For more information about these conditions, see the chapter on medical conditions.

### Recording Your Analysis

All of your observations during the skin analysis should be written down in a special chart for the client. Writing down of all observations and treatments is referred to as **charting**.

Analysis and treatment charts are available from many skin-care companies and are easy to fill out. These forms have places to mark skin types and conditions, along with their location. They also have places to record treatment procedures and home care recommendations and purchases.

You should take a special colored highlighter and highlight any contraindications so that any esthetician looking at the chart will notice the contraindication. Medical offices often use colored stickers to denote allergies, special warnings, or other contraindications. This will help prevent any accidental use of products or treatments that are contraindicated for your client.

**Charting** is the process of creating a written record of clinical observations and treatments in a client's or patient's chart.

At every visit you should record the exact treatment you performed and note any differences in the skin condition, along with any questions or issues discussed with the client. Also note any new products purchased or recommended.

Some estheticians take photos of the client's skin during the first visit and keep the photos in the client's chart. This is a good idea, but it is time consuming and sometimes expensive. However, it can be very helpful, as well as impressive, in showing clients their progress over time. It also can serve as a legal protective mechanism, in case there is ever any discrepancy about scars or other problems that existed before the client was ever seen by the esthetician.

## CLIENT CONFIDENTIALITY

You must always hold anything the client tells you in the strictest confidence. You should never show pictures of a client without the client's written permission. All files and charts should be kept in a secure location, only accessible by staff members. You must never discuss a client's condition with another client. All staff members should also be trained in client confidentiality.

## TOPICS FOR DISCUSSION

1. Explain Fitzpatrick Skin Typing. What does it indicate?
2. Why is esthetic skin type important when choosing products and treatments for the client?
3. What are the differences between skin type and skin condition?
4. What are some skin conditions that might be found on certain skin types?
5. What is client confidentiality and why is it important?

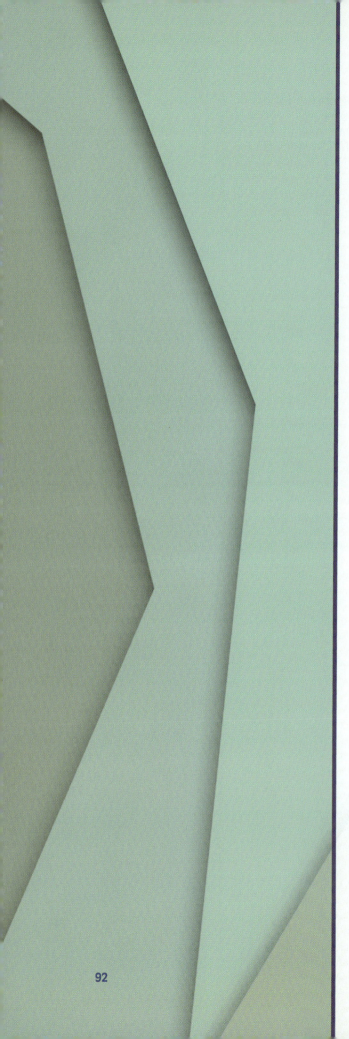

# CHAPTER 7

# Recognize and Refer Medical Conditions

## OBJECTIVES. . .

The esthetician should be trained to recognize common medical conditions and diseases of the skin and refer them to the proper medical authority—in most cases the dermatologist.

This chapter is designed to illustrate and briefly discuss some of the medical conditions that the esthetician may observe in routine practice. Although not all of these conditions are life-threatening, many skin conditions need to be referred to the dermatologist for proper medical treatment.

The esthetician will often have clients who come to the salon for treatment of what they may think is a cosmetic disorder but is actually a dermatological condition. The esthetician should never diagnose a medical condition, but he or she should be able to recognize conditions that require medical treatment. The esthetician should be well educated about the different types of common skin diseases and conditions and should be able to discuss conditions with the dermatologist. The esthetician should also be familiar with the cosmetic effects of certain skin disorders and know how they can help with cosmetic symptoms that the client may need to conceal.

This chapter will teach you about medical conditions that need medical referral. You should always refer any condition that you do not understand or that is obviously not just a minor cosmetic problem.

Before discussing the medical conditions in this chapter, it is important to discuss common medical terminology—specifically dermatological terminology. The medical community has very precise descriptions for symptoms of the skin. Using these specific terms, dermatologists can very accurately describe lesions and therefore diagnose illnesses more efficiently. (The author wishes to thank Rube Pardo, M.D., Ph.D., and the Department of Dermatology at the University of Miami for their assistance in preparing this section on dermatological terminology.)

## PRIMARY AND SECONDARY LESIONS

A **lesion** is any mark on the skin that is not a normal part of the skin. It does not necessarily mean that the skin is diseased. A freckle is a lesion; so is a wrinkle. However, lesions can also be symptoms of disease, such as melanoma, shingles, or measles. **Primary lesions** of the skin are lesions that are in the early stages of development.

**Secondary lesions** are lesions that primary lesions eventually become.

**Macules** are flat (nonelevated) marks on the skin in which there is only a change in the normal color of the skin. Again, a freckle can be an example of a macule, and the flat red mark left after a pimple has healed is also a macule. It is simply a descriptive term meaning that this is a flat area with a change in the normal color of the skin. The adjective used to describe a lesion is macular. Large macules, larger than 1 centimeter, are called **patches**. **Papules** are raised areas on the skin that are generally smaller than 1 centimeter. **Plaques** are papules that are larger than 1 centimeter.

**Nodules** are raised lesions that are larger and deep in the skin. A nodule looks like a lump, but the skin can be moved over the lesion. Very large nodules are called **tumors**.

A **pustule** is a lesion that is filled with pus, which is discussed in the chapter Acne and the Esthetician. Extremely deep infections with pockets of pus are called **abscesses**.

**Vesicle** is the medical term for blisters. They contain body fluids. A **bulba** is a large vesicle. A vesicle or bulba that has ruptured so that the fluid is exposed to the surface of the skin is said to be weeping or oozing.

A **wheal** is a hive. Wheals are caused by a concentration of the fluid in the tissue. Wheals are reabsorbed into the bloodstream via the lymphatic system.

**Erosion** refers to a shallow depression in the skin. Scratches on the skin are called **excoriations**, which we have already discussed in Chapter 15, Acne and the Esthetician. Deep erosions are called **ulcers**, in which part of the dermis has been lost.

Diseased skin often has remnants of body fluids, pus, or blood caked to a lesion. This is described as **crust**.

**Scales** are patches of dry, dehydrated skin without crust.

**Erythema** refers to any area of redness associated with a lesion. Bruises are known as **hematomas**. **Purpura** are hemorrhages of the blood vessels.

**Atrophy** means wasting away. Skin that has thinned from age or chronic sun exposure is said to have atrophied. **Hypertrophy** is thickening of a tissue. Hypertrophic scars are raised scars, due to thickening of a tissue. **Atrophic scars** are depressed scars, such as acne pocks, caused by loss of tissue.

---

**Lesion** is any mark on the skin that is not a normal part of the skin.

**Primary lesions** are lesions that are in the early stages of development.

**Secondary lesions** are lesions that primary lesions eventually become.

**Macules** are flat (nonelevated) marks on the skin in which there is only a change in the normal color of the skin.

**Patches** are large macules that are larger than 1 centimeter.

**Papules** are raised areas on the skin that are generally smaller than 1 centimeter.

**Plaques** are papules that are larger than 1 centimeter.

**Nodules** are raised lesions that are larger and deeper in the skin. A nodule looks like a lump, but the skin can be moved over the lesion.

**Tumors** are very large nodules.

**Pustule** is a clump of white blood cells that have formed and risen to the surface of the skin.

**Abscesses** are extremely deep infections with pockets of pus.

**Vesicle** is the medical term for blisters.

**Bulba** is a large vesicle.

**Wheal** is a raised red lesion associated with sensitivity or allergy. Wheals are also called hives.

**Erosion** refers to a shallow depression in the skin.

**Excoriations** are scratches on the skin.

**Ulcers** are deep erosions in which part of the dermis has been lost.

**Crust** is caked body fluids, pus, or blood remnants left from diseased skin.

**Scales** are patches of dry, dehydrated skin without crust.

**Erythema** refers to any area of redness associated with a lesion.

**Hematomas** are bruises.

**Purpura** are hemorrhages of the blood vessels.

**Atrophy** means wasting away.

**Hypertrophy** is thickening of a tissue.

**Atrophic scars** are depressed scars such as acne pocks, caused by loss of tissue.

**Linear** lesion is a line-like lesion.

**Annular** lesion is a ring-shaped lesion.

**Serpiginous** lesion is a lesion that has a snake-like pattern.

**Geographic** lesion looks like a map.

**Target**, or **iris**, lesion has a center with a round surrounding area, such as a pustule.

**Keratosis** is a general term meaning thickening of the stratum corneum, such as seborrheic keratosis.

**Eczematization** refers to a combination of symptoms, including erythema, weeping, crusting, and present vesicles.

**Nevus** is a mole.

**Lentigines** are freckles.

**Hyperpigmentation** refers to any condition that has more than a normal amount of melanin.

**Hypopigmentation** refers to any area with less than the normal amount of pigment.

**Impetigo** is a skin infection that is characterized by large, open, weeping lesions.

**Folliculitis** is a bacterial infection of the hair follicle.

**Pseudofolliculitis** is caused by irritation from shaving. Ingrown hairs are the main cause of pseudofolliculitis.

A number of terms are used to described the shapes of certain lesions. A **linear** lesion is a line-like lesion. A ring-shaped lesion is called **annular**. Lesions that have a snake-like pattern are called **serpiginous**. **Geographic** lesions look like a map. **Target**, or **iris**, lesions have a center with a round surrounding area, such as a pustule.

**Keratosis** is a general term meaning a thickening of a stratum corneum, such as seborrheic keratosis, described in Chapter 19, Sun and Sun Damage.

**Eczematization** refers to a combination of symptoms, including erythema, weeping, crusting, and present vesicles.

A **nevus** is a mole. More than one mole are described as nevi. **Lentigines** are freckles. Dyschromias are skin color abnormalities. **Hyperpigmentation** refers to any condition that has more than the normal amount of melanin. **Hypopigmentation** refers to any area with less than the normal amount of pigment.

## ACNE

Severe acne requires medical attention. Grade 4 acne is severe inflammatory acne with cystic lesions. Cysts should always be referred to the dermatologist. The medical treatment for cysts includes injections with steroids, which help to shrink the lesion. Some cysts may be lanced by the dermatologist and drained. Both topical and oral antibiotics may be used to help control inflammatory acne conditions. Common topical preparations may include the antibiotics erythromycin (trade name A/T/S®) or clindamycin (trade name Cleocin T®). These preparations are available only by prescription and are liquid roll-ons that are applied to the skin either daily or twice daily. The doctor may suggest that the client not use certain cosmetic products that will increase irritation. Frequently, dermatologists will prescribe prescription keratolytic products such as prescription-strength benzoyl peroxide treatments, retinoic acid (Retin-A®), adapalene (Differin®), azelaic acid (Azelex®), or other peeling and sloughing agents. These products are discussed in detail in the chapter on acne.

Other acne-related medical conditions include *acne rosacea, perioral dermatitis*, and *seborrheic dermatitis*, which are all also discussed in other chapters.

## COMMON INFECTIONS OF THE SKIN

Infections of the skin may be grouped into three types: bacterial, fungal, and viral.

### Common Bacterial Infections

**Impetigo** is a skin infection that is commonly seen on the face, particularly in the lower part of the face, but it can occur anywhere (Figure 7-1). This disease is characterized by large, open, weeping lesions. They look like large sores, similar to acne, except that impetigo lesions weep and appear damp. The lesions can range in size. Impetigo is frequently seen in children and is extremely contagious. Impetigo is caused by staphylococcus bacteria. The disease is treated by the use of antibiotics.

**Folliculitis** is a bacterial infection of the hair follicle. The infection results in irritation and is characterized by multiple pinpoint irritations around the pore openings (Figure 7-2). **Pseudofolliculitis** is caused by irritation from shaving. It also appears as irritated follicles but is not usually infected. Ingrown hairs are the main cause of pseudofolliculitis, seen frequently in the beard area of male clients, especially the neck.

A more severe infection of the hair follicle is called a **furuncle**, also known as a boil. Large boils often result in abscesses and are referred to as **carbuncles**. Folliculitis, furuncles, and carbuncles are treated with antibiotics. If a furuncle or carbuncle bursts on the inside of the lesion, the bacteria may enter the bloodstream, causing **septicemia**, also known as blood poisoning. Septicemia is characterized by a red

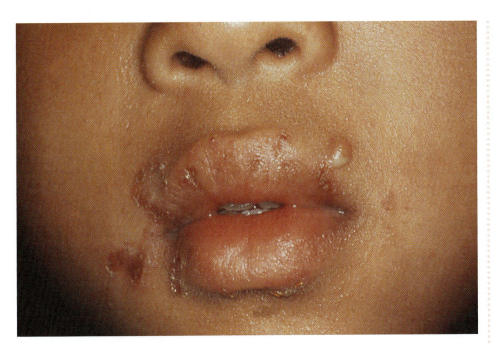

**Figure 7-1** Impetigo is a contagious bacterial skin infection that often affects the face especially in children. It must be treated by a physician (Reprinted with permission from the American Academy of Dermatology. All rights reserved.)

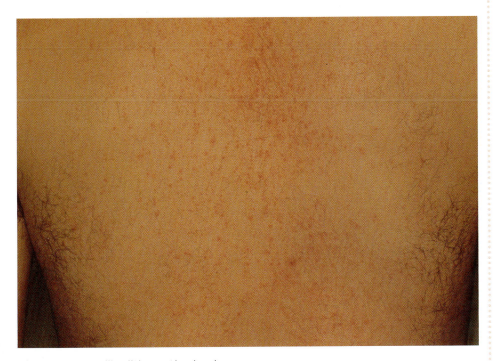

**Figure 7-2** Folliculitis on the back (Courtesy Rube J. Pardo, M.D., Ph.D.)

erythemic line running from the source of primary infection. Septicemia is extremely serious and should be treated immediately by a physician. **Cellulitis** is a deep infection of the dermis, caused by streptococcus (Figure 7-3). A severe form of cellulitis is called **erysipelas**, also known as St. Anthony's Fire. Again, this is extremely serious and should be seen immediately by a physician.

**Furuncle** is a severe infection of the hair follicle. It is also known as a boil.

**Carbuncles** are large boils that often result in abscesses.

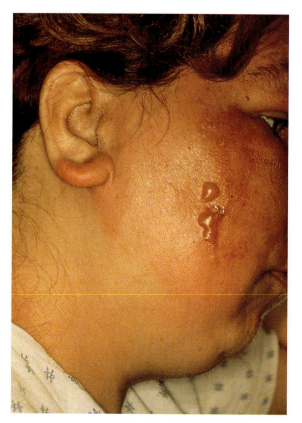

**Figure 7-3** Facial cellulitis. Note the severe swelling and inflammation
(Courtesy Rube J. Pardo, M.D., Ph.D.)

**Septicemia**, also known as blood poisoning, occurs when a bacterial infection enters the bloodstream.

**Cellulitis** is a deep infection of the dermis caused by streptococcus.

**Erysipelas**, also known as St. Anthony's Fire, is a severe form of bacterial cellulitis.

**Mycoses** are fungal infections.

**Tinea veriscolor** is what many refer to as sun "spots" or sun "fungus." These white splotches are a fungal condition.

**Tinea pedis** is commonly known as athlete's foot, which is a fungal infection of the skin on the foot.

**Tinea corporis** is better known as ringworm.

**Candidas** are yeast infections.

# Fungal Skin Infections

There are a number of fungal infections of the skin. Fungal infections are called **mycoses**.

**Tinea veriscolor** is sometimes called *sun fungus*. It is often seen on the backs and chests of persons who are tan. Tinea veriscolor inhibits the production of melanin in the skin, which results in its appearance as white patches. It is not actually directly related to sun exposure, but is often seen on tanned persons because the skin will not tan in the areas where tinea veriscolor is active. The disease is easily treated with the use of antifungal prescription medications.

**Tinea pedis** is commonly known as *athlete's foot*, which is a fungal infection of the skin on the foot. The disease is characterized by severe itching and scaling, particularly on the sole of the foot. Again, tinea pedis is easily treated by the use of antifungal prescription medications.

**Tinea corporis** is better known by the public as ringworm. It can occur on any area of the body and presents itself as a ring-like lesion (Figure 7-4).

**Candidas** are yeast infections. They can cause a variety of skin infections. Oral thrush, seen often in infants and persons with suppressed immune systems, such as patients with AIDS, is a yeast infection of the mouth characterized by white patches inside the mouth.

# Viral Skin Infections

**Herpes** refers to a group of viruses.

**Herpes** refers to a group of viruses. Herpes simplex is the cause of common cold sores, which generally appear on or around the mouth and often appear as oozing red ulcers

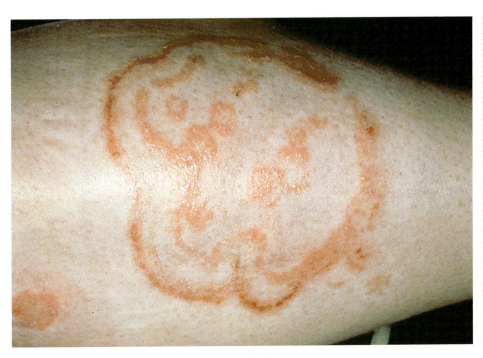

**Figure 7-4** Tinea corporis infection on the leg (Courtesy Rube J. Pardo, M.D., Ph.D.)

(Figure 7-5). They are very contagious and should be treated by a physician. Facial treatments should be avoided for clients with active lesions. Certain facial treatments such as chemical peels have been known to cause a flareup of the herpes virus.

**Herpes zoster**, better known as *shingles*, is caused by the same virus that causes chickenpox. Herpes zoster is harboured by the nervous system and generally follows a pattern along the nerves in the skin. The lesions of herpes zoster look like multiple red blisters (Figure 7-6). Subjective symptoms may include burning, tingling, or numbness, and severe cases can result in extreme pain. Minor infections can be only a nuisance, and the disease subsides by itself. However, the infection can reoccur and in some cases causes scarring and pain due to nerve inflammation. There is no cure for herpes zoster, although there are some prescriptions helpful in controlling it. Herpes zoster is another infection that may be a problem in immunosuppressed individuals, such as patients with AIDS.

**Molloscum contagiosum** is a viral infection frequently seen on the faces of children, which appears as groups of small, flesh-colored papules. They often resemble milia but are in groups or clusters and are hard to the touch (Figure 7-7). They must be treated by a physician.

The most frequent viral lesions seen are warts. **Warts** are caused by a variety of viruses known as *papovaviruses* or *veruccae*. Wart treatment varies with the lesion, including topical acid therapy using salicylic acid or trichloroacetic acid. Other dermatologic treatments include freezing the lesions with liquid nitrogen or cautery with an electric needle. Warts are contagious, especially to the same individual, and can be spread to another area of the body easily. Warts may be seen by the esthetician on the face, feet, and hands, especially the nails, and should be referred to a dermatologist for treatment (Figure 7-8).

**Pityriasis rosea** is a patchy, red, rashlike disorder. It can occur anywhere on the body but is frequently seen on the trunk. Groups of patches may develop. Many outbreaks resemble the pattern of a Christmas tree on the trunk. There is no real cure for pityriasis rosea, but it usually subsides after a few weeks. Itching associated with infection can be treated with topical prescription steroid creams (Figure 7-9).

**Herpes zoster**, better known as shingles, is caused by the same virus that causes chickenpox. The lesions of herpes zoster look like multiple red blisters.

**Molluscum contagiosum** is a viral infection frequently seen on the faces of children, which appear as groups of small, flesh-colored papules.

**Warts** are caused by a variety of viruses known as papovaviruses or verrucae.

**Pityriasis rosea** is a patchy, red, rashlike disorder.

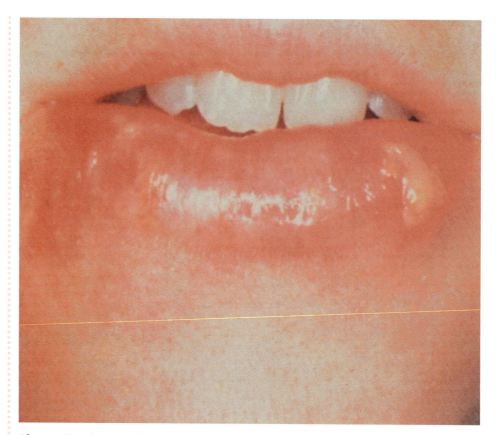

**Figure 7-5** Herpes simplex causes common cold sores (Courtesy Timothy G. Berger, M.D.)

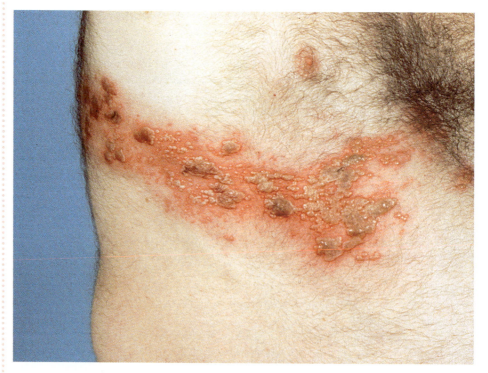

**Figure 7-6** Typical case of herpes zoster (shingles). Note the lesions follow a typical nerve-route pattern (Courtesy Rube J. Pardo, M.D., Ph.D.)

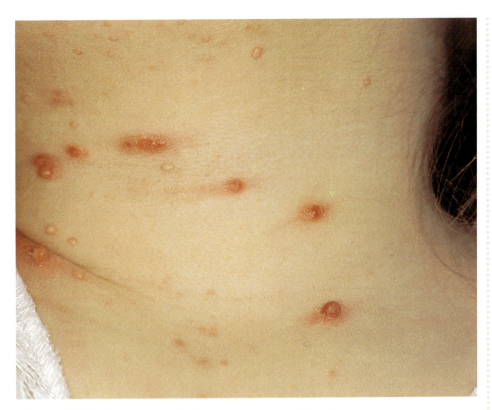

**Figure 7-7** Molloscum contagiosum (Courtesy Melvin L. Elson, M.D.)

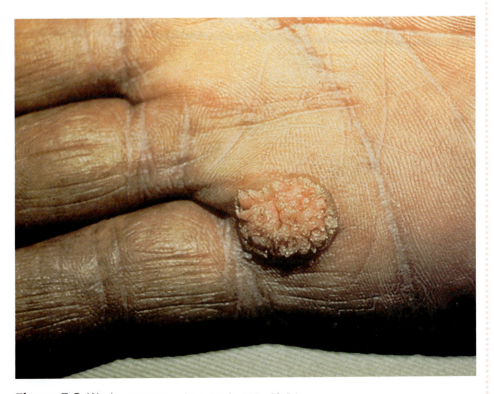

**Figure 7-8** Warts (Courtesy Rube J. Pardo, M.D., Ph.D.)

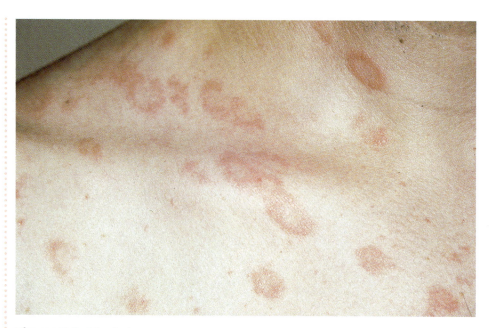

**Figure 7-9** Pityriasis rosea (Courtesy Mark Lees Skin Care, Inc.)

# COMMON REACTIONS, RASHES, AND IRRITATIONS

In the sensitive skin chapter we have discussed common allergies that the esthetician sees routinely. **Dermatitis** means inflammation of the skin. It is a descriptive term used to describe many different types of skin inflammation and irritation. Dermatitis is an irritation, rather than a disease. It is generally not caused by pathological organisms, such as infections caused by viruses, bacteria, and fungi. Many of the other terms already discussed in this chapter are used as adjectives to describe different types and patterns of dermatitis.

## Contact Dermatitis

**Contact dermatitis** is probably the most common form of dermatitis observed by the esthetician. Contact dermatitis is an irritation caused by either an allergic reaction or irritation to something or some substance touching the skin or coming in contact with the skin's surface. Cosmetics are a frequent cause of contact dermatitis. Other frequent causes of contact dermatitis include jewelry, laundry products, clothing fabrics and dyes, plants (such as poison ivy), and other substances (Figure 7-10A, 7-10B).

There are two basic treatments for contact dermatitis. The first, of course, is to avoid contact with the offending substance. This is sometimes hard to pinpoint, because we touch so many substances on a daily basis. Often the dermatologist can tell much about the source of irritation by the location of the dermatitis. Irritation of the hands is often caused by household products. Health and personal care professionals, including estheticians, often suffer from dermatitis related to substances they touch at work.

Irritation from hand washes, disinfectants, and antiseptics and even allergies to latex gloves are frequently seen in these professionals. Estheticians also come in contact with a large number of cosmetic products, which can also be a source of irritation.

The process of eliminating the offending substance is often a matter of trial and error, eliminating one or all substances and testing by slowly adding steps of substance

**Dermatitis** is inflammation of the skin.

**Contact dermatitis** is an irritation caused by either an allergic reaction or irritation to something or some substance touching the skin or coming in contact with the skin's surface.

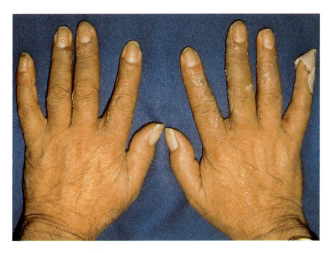

**Figure 7-10A** Contact dermatitis in a hairstylist due to parapheneline-diamine

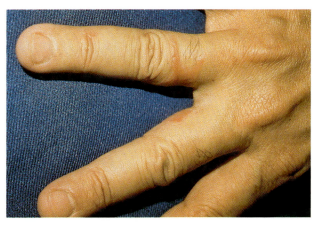

**Figure 7-10B** Contact dermatitis due to nickel allergy (Courtesy Rube J. Pardo, M.D., Ph.D.)

contact. Allergies are sometimes easier to detect. The dermatologist can often run allergy patch tests, and allergies have a tendency to be more acute, or sudden, than irritation dermatitis.

The second part of contact dermatitis treatment is to soothe and stop the inflammation. Topical steroid creams are often prescribed by the dermatologist to ease the symptoms of allergic or irritant dermatitis. These prescription creams usually work fairly quickly, assuming that the source of irritation has also been eliminated.

Dermatitis can have many characteristics visually, but it is usually red (erythemic), and often itchy or burning. The term *eczema* refers to the same condition as *dermatitis*.

## Atopic Dermatitis

**Atopic eczema** or dermatitis is a more complicated form of dermatitis. It is a more severe and chronic condition and is associated, in most cases, with heredity. It may be affected by illness, stress, and other changes. Some patients suffer from atopic dermatitis all their lives.

Atopic eczema can be controlled with the use of prescription steroid creams and oral antihistamines. Cosmetologically, the patient with atopic eczema will be more likely to have irritant reactions to cosmetics. If you have a client with atopic eczema, discuss any cosmetics with the client's doctor. In general, stick to fragrance-free, simple products—the simpler the better, and the fewer ingredients the better. Use the same care as discussed in the chapter on sensitive skin.

Occasionally, you may notice a rash following a pattern on the face that does not clear up. Rashes in a butterfly pattern across the cheeks can be a symptom of lupus erythematosus. We have already discussed lupus. If you notice a recurrent rash on a client's face, you should refer the client to a physician, as you should all rashes and chronic redness.

**Atopic eczema**, also known as atopic dermatitis, is a chronic inflammatory condition of the skin that is hereditary and may be related to respiratory allergies or asthma.

## Psoriasis

Psoriasis is an inflammatory disorder of the skin that is caused by the skin and epidermis "turning over" faster than it does in a normal individual. Largely hereditary, it can be chronic and last over a lifetime. The disorder is not contagious and is not related to any pathological organism. It is a disorder, not a disease (Figure 7-11).

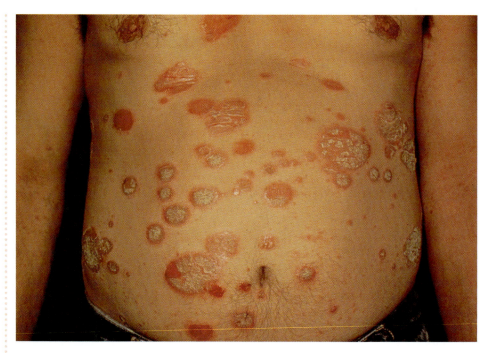

**Figure 7-11** Psoriasis (Courtesy Rube J. Pardo, M.D., Ph.D.)

Psoriasis primarily affects the skin on the body and is often symmetrical, which means it occurs simultaneously on both sides of the body in the same place. It often affects the elbows, the knees, and other extremities.

Treatments used to control psoriasis include steroid creams, antihistamines, and light therapy using controlled exposures of UVA (ultraviolet A). Some new oral drugs are also being used to treat chronic cases.

## Urticaria

An outbreak of **urticaria**, or hives, is due to allergies. Urticaria often quickly fades without treatment, but the source of the allergy should be identified. Dermatologists use topical steroids, oral steroids, antihistamines, and allergy testing to treat and identify causes of urticaria.

## Keratosis Pilaris

**Keratosis pilaris** is a condition in which the skin exhibits redness and irritation in patches, accompanied by a rough texture, and small pinpoint white papules that look like very small milia. Keratosis pilaris is often found on the cheeks and upper arms. It is often seen in children and teenagers, but it can affect any age group. In most cases, it is a nuisance disorder. Doctors have been successful in treating keratosis pilaris with glycolic or lactic acid solutions, but it often goes away by itself.

## VASCULAR LESIONS

**Vascular lesions** are visible conditions that involve the blood or circulatory system. Probably the most common forms of vascular lesion are **telangiectasias**, distended capillaries, commonly referred to as "broken capillaries" or **couperose**. In fact, the capillaries are not actually broken, they are simply dilated or new extensions of deeper capillaries that have developed near the surface of the skin. Telangiectasias

**Urticaria**, or hives, is due to allergies.

**Keratosis pilaris** is a condition in which the skin exhibits redness and irritation in patches, accompanied by a rough texture, and small pinpoint white papules that look like very small milia.

**Vascular lesions** are visible conditions that involve the blood or circulatory system.

**Telangiectasias** are small, red, enlarged capillaries of the face and other areas of the body.

**Couperose** refers to diffuse redness including telangiectasias of the face and other areas of the body.

are permanent and are caused by a variety of factors, including sun exposure, exposure to extreme temperatures, friction, or injury to the skin. They can be characteristic of rosacea.

Telangiectasias can be caused or worsened by vasodilators, which are drugs or substances that cause dilation of the blood vessels. Included in the category of vasodilators are tobacco and alcohol. Alcoholics often have many telangiectasias.

Telangiectasias are too deep in the skin to be affected or improved by ordinary esthetic treatment. Removal of irritants from the skin-care regimen, addition of soothing agents, improvement of the barrier function, and treatment with **LED light** may improve the appearance or severity of the visible telangiectasias, but to remove the lesion, medical treatment is required. Most telangiectasias are only a beauty nuisance, but clients with multiple telangiectasias should be referred to a dermatologist for treatment and evaluation.

**Spider angiomas** are similar to telangiectasias, but have a central "body" and branches of telangiectasias resembling a spider. They are also usually beauty nuisances and are treated by dermatologist in the same methods as telangiectasias.

Medical treatment often involves the use of a **hyfrecator**, an electric needle, or more commonly now, treatment with a **specialized laser** or **intense pulsed light** device. These devices cause a "drying up" of the vessel. When the flow of blood has been cut off to the telangiectasia, the capillary collapses. The results of these treatments are almost immediate and may involve some flaking or drying of the skin area.

Telangiectasias have a strong tendency to re-occur, even after medical treatment, or new telangiectasias can develop.

**Port-wine stains** are a form of vascular birthmark. They are large red or purple-toned patches, often involving as much as half the face. They are also treated with **vascular lasers**. Often many treatments are required over a period of time. Estheticians trained in camouflage makeup may be of great help to clients with port-wine stains.

## GROWTHS

Solar-induced skin growths and conditions that require medical referral are seen frequently by estheticians. These include hyperplasias, keratoses, sun-induced pigmentation disorders, and skin cancers. For much more information on these conditions, see the chapter on sun and sun damage.

You should review Chapter 19, Sun and Sun Damage, and be very familiar with identifying these growths, especially cancers and pre-cancers.

**Skin tags** are very small, threadlike growths. They are frequently seen on the eyelids, neck, and decollete. They are benign lesions, but frequently are irritated by jewelry or clothing rubbing against them. Most people find them unattractive, and they should be removed. They are easily removed by the dermatologist using freezing, electric needle, or scissors (Figure 7-12).

Skin tags are largely hereditary, and have been associated with obesity, pregnancy, post-menopause, diabetes, and intestinal disorders. These medical associations are another reason that skin tags should be seen by a physician.

**Xanthomas** or **xanthalasmas** are fatty pockets found on the eyelids. They look like large closed comedones and are frequently found on the upper and lower lids. They are somewhat flat and are usually oval or egg-shaped.

Xanthalasmas should be referred to a dermatologist for removal by extraction or excision. They are often associated with high cholesterol, and often the dermatologist will order tests to determine cholesterol levels.

We have only touched on the many disorders and diseases that can affect the skin. We have, however, discussed many conditions frequently observed by the practicing esthetician.

**LED light** is made up of light-emitting diodes, which are fast-flashing lights that emit energy to the skin and are used to treat sun damage and redness.

**Spider angioma** is a type of blood vessel distention that resembles a spider.

**Hyfrecator** is an electric needle used by a physician to remove small growths or treat certain vascular skin lesions.

**Specialized lasers** are designed for specific treatment uses such as vascular lesions and aging skin.

**Intense pulsed light** is a powerful medical light treatment used to treat pigmentation, vascular lesions, and aging skin.

**Port-wine stains** are hereditary vascular birthmarks.

**Vascular lasers** are designed specifically to treat vascular lesions.

**Skin tags** are very small, threadlike growths. They are benign lesions, but frequently are irritated by jewelry or clothing, rubbing against them.

**Xanthomas** are fatty pockets found on the eyelids.

**Xanthalasmas** are much flatter than milia, have a yellowish appearance, are below the skin's surface, and may have irregular shape.

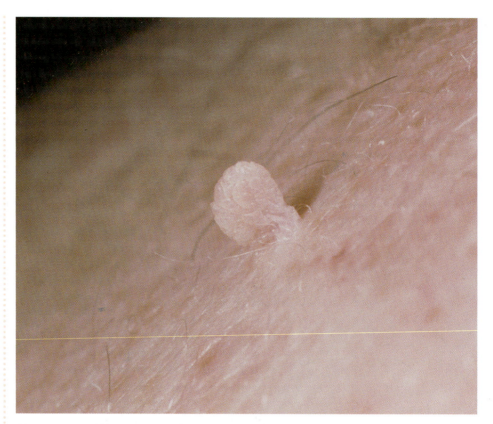

**Figure 7-12** Skin tags are often seen on the neck and in the chest area
(Courtesy Michael J. Bond, M.D.)

Again, this chapter should educate you to recognize symptoms that could indicate conditions that should be referred to a dermatologist or other appropriate physician. Estheticians treat cosmetic disorders of the skin. They should never attempt to diagnose or treat a disease or medical disorder. Always refer any suspicious rash, growth, or other abnormality to a dermatologist.

## COMMONLY USED PRESCRIPTION DERMATOLOGICAL DRUGS

It is important for practicing estheticians to have a working knowledge of both topical and internal drugs frequently used in dermatology. The main reason why it is important to have a basic understanding of these drugs is that they may have contraindications for types of esthetic or cosmetic treatments and side effects that affect esthetic treatment.

### Keratolytic Drugs

Keratolytic drugs are topical medications applied directly to the skin. They cause rapid exfoliation of the skin and are actually peeling agents. They are primarily used to treat acne, but they also can be used to treat sun-damaged skin, actinic keratoses, and other dermatological problems.

Many of these drugs are **retinoids**, or vitamin A derivatives. **Tretinoin (Retin-A®, Renova®, Avita®), adapalene (Differin®),** and **tazarotene (Tazorac®)** are all retinoids. They cause peeling of the skin; thin the surface layers; and can cause inflammation, redness, and flaking.

**Retinoids** are drug or skin-care ingredients that are vitamin A derivatives.

**Accutane**® is thoroughly discussed in the acne chapter. This oral drug has many side effects and cosmetic effects. Use the same precautions as for the retinoids. For patients taking Accutane, *no waxing should be administered anywhere on the body*. Review the chapter on acne for more information.

**Azelex**® and **Finacea**®, generically known as azelaic acid, are used to treat acne, rosacea, sun damage, and hyperpigmentation. Azelaic acid is not a retinoid, but it has similar but milder side effects.

Contraindications for keratolytic drugs mainly involve the avoidance of other peeling agents and exfoliation procedures such as AHA and other peels and microdermabrasion. Waxing on or around the areas being treated should also be strictly avoided. Fragranced products, essential oils, and other stimulating treatments, including aggressive massage, should be avoided. Drying alcohols may cause or worsen flaking and inflammation in clients using these drugs.

**Triluma**® is a combination of tretinoin, hydroquinone, and a steroid called fluocinolone acetonide. It is used to treat melasma and hyperpigmentation. Contraindications are the same for other keratolytics.

Prescription strength **hydroquinone**, usually at 4% concentration, is also used to treat hyperpigmentation. Commercially known as **Melanex**®, **Solaquin Forte**®, and other names, often these drugs are used in conjunction with tretinoin. Again the same esthetic and waxing treatments should be avoided.

**Hydroquinone** is an active topical ingredient that inhibits the production of melanin.

## Rosacea Drugs

**Metronidazole**, commercially known as **Metrogel**®, **Metrocream**®, **Metrolotion**®, and **Noritate**®, are actually antibiotic topicals. **Finacea**® (azelaic acid), **Sulfacetamide (Sulfacet-R**®, **Klaron**®, and **Novacet**®) are also used for rosacea treatment.

The list of contraindications for rosacea is extensive. Please review the chapter on rosacea.

**Metronidazole** is a prescription anti-yeast antibiotic that is used topically to treat rosacea.

## Cortisone

**Hydrocortisone** is a hormone that helps relieve inflammation, redness, rashes, and other skin irritations. Up to 1% hydrocortisone can be obtained as an over-the-counter drug, but prescription cortisone drugs are much stronger. Repetitive use of strong cortisone creams can cause thinning of the skin. Again, peeling agents, waxing, drying alcohols, fragranced products, and stimulating treatments should be avoided if the client is using a hydrocortisone topical drug. For more information on all these drugs, please see the pharmacology section of *Milady's Comprehensive Training for Estheticians*.

**Hydrocortisone** is a hormone that helps relieve inflammation and skin irritation.

## TOPICS FOR DISCUSSION

1. What is the difference between a primary and a secondary lesion?
2. What are some common infections of the skin? What are their causes?
3. What are some common fungal infections?
4. Use your knowledge of dermatological terminology to describe a grade 3 acne condition.
5. Why should estheticians be familiar with common forms of skin disease?

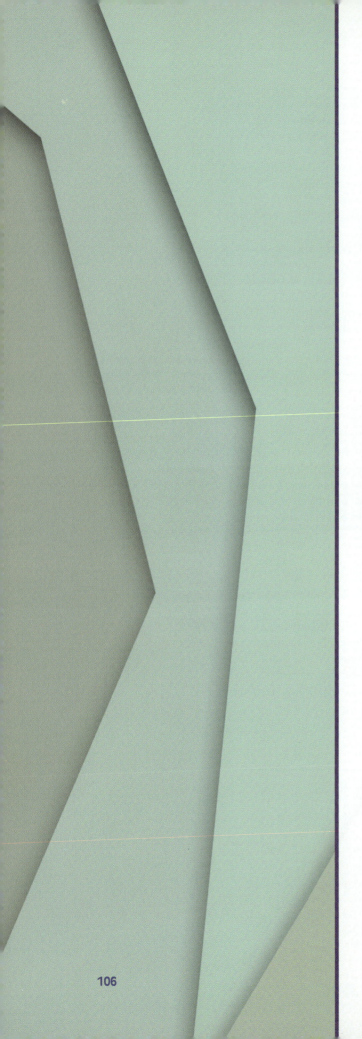

# CHAPTER 8

# Essential Knowledge of Chemistry

## OBJECTIVES. . .

The esthetician is not really a chemist. The esthetician specializes in applying cosmetic chemicals and teaching clients about their uses. However, it is extremely important that the esthetician have a working knowledge of basic chemistry to better understand the biochemical functions of both the skin's cells and the cosmetics and products used in the practice of esthetics. This chapter focuses on basic principles of chemistry, providing the practicing esthetician with the basic knowledge needed to communicate better with clients about skin-care and cosmetic products.

# PRINCIPLES OF CHEMISTRY

Chemicals make up our whole world, from the ink on this page to the tip of your finger. Everything is made of chemicals. In the practice of esthetics, estheticians handle many chemicals on a daily basis. When you prescribe a product, or use galvanic current, or clean a steamer with vinegar, you are dealing with chemistry. Because our lives, as well as our jobs, involve a series of chemical reactions and procedures, it is important that the esthetician understand the basics of chemistry.

An **element** is a chemical in its simplest form. In other words, it cannot be changed to be any purer by practical purposes and means. There are about 110 elements that make up all chemicals and all matter.

**Matter** is anything that takes up space and has substance. You are matter. This book is matter. Your products are matter. Essentially everything is matter! And therefore everything is chemicals!

Examples of elements are silver, gold, carbon, oxygen, nitrogen, silicon, hydrogen, sodium, chlorine, and so on. Remember, these chemicals (elements) cannot be broken down by ordinary means. The chart of all the elements is called the **periodic table** (Figure 8-1).

The smallest measurable unit of an element is called an **atom**. An atom is made up of a **nucleus**, which is the center of the atom, and **electrons**, which orbit around the nucleus. An atom resembles planets orbiting the sun. The "planets" are the electrons and the "sun" is the nucleus. The nucleus of an atom is made up of protons and neutrons. **Protons** are very small positively charged particles, whereas **neutrons** are very small particles with no real charge.

Electrons, which orbit the nucleus, are negatively charged. Remember from basic science how positive and negative charges are attracted to one another? This principle is what keeps electrons orbiting around the nucleus. The electrons, which are extremely light (it takes about 1,800 electrons to equal the mass of one proton), are attracted to the nucleus because they are negative. The nucleus, of course, is positive,

**Element** is a chemical in its simplest form.

**Matter** is anything that takes up space and has substance.

**Periodic table** is the chart of all the elements.

**Atom** is the smallest measurable unit of an element.

**Nucleus** of the cell is made up largely of protein and is also responsible for building certain proteins.

**Electrons** are negatively charged particles that orbit the nucleus of an atom. The exchange of these particles causes chemical reactions.

**Protons** are very small positively charged particles within the atom.

**Neutrons** are very small negatively charged particles within the atom.

| ACTIVE METALS | | | | | | | | | | | | | | NONMETALS | | | | | | |
|---|---|---|---|---|---|---|---|---|---|---|---|---|---|---|---|---|---|---|---|---|

ACTIVE METALS / NONMETALS

TRANSITION METALS

| 1A | 2A | 3B | 4B | 5B | 6B | 7B | | 8B | | 1B | 2B | 3A | 4A | 5A | 6A | 7A | 8A |
|---|---|---|---|---|---|---|---|---|---|---|---|---|---|---|---|---|---|
| | | | | | | | | | | | | | | | | 1 H | 2 He |
| 3 Li | 4 Be | | | | | | | | | | | 5 B | 6 C | 7 N | 8 O | 9 F | 10 Ne |
| 11 Na | 12 Mg | | | | | | | | | | | 13 Al | 14 Si | 15 P | 16 S | 17 Cl | 18 Ar |
| 19 K | 20 Ca | 21 Sc | 22 Ti | 23 V | 24 Cr | 25 Mn | 26 Fe | 27 Co | 28 Ni | 29 Cu | 30 Zn | 31 Ga | 32 Ge | 33 As | 34 Se | 35 Br | 36 Kr |
| 37 Rb | 38 | 39 Y | 40 Zr | 41 Nb | 42 Mo | 43 Tc | 44 Ru | 45 Rh | 46 Pd | 47 Ag | 48 Cd | 49 In | 50 Sn | 51 Sb | 52 Te | 53 I | 54 Xe |
| 55 Cs | 56 Ba | 57 La | 72 Hf | 73 Ta | 74 W | 75 Re | 76 Os | 77 Ir | 78 Pt | 79 Au | 80 Hg | 81 Tl | 82 Pb | 83 Bi | 84 Po | 85 At | 86 Rn |
| 87 Fr | 88 Ra | 89 Ac | 104 Rf | 105 Ha | | | | | | | | | | | | | |

| LANTHANIDE SERIES | 58 Ce | 59 Pr | 60 Nd | 61 Pm | 62 Sm | 63 Eu | 64 Gd | 65 Tb | 66 Dy | 67 Ho | 68 Er | 69 Tm | 70 Yb | 71 Lu |
|---|---|---|---|---|---|---|---|---|---|---|---|---|---|---|
| ACTINIDE SERIES | 90 Th | 91 Pa | 92 U | 93 Np | 94 Pu | 95 Am | 96 Cm | 97 Bk | 98 Cf | 99 Es | 100 Fm | 101 Md | 102 No | 103 Lw |

**Figure 8-1** Periodic table of the elements

because it is made up of positive protons and neutrons that have no charge. Electrons orbit the nucleus in circular patterns. These patterns are called electron shells or energy levels. We refer to these orbital patterns as shells or levels. There may be one shell or many shells, depending on the size of the particular atom (Figure 8-2).

All atoms of the same element are exactly alike. They are the same size, weigh the same, and have the same number of protons. Atoms also have the same number of protons and electrons. The atomic weight of an element is the number of protons in one of that element's atoms. So if the number of protons in an atom is the same as the number of electrons in that atom, and you know the atomic weight of that element, you know exactly how many protons and electrons an atom of that element has. For example, hydrogen is a very small atom. It has a molecular weight of 1. That means that it has one proton in its nucleus and one electron orbiting the nucleus. Carbon is a bigger atom. It has an atomic weight of 6. Therefore, it contains six protons orbited by six electrons.

It takes a certain number of electrons to fill one of the shells, which are also called energy levels. The bigger the element, the more levels of electrons will be present. The first energy level holds two electrons; the second level holds eight electrons; the third level holds eight electrons. The reason this is important is because each level has a certain capacity of electrons it can hold, sort of like the capacity of a room. Atoms have a physical need to have full outer levels.

What this means is that if an outer level of electrons is almost full, the level will "want" to fill itself up. If the outer lever is almost empty, it will "want" to get rid of its few outer electrons. For example, chlorine has seven electrons in its outer level. It needs eight to complete the level. Chlorine will have a tendency to "want" to fill that level. Sodium, however, has only one electron in its outer level; it will have a tendency to "want" to get rid of that one electron, so its next level will be full. Remember, the normal configuration of atoms is to have "full" outer levels of electrons. Where can the chlorine atom find that extra electron it needs to fill its outer level? Maybe it can get one from the sodium atom that wants to get rid of its outer electron! So chlorine "steals" the electron from sodium, which sodium is glad to get rid of. Both atoms now have full outer levels of electrons. However, remember that we said earlier that each atom had the same number of positive protons in its nucleus as negative electrons orbiting the atom. Now that chlorine and sodium have exchanged electrons, doesn't that change their positive–negative electrical charges? Now that chlorine has an extra electron, it has one more electron than it has protons. That means that it has one more

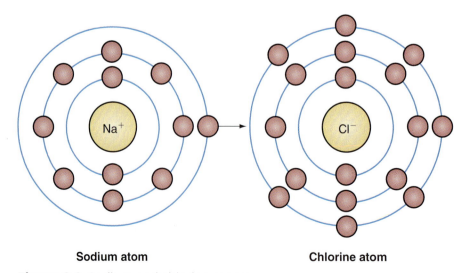

**Sodium atom**                    **Chlorine atom**

**Figure 8-2** Sodium and chlorine atoms

negative charge than it did before. Sodium has lost an electron, so it now has one more proton than it has electrons, giving it a positive charge. It has one more positive charge (protons) than it has negative charges (electrons).

When atoms "steal" or "give away" electrons to each other, the resulting atoms with new charges (and number of electrons) are called **ions**. Ions are charged atoms. The chlorine is now negative, and the sodium is now positive (Figure 8-3).

Positive and negative charges are attracted to one another. So chlorine, with its negative charge, will be closely attracted to sodium, with its positive charge. They are so closely attracted they become "locked" together because of their charges. When two or more atoms become "locked" together in this manner, they become a molecule. A **molecule** is two or more atoms joined together. Molecules have completely different properties than individual atoms. Chlorine is a gas, and sodium is a solid. Together in this molecule they are called **sodium chloride**, which is actually table salt! When two ions form a molecule by being attracted to each other's charge, the bond is said to be an **ionic bond**.

Therefore, the way atoms are joined together has a lot to do with how many electrons are present in the outer electron levels. The number of electrons in the outer level is known as that atom's or element's **valence**. Low-valence atoms are, in general, attracted to high-valence atoms.

What happens if an atom has a medium number of electrons in its outer shell? In other words, if the shell is half full, will the atom try to get more electrons or lose outer electrons? Elements with a medium-filled outer level of electrons share electrons, rather than trade electrons like ionic bonds. When atoms share electrons, the bond between the atoms is called a **covalent bond**. For example, carbon has four electrons in its outer level. It needs four more electrons to fill its outer level. So it shares electrons with other atoms. Often it shares with four other carbon atoms (Figure 8-4).

Let's go back and look again at the periodic table of the elements. The elements in vertical columns are called families of elements. The elements that are in the same horizontal column are called a period. The elements are listed from left to right in order of their atomic numbers, or the number of protons in each element's atoms. Also listed is the atomic mass, which for the purposes of this discussion is the weight of an atom of that element.

**Ions**, or charged atoms, are the resulting atoms with new charges when atoms "steal" or "give away" electrons to each other.

**Molecule** is two or more atoms joined together.

**Sodium chloride** is the compound created by combining sodium and chloride and commonly known as table salt.

**Ionic bond** is the bond of two ions joining to form a molecule.

**Valence** is the number of electrons in the outer level.

**Covalent bond** is the bond between atoms sharing electrons.

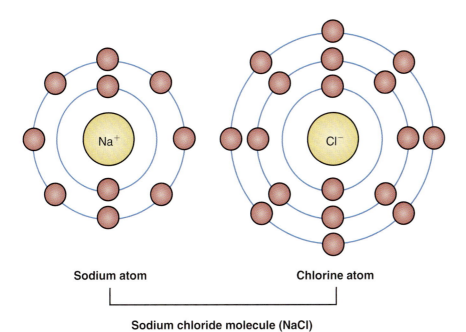

Sodium atom         Chlorine atom

Sodium chloride molecule (NaCl)

**Figure 8-3** Sodium and chlorine ions

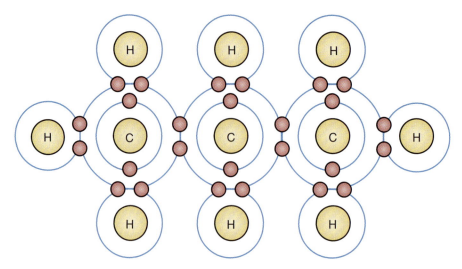

**Figure 8-4** Carbon atoms "sharing" electrons with other carbon and hydrogen atoms

Each element has its own abbreviation, or symbol. Some symbols are the first letter or the first two letters of the element. Some abbreviations are taken from the Latin word for that element. For example, the symbol for carbon is C, but the symbol for iron is Fe, which stands for *ferrous*, the Latin term for iron.

When atoms join together to form molecules, the number of atoms of each element in the molecule is listed beside the symbol for the element. For example, $H_2O$ is made of one atom of oxygen and two atoms of hydrogen. Hydrogen atoms need one electron to fill the outer level. Oxygen needs two electrons to fill its outer ring. Each hydrogen atom shares an electron with the oxygen atom (Figure 8-5).

When a molecule joins two different elements together, the reaction produces what is known as a **compound**. A compound is two or more elements joined chemically to produce an entirely different substance. The new substance has completely new chemical and physical characteristics.

A **mixture** is produced when different elements or compounds are mixed together physically but still retain separate characteristics. Most cosmetic formulas are mixtures. In other words, the ingredients do not change when mixed with other chemicals. We will discuss cosmetic formulations in more depth in Chapter 9, Cosmetic Chemistry and Functional Ingredients.

A **solution** is a mixture of other chemicals. It is an even mixture, which means the various chemicals are evenly dispersed throughout the mixture. An example of this is salt water. If you mix salt in water, the salt will distribute itself evenly throughout the water. If you keep adding more salt to the water, the salt will begin to pile up on the bottom. This means that no more salt can be dispersed evenly in that amount of water. The point at which mixtures no longer mix evenly is known as the point of saturation.

The liquid part of a solution is called a **solvent**. A **solute** is the solid part of the solution. So, in the example of salt water, salt is the solute, and water is the solvent. Salt water is a mixture, not a compound. The salt has not changed chemically; it is simply dispersed through the water. Salt (sodium chloride) is compound, and so is water ($H_2O$). The two compounds are mixed together but do not react chemically with one another (Figure 8-6). Many cosmetics are solutions. Makeup is a good example of pigments evenly distributed through a solvent of oil or water or both. This, too, is a solution.

**Compound** is produced when molecules of two different elements join.

**Mixture** is produced when different elements or compounds are mixed together physically.

**Solution** is a mixture of chemicals.

**Solvent** is the liquid part of a solution.

**Solute** is the solid part of a solution.

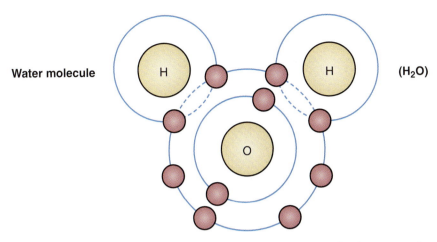

**Figure 8-5** $H_2O$ molecule "sharing" electrons between hydrogen and oxygen atoms

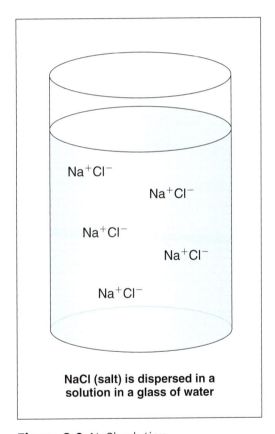

**NaCl (salt) is dispersed in a solution in a glass of water**

**Figure 8-6** NaCl solution

## HOW CHEMICAL REACTIONS TAKE PLACE

Reactions between two elements or two compounds that result in chemical changes are called **chemical reactions**. During a chemical reaction, electrons of the elements or compounds involved begin either to share energy levels in a covalent bond, or form ionic bonds.

Some chemical reactions take place simply by mixing two chemicals together. Sodium, for example, is very reactive with water. In fact, sodium is violently reactive

**Chemical reactions** are reactions between two elements or two compounds that result in chemical changes.

with water. The sodium bonds with hydrogen and oxygen to form sodium hydroxide (lye) and allows hydrogen gas to escape. In the process much energy is given off in the form of heat. The reaction is as follows:

$$2Na + 2H_2O = 2NaOH + H_2 + energy \text{ (heat)}$$

Let's talk about this equation, or symbol, for the chemical reaction taking place. Remember the chemical symbols from the periodic table. Na is the symbol for sodium; O is for oxygen; and H is for hydrogen. The number in front of each chemical stands for the number of molecules of each chemical. Numbers below a chemical symbol stand for the number of atoms of that element in a particular molecule. So, getting back to the reaction, 2Na stands for two atoms of sodium, and $2H_2O$ stands for two molecules of water, which equals 2NaOH, two molecules of sodium hydroxide, plus $H_2$, one molecule of hydrogen.

Notice that the same number of atoms are present before and after the reaction. Before the reaction, there were two sodium atoms, four hydrogen atoms, and two oxygen atoms, $2Na + 2H_2O$. After the reaction there are the same number of atoms, only with a different chemical structure. Because of the electron changeovers, we now have two totally new chemicals, lye and hydrogen. Hydrogen, of course, is a gas, and generally escapes into the air. 2NaOH, or two molecules of sodium hydroxide, have two atoms of sodium, two atoms of oxygen, and two atoms of hydrogen. The other two hydrogen atoms are given off as $H_2$ (hydrogen gas). So, equal numbers of the same atoms are on either side of the reaction. This is why the reaction is called an **equation**.

Some reactions such as the one discussed here occur very naturally, by simply combining two chemicals. Other reactions do not happen as naturally. These types of chemical reaction require what is called a catalyst. A catalyst is a substance that helps to cause the reaction, or speed up the reaction, without its atoms becoming a direct part of the reaction's products.

Another condition required for some chemical reactions is heat. Heat can trigger chemical reactions. Some reactions require exposure to ultraviolet light or pressure to take place.

## CHEMICALS FOUND IN THE SKIN AND BODY

When we discuss chemicals and chemical reactions within the body, we are talking about a subject called **biochemistry**. Biochemistry is a highly complex subject that we will barely touch. So many complex chemical reactions take place in the body. Many reactions are still not fully understood.

As discussed in previous chapters, almost every body function involves chemical reactions. The hormones that tell our cells what to do are chemicals that react with receptor sites. The pituitary hormones that signal other glands to manufacture other hormones is another example of chemical reactions within the body.

Most of the chemical reactions within the body are called organic reactions. Organic chemistry does not mean natural chemistry. Organic chemistry is the chemistry of compounds containing carbon atoms. Carbon is an element that is a large constituent of almost all the many chemicals in the body. The chemicals that the body uses most are oxygen, carbon, hydrogen, and nitrogen. Carbon and hydrogen frequently bond together in chains. These chains of carbon–carbon and carbon–hydrogen bonds are known as **polymers**. Polymers are found in many of the body's chemicals. Proteins, DNA, sugars, and carbohydrates are just a few of the examples of polymers in the body's chemistry.

**Protein** is made of carbon, oxygen, nitrogen, hydrogen, and sulfur. The basic unit of a protein molecule is called an **amino acid**. Think of amino acids as modules or cars of a toy train. When many different modules are placed together, a protein

**Equation** is a chemical reaction such that equal numbers of the same atom are on either side of the reaction.

**Biochemistry** is the study of chemicals and chemical reactions within the body.

**Polymers** are chains of carbon–carbon and carbon-hydrogen bonded together.

**Protein** is made of carbon, oxygen, nitrogen, hydrogen, and sulfur.

**Amino acid** is a protein that helps break down simple sugars, fats, and parts of proteins.

molecule results. Simple proteins are groups of amino acids linked together. Sometimes the amino acids will have another chemical linked to them that is not an amino acid. These proteins with a non-amino-acid group are called conjugated proteins. Conjugated proteins make up most of the substances found in intercellular cement. Glycoproteins are amino acid chains with a carbohydrate group attached to it. Lipoproteins are amino acid chains with lipids or fats attached to the chain. Phosphoroproteins have a phosphorus or phosphate group attached to the protein chain.

The bond between amino acid groups is called a **peptide bond**. When many amino acids are in long chains, there are obviously many bonds. A chain of amino acid molecules is known as a **polypeptide**.

Simple proteins make up basic material for the body's tissues. The skin, hair, and connective tissue are made up of a protein called schleroprotein. The protein that makes up the blood and lymph are called globulins. Albumin is another type of simple protein used in the blood. Nucleic acids with protein DNA structures are another type of simple protein product. The carbohydrate groups include sugars and other compounds. Carbohydrates are formed by a chain of carbon atoms united with oxygen and hydrogen. They form units, similar to protein and amino acid units. A simple unit of a carbohydrate is called a **saccharide**. One saccharide by itself is called a monosaccharide. Two saccharides together are called a **disaccharide**. Many saccharides bonded together are called a **polysaccharide**. Examples of the various carbohydrates are illustrated (Figure 8-7).

Monosaccharides are simple sugars like glucose (blood sugar). Disaccharides include sucrose or table sugar, and maltose, the sugar used to make malted milk.

Polysaccharides are the more complex carbohydrates. They include the sugars in starch and the carbohydrates that make up vegetables and cellulose-type substances.

Lipids are basically fats. They are a third major chemical group within the body. Lipids are made up of carbon, oxygen, and hydrogen. Lipids do not form in units like proteins and carbohydrates. They are more complex. Triglycerides are the best known type of lipid. Other lipids include waxes, fats, and steroids.

Again, lipids are very important chemicals in cosmetology. They can bind with proteins to form proteolipids, which are a major part of the intercellular cement. Phospholipids and glycolipids are two examples of lipid-protein compounds found in the intercellular cement.

**Peptide bond** is the bond between two amino acid groups.

**Polypeptide** is a chain of amino acid molecules.

**Saccharide** can refer to any carbohydrate group.

**Disaccharide** means two saccharides are bonded together.

**Polysaccharide** means many saccharides are bonded together.

## pH, ACIDS, AND BASES

When water is added to certain compounds like acids, the water ($H_2O$) breaks up and restructures, with certain atoms joining the acid chemicals. Hydrogen chloride (HCl), for example, becomes hydrochloric acid when mixed with water. The hydrogen ions float separately in the acid. The measurement of these hydrogen ions is known as the pH of the substance. pH is an abbreviation for the negative logarithm of hydrions (positively charged hydrogen ions). Acids have a low pH, which actually means that they have a large number of hydrogen ions. Alkaline substances, or **bases**, have a low concentration of hydrogen ions. They have high pH values. Acids all have similar chemical characteristics. Bases, or alkaline substances, are also similar to each other.

The pH scale ranges from 0 to 14. The lower the pH, the more acidic the substance. The higher the pH, the more alkaline the substance. Figure 8-8 gives examples of various substances and their pH values.

**Bases** have a low concentration of hydrogen atoms and high pH values.

## Why pH Is Important in Cosmetics

The skin has an acid mantle on its surface, made of a mixture of lipids, sebum, and sweat. This acid mantle has a pH of about 5.5. Therefore, it has a slightly acidic pH.

**A** D-Fructose (levulose)

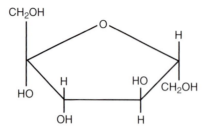

**B** Sucrose (glucose + fructose)

**C** Amylopectin

**Figure 8-7** Examples of (A) monosaccharide, (B) disaccharide, (C) polysaccharide

Cosmetics should also have a slightly acidic pH. Higher pH values tend to swell the skin and make it more permeable. This can be good or bad, depending on the circumstances. For example, desincrustant solutions and "pre-masks" used for treating clogged pores and oily areas need to have a slightly alkaline pH to slightly dilate the pores for easier extraction. They also help to conduct electricity (galvanic current) better for desincrustation.

Cleansers for oily skin may also have a slightly higher pH than that of the acid mantle. This enables these cleansers to perform a more efficient job of cutting the sebaceous secretions of oily or problem skin. Most of these high pH cleansers are followed by low pH toners. A cleanser with a pH of 6.5 or 7.0 is often followed by a toner with a pH of 4.0 or 4.5. High pH values, however, can be harmful to the skin also, particularly if they are not controlled. High pH increases the permeability of the skin, making it easier for bacteria, microorganisms, and other harmful substances to enter the body. Harsh, high pH soaps can be very irritating and can severely overdry the skin.

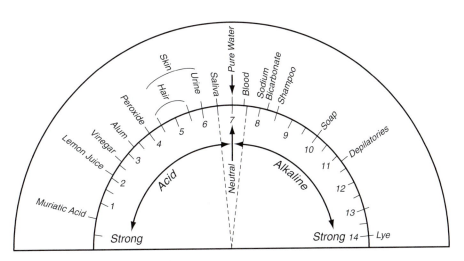

**Figure 8-8** Average pH values

Being aware of pH values is very important in chemical exfoliation and peeling procedures. Alphahydroxy acid (AHA) and betahydroxy acid (BHA) professional esthetic exfoliation treatments have lower pHs. The lower the pH, the more acidic the product is. The ideal pH for AHA professional esthetic treatments is 3.0 with an AHA concentration of not greater than 30%. When the pH is less than 3.0, the irritation potential of these exfoliation treatments increases. Likewise, concentrations of greater than 30% can also increase irritation potential.

Exposure to pHs less than 3.0 increase chances of barrier function damage and therefore increase the possibility of inflammation. Frequency of application can also increase irritation potential. Generally, AHA treatments with a pH of 3.0 should not be administered more than once or twice a week to begin treatment, and not more than twice a month after an initial series of 6–12 treatments. Should irritation such as peeling skin or redness develop, exfoliation should be discontinued, at least until the irritation subsides.

Combining chemical exfoliation treatments with mechanical exfoliation such as microdermabrasion further increases irritation chances and is not advisable.

The ideal pH for at-home AHA exfoliation products is 3.5. Again, repeatedly using products with a pH less than 3.5 on a daily basis can lead to irritation. Other products, such as certain vitamin serums can also have very low pHs.

Clients using AHA or BHA products should always use a daily broad-spectrum sunscreen with an SPF of at least 15.

BHA exfoliation treatments cannot be performed as frequently. Always follow the manufacturer's instructions when using any exfoliation product. Do not attempt chemical exfoliation procedures unless you have been properly trained. For much more information about chemical exfoliation, see the chapter on chemical peeling.

## CHEMICAL TERMS ESTHETICIANS SHOULD KNOW

There are a variety of chemical terms besides those already mentioned that estheticians should know to better interpret ingredient labels and understand more about cosmetic chemicals. Some of these words are actually suffixes or prefixes that you will see attached to different chemical names. Most of these are derived from Latin.

**Proteo**—(prefix) refers to protein. *Proteolytic*, as in proteolytic enzyme peelings, means protein-dissolving.

**Lipo**—(prefix) refers to fats, lipids, or waxes. Examples are lipoproteins, found in the intercellular cement, or liposuction, the surgical procedure used to remove fat.

**Saccharides**—can refer to any carbohydrate group. An example is mucopolysaccharide, a popular moisturizing ingredient.

**Saturated**—can either mean that a solution has absorbed as much solute as possible, or that a molecule has taken on as many hydrogen atoms as it can hold, as in saturated fat.

**Aqueous**—water-based, as in an aqueous solution.

**Aerobic**—refers to a reaction that takes place in the presence of oxygen. *Anaerobic* means without oxygen.

**Hydration**—water is added.

**Homogenous**—a mixture that is even. The solute is evenly dispersed throughout the solvent.

**Suspension**—the solute is suspended throughout a solvent. Suspension is usually not homogenous. A separating makeup foundation is an example of a suspension.

**Alcohol**—is a molecule that has a hydroxy (OH) group bonded to it. The molecule must be a hydrocarbon made of carbon and hydrogen atoms.

**Amino**—(prefix) refers to compounds that have an amino acid group attached; may also indicate protein derivation.

**Mono**—(prefix) means *one*. Example: monosaccharide, which is a simple sugar with one saccharide group.

**Di**—(prefix) means *two*. Disodium means two sodium atoms that are included in a molecular structure.

**Carbo**—(prefix) has carbon as a base in the molecule. Example: carbohydrate.

**Distilled**—heated to remove one chemical from another. Water, for example, is distilled by boiling water and allowing the gas to condense back into liquid, separating the water from impurities and other contaminant chemicals.

**Enzyme**—a protein that is involved as a catalyst in a chemical reaction. Enzymes in cosmetics are often used to break down substances, as a proteolytic enzyme breaks down keratin protein in dead cells. The chemical names of enzymes generally end in the suffix *-ase*. Examples are *lipase* (fat-dissolving enzyme) and *maltase*, which breaks maltose, a disaccharide, into two simple glucose (sugar) molecules.

**Ionized**—substance has been charged by changing atoms to ions. *Deionized* means that ions have been neutralized and do not have a charge.

**Poly**—(prefix) means *many*. Example: *polymer, polysaccharide*.

**Tri**—(prefix) means *three*. Example: *tridecyl trimellitate*, an emollient.

**Cyclo**—(prefix) means that the molecule is in a ring structure. The carbon atoms are joined in a ring formation.

**Aldehyde**—a compound made of carbon and hydrogen, with a carbon, hydrogen, and oxygen group on the end of the molecule.

## TOPICS FOR DISCUSSION

1. What is an element?
2. Explain why electrons orbit the nucleus.
3. What is the difference between an element, a compound, and a mixture?
4. Describe pH. Give some pH values for various substances.
5. Explain how variations in pH affect the skin.

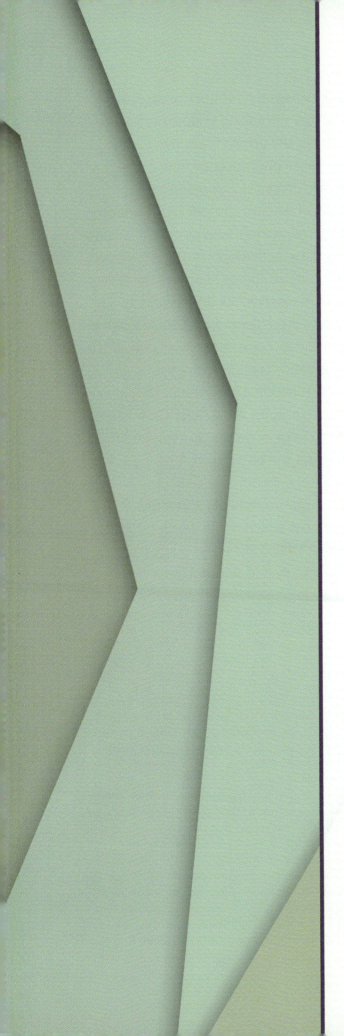

# CHAPTER 9

# Cosmetic Chemistry and Functional Ingredients

## OBJECTIVES. . .

It is very important that the esthetician be well informed about cosmetic ingredients. This chapter is an overview of common types of cosmetic ingredients. Discussion of their chemical functions in formulations is also included. The esthetician will learn about vehicles, including surfactants, emulsifiers, and emollients. We will also discuss preservatives, coloring agents, and other chemicals necessary to produce cosmetics.

Cosmetic chemistry is a highly complex field. Cosmetic chemists work very closely with cellular function and must be well versed in medicine, biology, chemistry, pharmacology, and cosmetology. They must be aware of the beauty needs of people but at the same time be well trained in chemistry in order to make beauty products.

Making cosmetics is not as simple as many people think. Cosmetics vary greatly in formula. One slight variation in chemical makeup can create a whole new product texture, color, or other property. Cosmetic chemicals are divided into two basic groups. The first group is known as the functional ingredients. **Functional ingredients** make up the main part of any

**Functional ingredients** are cosmetic ingredients that are used primarily to spread, preserve, or affect the feel of look of a product.

**Performance ingredients** are cosmetic ingredients that cause the actual physical appearance to change.

**Active agents** are chemicals that cause physical changes in the skin's appearance or alter the appearance in any way.

**Active ingredients** are ingredients in drug products that cause a change in the function of the human body.

**Vehicles** are ingredients used as spreading agents.

**Water** is the most common vehicle ingredient.

**Deionizing** is the process of neutralizing ions in water that can cross-react in a product.

**Distillation** is the process of purifying water.

cosmetic or skin-care product. They help the product to spread across the skin, help the product stay mixed and uniform in texture, adjust the pH of the product, or help the product stay fresh. Functional ingredients do not usually cause physical appearance changes associated with the use of skin-care products and cosmetics.

Ingredients that cause the actual physical changes to the appearance of the skin are known as **performance ingredients** or **performance agents**. They occasionally are also called **active agents**. There is a trend toward not calling these chemicals "active agents," because the similar-sounding term **"active ingredients"** is reserved for drug products. Saying a skin-care product has an "active ingredient" would imply that it is a drug. For more information about the technical differences between drugs and cosmetics, see the chapter on claims in cosmetics.

In this chapter, we will discuss functional ingredients, which include a large number of cosmetic chemicals. We will learn about how ingredients are used to stabilize, thicken, preserve, and spread other ingredients across the skin that cause the physical changes we see when we use skin-care products.

The biggest category of functional ingredients is **vehicles**. Vehicles are spreading agents. They are the substance in which the performance ingredients are "floating." They make up the largest actual amount of any skin-care product or cosmetic. Without vehicles, we could never apply the performance ingredients and cause the changes we see to the skin's appearance.

## ABOUT WATER

**Water** is the most common vehicle ingredient. You will notice that water is listed first on the ingredient label of most products. That means that there is more water than any other ingredient in the product. The thinner the product, the more water is present.

Cosmetic factories have large tanks to purify water before using it in a formulation. This purification process is accomplished by filtering, distilling, deionizing, and sterilizing water before it is used in a formula.

**Deionizing** water neutralizes ions that can cross-react with other ingredients or make a product unstable. Deionization is important in the process of emulsification, or keeping the product well blended. **Distillation** means that the water has had minerals and other trace elements removed from it.

Water is both a functional and a performance ingredient. As a functional ingredient it is an excellent spreading agent and is important to rinse and remove certain products. It works as a performance ingredient in moisturizers, helping to hydrate the skin. Water is the real magic ingredient in moisturizers because it is attracted to and binds to humectants used in moisturizers. We will discuss much more about these ingredients in the chapter on performance ingredients and active ingredients.

# EMOLLIENTS

**Emollients** are also can be both functional and performance ingredients. Emollients are ingredients that lubricate the skin; work as vehicles to help to spread other performance ingredients; and give cosmetics a soft, smooth feeling. Emollients also significantly help skin-care products and cosmetics adhere or stick to the skin surface. Emollients also help to fill in texture gaps in the skin surface, making the skin look smoother and feel softer. There are many types and textures of emollients.

As performance ingredients, emollients sit on the skin surface and prevent water loss (dehydration). They help trap water in the skin. Because they are larger molecules, water has problems evaporating through the emollient. Chemists often refer to chemicals that stop water evaporation from the skin as **protectants**. Protectants can also help prevent other agents from entering the skin.

A really good example of an emollient is mineral oil. Mineral oil with fragrance is commonly known as baby oil. Applying baby oil to a baby's bottom helps keep the skin protected from dryness (dehydration) and prevents human waste from penetrating the skin and causing irritation known as diaper rash.

**Petrolatum**, commonly known as petroleum jelly, has similar properties and benefits. Commonly used in ointments, petrolatum is used as a vehicle, protectant, and lubricant.

**Silicones** are a multi-purpose group of different chemicals very commonly used in many skin care and makeup products as protectants and vehicles. Silicones leave a protective film on the skin surface, preventing water evaporation. Known as "breathable barriers," they help protect the skin from dehydration without being heavy or completely occluding the skin surface. They can vary in molecular size and concentration in a formula, and have many different feels and textures. Silicones generally feel very soft and silky, improving the texture and feel of many skin-care products. They help creams and makeup products glide across the skin and fill in rough textures for a smoother skin appearance. Silicones are also used to more evenly apply sunscreen ingredients.

**Dimethicone**, **cyclomethicone**, and **phenyl trimethicone** are three examples of silicone compounds frequently used in moisturizers, sunscreens, serums, and foundations. They are also used in pressed powders and blushes, helping to keep the powdered makeup in a cake form and helping it adhere to the skin when applied.

One of the best features of silicones is that they are noncomedogenic (not pore-clogging) and nonacnegenic (do not cause acne flares).

Petrolatum, silicone compounds, and mineral oil are **biologically inert**, which means that they will not react with normal skin reactions within the skin, making them extremely unlikely to cause allergic or irritant reactions. Therefore they are excellent ingredients and are frequently used in formulations for sensitive skin, including use for drug vehicles for dermatological conditions such as eczema and psoriasis.

Unfortunately, all three of these emollient ingredient types have been erroneously accused of causing problems because they are not "natural," having been purified or derived from other sources in the laboratory. The truth is that many natural substances, including plant oils, are much more likely to cause allergies.

## Other Types of Emollients

Emollients also include the categories of **natural oils**, such as sunflower, safflower, jojoba, palm, and coconut oils. **Waxes** such as paraffin are also emollients. Natural oils and waxes are fatty emollient materials derived from plant sources.

**Polymers** are synthetic molecular structures used as state-of-the-art spreading agents that help many ingredients adhere to the skin surface or help penetrate performance ingredients. Polymers are used for texture to help deliver performance

**Emollients** are somewhat like occlusives in that they mostly lie on the surface of the skin and prevent water loss. They also help to "fill in the cracks" of dry, dehydrated skin.

**Protectants** are chemicals that stop water evaporation.

**Petrolatum** prevents urine and soggy diapers from irritating the baby's sensitive skin.

**Silicone** is an emollient that leaves a protective film on the surface of the skin.

**Dimethicone** is a smaller, lighter version of silicone.

**Cyclomethicone** is a type of silicone used primarily as a vehicle or emollient.

**Phenyl trimethicone** is a type of silicone emollient.

**Biologically inert** means will not react with chemicals in the human body.

**Natural oils** occur in nature, primarily in plants.

**Waxes** are thick, fatty substances that are derived primarily from plants and are used as emollients in skin-care products.

**Polymers** are chains of chemical structures used a delivery systems.

ingredients more effectively; improve efficacy of sunscreens and other drug ingredients; and avoid irritant, allergic, and acnegenic reactions. Polymers are often referred to as delivery systems.

## FATTY ACIDS

**Fatty acids** are derived from plant or animal sources. They are not corrosive acids like hydrochloric acid, and they are not inflammatory to the skin. They are triglycerides that have been broken down by removing glycerin from fat. They help to give a soft, firm texture to lotions and creams. They are good emollient lubricants and smooth across the skin evenly. Fatty acids also add stability to formulations. They are also major ingredients in many soaps. When fat is mixed with sodium hydroxide, soap forms.

Fatty acids are also often used in creams, lotions, shaving creams, and lipsticks and are used as pressing agents in pressed powders and blushes. They are also used in foundations and cleansers. Each cosmetic use of fatty acids may be somewhat different.

In lipstick, for example, the fatty acid may be used to improve creaminess or adherability. In shaving creams, stearic acid is frequently used because it adheres well to the skin and allows the razor to move smoothly across it. It is also a good protectant against razor burns and accidental cuts to the skin.

In makeup, fatty acids may be used for improving spreadability and texture. In pressed powders and blushes, fatty acids are used to "press" the powder into a cake, which keeps the product in a solid form until it is used.

Common fatty acids used in cosmetic formulations are as follows:

◆ Stearic acid—derived from animal fats and some plants.

◆ Caprylic acid—derived from coconut oil, palm oil, or animal sources.

◆ Oleic acid—from animal fats and vegetable oils.

◆ Myristic acid—occurs in coconut oil, animal fat, palm seed, and other vegetable fats.

◆ Palmitic acid—derived from plant and animal sources.

◆ Lauric acid—derived from laurel oil and coconut oil.

All of these acids are derived from fats (triglycerides) from natural sources.

Although fatty acids have many good properties for cosmetic use, many can be comedogenic. For more details, see the chapter on comedogenicity.

## FATTY ALCOHOLS

When most people think of alcohol, they think of isopropyl alcohol, poured on cuts as an antiseptic when they were children. They may also think of alcoholic beverages. All of these forms of alcohol have negative connotations. This may explain the notorious (and undeserved) reputation that alcohol has in the cosmetic industry. Although isopropyl (rubbing) alcohol can be very drying to the skin's surface, this is only one type of alcohol. Most types of alcohol used in the cosmetic industry are actually more like oils or waxes. The term *alcohol* is a chemical term that simply means that an oxygen atom and a hydrogen atom have attached themselves to the end of a carbon chain.

There are many types of **fatty alcohols**, which are fatty acids that have been exposed to hydrogen. They have a slightly waxy feel as a raw ingredient. They are used as emollients in moisturizers. They are less sticky and less heavy than many fats. Fatty alcohols are also frequently used to improve the viscosity of lotions and creams. **Viscosity** is the thickness and liquidity of a solution. There are many types of fatty alcohols:

◆ Cetyl alcohol—a widely used fatty alcohol. Cetyl alcohol is used as an emollient, an emulsifier, an **opacifying agent** (helps to turn a cream an opaque color, which helps protect the product from light exposure), and a spreading

**Fatty alcohols** are fatty materials used as vehicles and emollients in skin-care products and cosmetics.

**Viscosity** is the thickness and liquidity of a solution, skin-care product, or cosmetic.

**Opacifying agent** is a functional ingredient that helps a product be opaque in color.

agent. Cetyl alcohol is derived from animal tallow but can also be made synthetically.

- ◆ Lauryl alcohol—derived from coconut and palm seed oils, is used as an emollient and spreading agent.
- ◆ Stearyl alcohol—derived from stearic acid, used as a foam-booster in detergent cleansers, as an emollient, and as a viscosity-opacity builder.
- ◆ Cetearyl alcohol—a mixture of cetyl and stearyl alcohols, its uses are the same as its parent alcohols.
- ◆ Oleyl alcohol—derived from oleic acid, is somewhat fattier and greasier than other alcohols. It is often used in superfatted soaps and dry skin emulsions.

# FATTY ESTERS

An **ester** is formed when an organic (carbon chain) acid combines with an alcohol. Fatty esters are frequently used in skin-care products and cosmetics as emollients and conditioning agents. One of their best qualities is that they do not feel as oily to the touch as some other types of emollient fatty ingredients.

**Esters** are modified fatty substances that are primarily used as vehicles and emollients in skin-care products and cosmetics.

Both functional and performance ingredients, they can be used to smooth the surface of the skin or hair; to serve as a protectant; to help replace natural fatty esters that are missing from older, drier skin types; and sometimes as emulsifiers.

The easiest way to spot fatty esters in an ingredient label is that they have the suffix *-ate*. An example is isopropyl palmitate. Isopropyl palmitate is a palmitic acid molecule that has been attached to the carbon chain of an alcohol, propanol.

Fatty esters vary greatly in molecular weight and size. The size can have an effect on how the ester is used in cosmetics and skin-care formulations. Again, fatty esters, like fatty acids and alcohols, are often comedogenic, and many should be avoided in formulations for oily and acne skin. (See the chapter on comedogenicity.)

Frequently used fatty esters in skin-care and cosmetic formulations are the following:

Isopropyl myristate
Isopropyl palmitate
Ethylhexyl palmitate
Ethylhexyl stearate
Isopropyl isostearate
Glyceryl stearate
Propylene glycol dicaprate/dicaprylate
Cetyl palmitate
Decyl oleate

# SURFACTANTS

**Surfactants** are chemicals in cosmetics that cause the cosmetic to be able to slip across or onto the skin. Surfactants lower surface tension on the surface of the skin to allow cosmetic products to slip across and adhere to the skin. They are one of the biggest categories of cosmetic chemicals.

**Surfactants** are chemicals in cosmetics that cause the cosmetic to be able to slip across or onto the skin.

Surfactants also include detergents and soaps. **Detergents** are surfactants that are used for cleansing. They break up oils, fats, and other debris, and cause the debris to separate from the skin. When detergents are applied to the skin and are mixed with water, they begin to bubble. This bubbling is a good example of how surfactants and detergents reduce surface tension and allow water to spread more easily across the skin. Bubbling is air that has come between the surfactant and the surface of the skin. The surfactant removes surface oils from the skin, as well as makeup, dirt, pollutants, and other agents that have come in contact or adhered to the skin during the day.

**Detergents** are surfactants that are used for cleansing.

Another good example of reduction of surface tension by a surfactant is in your kitchen. You cooked hamburgers for dinner and you left the pan with the hamburger grease on the stove while you ate dinner. During that time the grease, which is fats and fatty acids, has solidified in the pan. After dinner, you add hot water to the pan, which liquifies the fat. It is the temperature, not the water, that liquifies the fat. If you leave the water in the pan, the grease will remain nonsolid for the most part. But we know that hot water alone will not remove beef grease from a pan.

So you pour in some dishwashing liquid. If you look closely while you are pouring in the dishwashing liquid, you will notice that the fat has a tendency to "run" from the dishwashing liquid. This "running" is actually the surfactant or detergent improving the water's ability to remove the grease from the pan's surface. The grease will break up much faster with the detergent added to the pan.

During the process of cleaning the pan, you accidentally rubbed grease from the hamburgers on your hand. When you remove your hand from the sink, you discover that your hand is greasy. Dipping your hand into the dishwater seems to loosen the grease from your hand. This is because the surfactant (detergent) works on skin in the same way that it works on the dishes or pan.

Of course, the surfactant used in dishwashing is much too strong a detergent to use routinely on your skin. Similar detergent agents may be used in dishwashing liquids, but the concentration of detergent in the formula is far greater than that used in a facial cleanser. Detergent facial cleansers also may vary in strength and concentration. The four major types of surfactants vary with the pH of the water being used in the formulation. The four basic types of surfactants are as follows:

**Anionic surfactants** are strong cleansers and are frequently used in household products.

**Cationic surfactants** have a positive ionic charge. They are frequently used in cosmetics and hair shampoos.

**Amphoteric surfactants** may have either a positive or negative ionic charge. They are frequently used in facial lotions and creams.

**Nonionic surfactants** are used in heavier creams such as hand creams.

1. **Anionic surfactants**, which have a negative ionic charge. Anionic surfactants are strong cleansers and are frequently used in household products.

2. **Cationic surfactants** have a positive ionic charge. They are frequently used in cosmetics and hair shampoos.

3. **Amphoteric surfactants** may have either a positive or negative ionic charge. They will adapt to the pH of the water used in the solution. Because they are so adaptable to both acid and alkaline water, they are frequently used in facial lotions and creams. The neutrality of the surfactant is important to the mildness of the cosmetic product.

4. **Nonionic surfactants** are used in heavier creams such as hand creams.

Some surfactant ingredients are very frequently used in cosmetic cleansers. Some of these are as follows:

> Sodium lauryl sulfate
> Sodium laureth sulfate
> Disodium lauryl sulfosuccinate
> Ammonium lauryl sulfate
> Cocoamphocarboxyglycinate
> Cocamidopropyl betaine
> Alpha-olefin sulfonate
> Decyl polyglucoside

All of these surfactants can help remove oils, dirt, and other debris from the skin's surface. How much they remove depends on the amount of surfactant in the individual cleanser.

For sensitive and drier skin types cosmetic manufacturers often add a fatty acid, oil, or wax to cut the contact of the surfactant with the skin. The fatty substance prevents too much of the surfactant from coming in contact with the skin. Too much detergent can be irritating or dehydrating to sensitive, dry, or thin skin.

Cleansers can also vary in strength directly from the amount of surfactant that is in the formula. A cleanser for oilier skin will, in general, contain more surfactant than a cleanser for dry skin. Most cleansers are carefully prepared so that they prevent irritation on most skin types. Surfactants are also added to creams to improve the cream's slip and adhesive qualities. Some surfactants may be very irritating to the skin when used in creams.

## EMULSIFIERS

**Emulsifiers** are chemicals that keep water and oil solutions well mixed. Let's go back to the kitchen for a moment. Remember that greasy pan? Let's pretend that the grease is in a mayonnaise jar. If you add water to the jar with grease in it, what happens to the oil? It floats to the top. This is because water and oil will not mix under normal circumstances.

If we add some dishwashing detergent to the jar, the oil will start to "break up." If we put a top on the jar and shake it, the oil will be dispersed throughout the water evenly. The water will become cloudy because the oil has saturated the water in small droplets.

The detergent is what made the oil break into small droplets and disperse throughout the water. But didn't we add a *detergent* to the water? You thought that this section was about emulsifiers? Well, it is. It just so happens that surfactants, detergents included, are also emulsifiers. They reduce the tension of the water in a cleanser and also reduce the tension of the water in a solution, or even a cosmetic lotion!

Emulsifiers work by forming a sort of "shell" around the very small oil droplets, allowing them to remain suspended in a solution of water. When a solution of water and oil is mixed, and it is mostly water, the solution is called an **oil-in-water solution**. When the solution is mostly oil, it is called a **water-in-oil** solution (Figure 9-1).

Most lotions available today are oil-in-water emulsions. They are much lighter in weight and texture, feel much less greasy, and are easier to remove. Most bottled moisturizers are oil-in-water (abbreviated o/w) emulsions. Old-fashioned cold creams

> **Emulsifiers** are chemicals that keep water and oil solutions well mixed.

> **Oil-in-water solution** is a solution of water and oil that is mostly water.

> **Water-in-oil** is a solution of oil and water that is mostly oil.

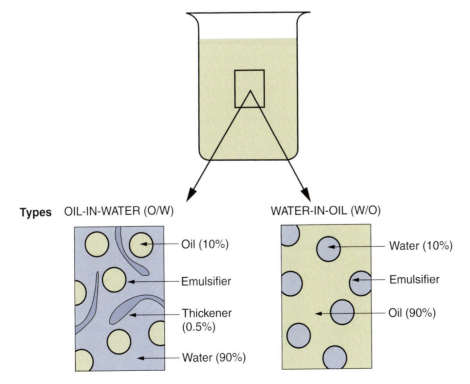

**Types** OIL-IN-WATER (O/W)        WATER-IN-OIL (W/O)

Oil (10%)
Emulsifier
Thickener (0.5%)
Water (90%)

Water (10%)
Emulsifier
Oil (90%)

**Figure 9-1** Types of emulsions

are a good example of a water-in-oil emulsion. Some heavy night creams are also water-in-oil.

Have you ever found an old bottle of lotion in your cabinet? Did it look "watery"? Over time, generally a year or more, emulsifiers can stop working in an emulsion. When this happens, the lotion begins to separate back into its water and oil phases.

As a general rule, almost anything in a bottle is an oil-in-water emulsion. Almost all water-in-oil emulsions are packaged in jars. They are often too heavy and thick to be poured out of a bottle. Another way to determine a particular product's emulsion type is to check the ingredient label. The FDA requires that cosmetics list their ingredients in descending order. If oil is listed before water, it is a water-in-oil emulsion. If water is listed first, then it is oil-in-water.

Emulsifiers help to provide stability and texture to lotions and creams. They make the cream feel even and smooth. If they were not used in moisturizers the lotion would feel wet and oily when applied. Some frequently used emulsifiers are as follows:

Amphoteric 9
Ceteth-20
Beeswax
Polyethelene glycol (PEG)
Polysorbate
Carbomer
Carbopol
Stearamide

"Water-based" generally means that the emulsion or lotion is an oil-in-water emulsion. It does not necessarily mean that the emulsion is oil-free. The main reason cosmetic companies refer to a product as being water-based is to appeal to the consumer. Consumers who have oily or problem skin and consumers who do not like greasy products look for products that are watery textured because they are lighter weight and nongreasy.

How can you tell the difference among the three basic types of surfactants? Surface active agents (which reduce surface tension of water for spreading of cosmetic products), detergents (cleansing and foaming agents), and emulsifiers (which keep water and oils in emulsion state) are all surfactants.

The difference among the three has to do with their molecular structures. The size of the molecule determines the different properties that the particular surfactant will have in a cosmetic solution. Surfactants are polymer molecules. This means that there is a chain of carbon atoms that are connected to one another. Surfactant polymer molecules have two ends. One end is attracted to water; the other end is repelled by water. The end that is repelled by water is instead attracted to fatty substances. **Lipophilic** means *fat-loving*. **Hydrophilic** means *water-loving*. The size of the lipophilic end of the polymer determines which kind of surfactant group the molecule will be. Shorter chain carbon polymers, chains with eight or ten carbon atoms, have a shorter lipophilic end and are surface active agents used in creams to improve slip (how well the product flows across the skin) and spreadability.

Medium-length chain molecules with a medium-size lipophilic end are the detergents used in cleansers that help foam and remove surface debris. Long chain polymers, which have a large lipophilic end, are the emulsifiers. This makes sense, because these molecules must have a strong attraction to fat. Remember, these molecules are the ones that "surround" or form the "shell" around the oil droplets and spread themselves throughout the water solution. The other end of the emulsifier (the hydrophilic end) is attracted to the water in the solution. So the molecule produces a "tug-of-war" between the oil and the water. The emulsifier is attracted to the oil and is more or less wrapped around the oil, but the other end is attracted to the water in which it is floating. This constant "pulling" keeps the oil or fat evenly suspended in the water solution, or vice versa in the case of a water-in-oil suspension. The oil droplets in an

**Lipophilic** means fat-loving.

**Hydrophilic** means water-loving.

oil-in-water emulsion are referred to as **globules**. They are the dispersed part of the emulsion and are referred to as the **internal phase**. The water in an oil-in-water emulsion is called the **external phase**. A **suspension** is a liquid solution in which the internal and external phases do not stay mixed for any period of time.

We have only talked here about lotions. Many types of cosmetic emulsions are not lotions and contain other components besides water and oils. Makeup, for example, is a solid such as talc that is emulsified in a liquid. The external phase of a makeup base is usually water, possibly mixed with propylene glycol or another solvent. Aerosol hair spray is an example of a liquid that is emulsified within a gas. Mousse is an example of a gas that is emulsified within an external phase liquid.

## PHYSICAL EMULSIONS

Emulsifiers can sometimes cause problems for thin, sensitive, or dry skin types. What happens in these cases is that the emulsifiers actually start breaking down the natural intercellular lipids that form the barrier function of the skin. Although this is not a problem for all types of skin, it can cause sensitivity for already thin sensitive skin with impaired barrier function.

There is a relatively new technology that uses high-speed mixers, called **homogenizers**, to emulsify products. Most of these products are creams and lotions for sensitive skin. These products use special blends of emollients and nonsurfactant emulsifying agents that are then mixed at high speeds under pressure. This process produces a suspended effect without the use of traditional surfactant emulsifiers, eliminating further disturbance of the barrier function. These types of products are **physical emulsions** and are known as excellent moisturizers for sensitive skin.

## SOLVENTS

Solvents have already been discussed in Chapter 8, Essential Knowledge of Chemistry. Solvents are used in cosmetic formulations either as vehicles for the product or as vehicles for other ingredients.

Plant extracts used in cosmetics, for example, have to be extracted from the actual plant. The solvent normally used for extraction is propylene glycol. So, if you see "arnica (arnica montana) extract" on a cosmetic label, it often means that the arnica extract is present in a solution of propylene glycol or another solvent. Both the extract and the solvent must be listed on the cosmetic product label. However, both ingredients still must be listed in the exact order of predominance in the final formulation. Alcohols of various types are also often used as solvents for plant extracts.

## ANTIMICROBIALS AND PRESERVATIVES

**Preservatives** are chemical agents that inhibit the growth of microorganisms in creams or cosmetic products. Because of the many fats used in cosmetics, formulations are more susceptible to invasion by microorganisms than other types of chemical formulations.

The three main types of microorganisms present in cosmetic formulations are bacteria, fungi, and yeast. Cosmetics may become contaminated because of cross-contamination by the user. The user will apply the cream to the skin, re-dipping the same hand that has touched the skin into the jar of cream. When the fingers touch the cream, bacteria and other microorganisms come in contact with the product in the jar.

Preservatives must be added to cosmetics to kill these contaminating bacteria. Bacteria are also present in small amounts in the raw ingredients used to make the cosmetic. In the making of cosmetics, preservatives are usually the first or one of the first

---

**Globules** are oil droplets in an oil-in-water emulsion.

**Internal phase** is the dispersed part of the emulsion.

**External phase** is the water in an oil-in-water emulsion.

**Suspension** means the solute is suspended throughout a solvent. Suspension is usually not homogenous. The internal and external phases do not stay mixed for any period of time.

**Homogenizers** are high-speed mixers used to emulsify lotions and creams.

**Physical emulsions** are lotions or creams that use physical rather than chemical techniques to blend and suspend oil and water mixtures.

**Preservatives** are chemical agents that inhibit the growth of microorganisms in creams or cosmetic products.

ingredients used in the production process. This is because, if the preservative is already in the mixing tank, any bacteria introduced into the formula will be killed as ingredients are added.

Preservatives work by either directly poisoning bacteria or releasing other chemicals that poison the microorganisms. We have already discussed the allergy and irritation possibilities associated with preservatives. It is important that enough preservative be used in the cosmetic formulation to kill microorganisms without adding so much preservative that allergies will be more likely to flare.

Another trend in skin-care products is the use of botanical (plant) ingredients and other natural materials. Natural materials are more likely to break down than synthetic materials and are more likely to be contaminated with microorganisms such as fungi. Therefore, the use of natural materials actually increases the need for more preservatives!

The most commonly used preservatives are methylparaben, propylparaben, and imidazolidinyl urea. Other paraben groups such as ethyl and butyl paraben are also used.

There are many preservative agents besides those already mentioned used in cosmetic formulations. Some of the more frequently used preservatives are as follows:

Methylparaben
Propylparaben
Ethylparaben
Butylparaben
Imidazolidinyl urea
DMDM hydantoin
Methylchloroisothiazolinone
Methylchlorothiazolinone
Quaternium-15
Diazolidinyl urea
Phenoxyethanol

Preservatives are used in very small quantities so they do not cause unnecessary irritation. Because they are present in small quantities, they are almost always some of the very last ingredients to be listed on an ingredient label. Remember, federal law says that ingredients must be listed in descending order of their presence amount.

## OTHER TYPES OF PRESERVATIVES

Besides microorganisms, chemical reactions can take place that can alter or even ruin cosmetics. Oxidation is one of these chemical reactions. **Oxidation** is the process by which oxygen is exposed to certain ingredients, which results in a breakdown of the ingredient. It is also the process by which free radicals form! Fats and fatty substances are particularly vulnerable to oxidation. Have you ever been to a picnic and noticed that the potato salad was a yellowish color on the top, but when you spooned some onto your plate, noticed that the potato salad below the surface was lighter?

This is oxidation. One of the main ingredients in potato salad is mayonnaise, which is mainly oil. The oil in the mayonnaise oxidizes very quickly, causing the yellow color on the top of the potato salad.

The exact same reaction takes place in the fats, fatty acids, and esters in cosmetic products. Oxygen constantly comes in contact with the cream during the manufacturing process. After the product is opened by the consumer, the product is exposed to more oxygen. Every time the consumer opens and shuts the container, the product is exposed to oxygen.

**Antioxidants** are chemicals that are added to cosmetic formulas to prevent oxidation. They also keep creams and other products from developing color and odor changes caused by oxidation. A bad odor may develop in creams that do not contain

**Oxidation** is the process by which oxygen is exposed to certain ingredients, which results in a breakdown of the ingredient.

**Antioxidants** are topical free-radical scavengers that help neutralize free radicals before they can attach themselves to cell membranes, eventually destroying the cell. They are added to cosmetic formulas to prevent oxidation.

enough antioxidant. An oxidized cosmetic product that has discoloration and/or odor due to oxidation is said to be **rancid**. Commonly used antioxidants are as follows:

Butylated hydroxyanisole (BHA)
Butylated hydroxytoluene (BHT)
Tocopherol (Vitamin E)
Benzoic acid

Antioxidants can also be used as skin protectants. This will be discussed in Chapter 10, Active Agents and Performance Ingredients.

## CHELATING AGENTS

A **chelating agent** is a chemical that is added to cosmetics to improve the efficiency of the preservative. Chelating agents work by breaking down the cell walls of bacteria and other microorganisms so that the preservative is more easily absorbed by the microorganism.

Common chelating ingredients are disodium EDTA, trisodium EDTA, and tetrasodium EDTA. EDTA stands for the chemical name *ethylenediaminetetraacetic acid*. Again, you will see these ingredients further down on the ingredient list because they are not used in large quantities.

## BUFFERING AGENTS

**Buffering** refers to adjusting the pH of a product to make it more acceptable to the skin. Sometimes, when products are made, the pH of the end product may be too high or too low. These pH levels may be irritating to the skin if they are not adjusted.

To remedy this problem the chemist will add a small amount of an acidic or basic chemical to bring the pH up or lower it appropriately. Citric acid is commonly used to lower the pH of a product. Tartaric acid is another acidic agent used in small quantities to bring the pH down to an acceptable acid level.

Some products have the opposite problem. The product turns out to be too acid for the skin. Ammonium carbonate, calcium carbonate, potassium, sodium, or ammonium hydroxide is sometimes added to a product to raise the pH. These buffering agents are added in very small quantities and again will be seen lower on the ingredient label, indicating their small concentration in the product.

## GELLANTS AND THICKENING AGENTS

A **gellant** is an agent that is added to a product to give it a gel-like consistency. It improves the appearance of the product and gives it more body, making it stiffer and less runny. Thickening agents make the product thicker so that it spreads more easily, is easier to handle, and is more acceptable to the eye.

Examples of thickening and gellant agents are methyl cellulose, xanthum gum, beeswax, and carbomer. Many thickening agents can also be used as emulsifiers.

## COLORING AGENTS

Colors are added to products to make them more appealing to consumers. There is no other legitimate reason to use color agents in skin-care products.

In makeup, of course, color agents are extensively used. Color agents appear on the ingredient label as a variety of different names. There are two types of regulated colors, certified and noncertified.

**Rancid** means discoloration and/or odor due to oxidation.

**Chelating agent** is a chemical that is added to cosmetics to improve the efficiency of the preservative.

**Buffering** refers to adjusting the pH of a product to make it more acceptable to the skin.

**Gellant** is an agent that is added to a product to give it a gel-like consistency.

**Lakes** are certified colors and are regulated by the Food and Drug Administration.

Certified colors are pigments, also called **lakes**, that are certified and regulated by the Food and Drug Administration (FDA). They are named by listing the color name, the number assigned to that color agent by the FDA, and the metal associated with the chemical structure. An example would be *D & C* (stands for Drug and Cosmetic) *Red No. 4 Aluminum Lake*. On food packages, you may see listed on the ingredient label *F, D, & C Yellow*, for example. Some colors are approved for use in drugs, cosmetics, and foods. However, in general, you will rarely see *F, D, & C* listed on a cosmetic ingredient label.

The colors certified by the FDA are blue, green, orange, red, and yellow. Noncertified colors are not metal salts. Most of these are natural plant or animal extracts, mineral pigments, and sometimes synthetic colors. Although these colors are regulated by the FDA, they do not have a specific certification number. They include a variety of common cosmetic color agents, including iron oxide, zinc oxide, carmine, beta-carotene, chlorophyllin-copper complex, annatto, ferric ferrocyanide, mica, the ultramarine colors, henna, and others.

Iron oxides are used extensively in the development of foundations. Iron oxide is frequently used to give makeup its color. There are various shades of iron oxide, and, of course, they can vary with the amount used in a particular solution. Iron oxide is actually rust, but it is used in scientific formulations in makeup production.

Color agents are used extensively in the formation of foundations, mascara, eyeshadows, eye pencils, lip pencils, powders, blush, lipstick, and contour and camouflage products. Certified colors are not permitted by the FDA to be used in any cosmetics intended for the eye area. Chemists must use noncertified colors in eyeshadow, eyeliner, and other cosmetics intended for the eye area.

When the FDA first began regulating colors, there were about 116 certified colors. Over the years the FDA has determined that many of these colors are not safe for continual use, and therefore the list has dwindled to about 35 certified color agents. Some individuals are allergic to certain of the color agents. You must be careful to notice if a client tells you she is allergic to a particular color. You must check the ingredient labels of any products you wish to use on her or sell her for that particular color agent.

As discussed previously, there is no reason other than esthetics to put color agents in skin-care products. The one exception to this rule would be a moisturizing bronzer, designed to moisturize or protect and still give a slight hint of color to the skin's surface.

Many cosmetic companies now totally eliminate color from their skin-care products, because the public is becoming more aware of the lack of need for these chemicals in skin-care formulations. Also, because color agents can occasionally cause allergic reactions, eliminating the coloring agents from skin-care products cuts down on the likelihood of allergic reaction to the product.

If you use imported cosmetics, you must check to see if the import company has complied with FDA rules concerning color. Some countries do not have strong laws governing the use of color agents and therefore may use color agents that are not permitted in cosmetics in the United States. The European Economic Community, EEC, also known as the EU, European Union, Germany, and Japan all have regulations regarding color, but even they may differ significantly from those of the United States.

## HIGH-TECH VEHICLES

As we learn more about the skin's anatomy and physiology, the intercellular cement, and penetration of the skin, we learn more about formulating products that are more easily accepted by the skin and that penetrate the skin's surface better.

We know, for example, that the intercellular cement is made of various lipids. Making products and using vehicles that are compatible with the intercellular lipids can increase the product's permeability and efficacy. Lipid-based products are good examples. Of course, not every product should easily penetrate the skin. There are many examples of ingredients that would be irritating if they penetrated deeper, and there are many that are too large in molecular size to penetrate, regardless of what type of vehicle is used.

## MICELLES

If you overemulsify an ingredient, the result is called a **micelle**. When you add emulsifier to a solution of water and oil, the emulsifier surrounds the internal phase of the solution. As the emulsifier lines up around the oil, as an example, there are small spaces between emulsifier molecules (Figure 9-2).

In a micelle, the emulsifier completely surrounds the oil, creating a sort of bubble. The bubble encloses the oil, or whatever internal phase ingredient is being emulsified. A cosmetic that has micelles present in it is said to be micellized.

## LIPOSOMES AND MICROENCAPSULATION

**Microencapsulation** is the process of using barrier and intercellular-compatible materials like lipids to form special microshells to protect and better penetrate certain ingredients. Many ingredients that are unstable or highly reactive can be protected from becoming unstable and can be delivered in a more effective way through microencapsulation. A good example is tocopherol, or vitamin E. Vitamin E, if unprotected, will serve as an antioxidant for the product. But if tocopherol is microencapsulated, it will serve as an antioxidant for the skin's protection, instead of the product's protection! A good example of microencapsulation is the liposome.

**Liposomes** are hollow spheres made of phospholipids. You can think of a liposome as a balloon, made out of lipids that are compatible with the lipids making up the intercellular cement.

Liposomes may be used to transport other agents, which may include moisturizers, conditioning agents, or drugs. Drugs, of course, are not used in cosmetic formulations.

The liposome may be **loaded**, which means that the liposome may be implanted with an ingredient. This ingredient, theoretically, will penetrate the skin. Eventually, the liposome will begin to dissolve, releasing the ingredient into the intercellular cement, to carry out whatever function it is meant to complete (Figure 9-3).

What you can put into a liposome depends on many factors. These include the size of the liposome, the size of the ingredient to be carried by the liposome, the shape of the liposome, the ionization of any components, and the purpose of the product. Many ingredients are simply too big to put inside a liposome.

Empty liposomes, or unloaded liposomes, are sometimes used in cosmetics to improve the penetration of a cream or moisturizer. Liposomes are not listed as such on

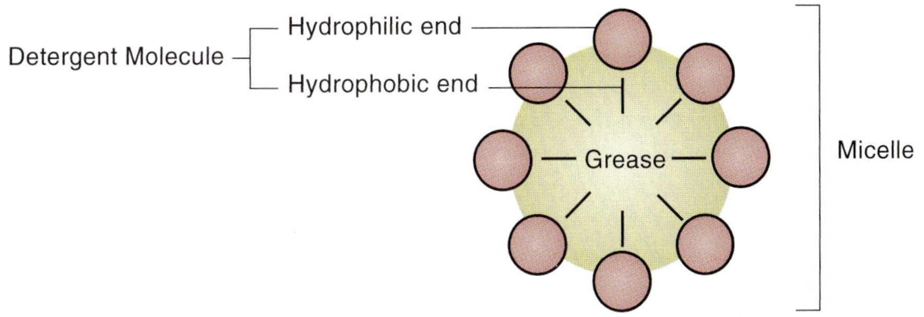

**Micelle** is an overemulsified ingredient.

**Microencapsulation** is the process of using barrier and intercellular-compatible materials like lipids to form special microshells to protect and better penetrate certain ingredients.

**Liposomes** are hollow spheres made of phospholipids that are used to transport other agents.

**Loaded** is the term to describe a microencapsulation unit, such as a liposome, that contains a performance ingredient, such as an antioxidant.

**Figure 9-2** Detergent micelle

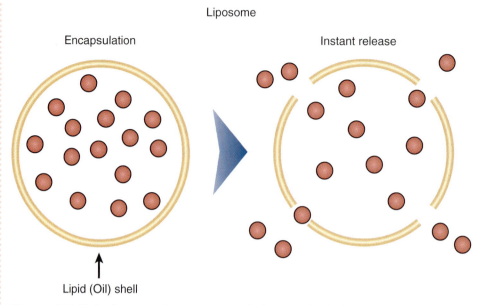

**Figure 9-3** This diagram shows encapsulation methods in the liposome and the nanosphere or microsponge (Courtesy Thibiant International/Guinot-Paris)

ingredient labels—ingredients of the liposome are listed. These may include soya lecithin, lecithin, phospholipids, ceramides, or others.

The theories behind liposome functions are still being confirmed. Although chemists have a good idea of how liposomes work, more is being learned all the time about their value in cosmetics.

## OTHER INNOVATIVE VEHICLES

Other new vehicles similar to liposomes are currently being investigated. One type involves a "microsponge" that releases an active ingredient once inside the skin. Another is the nanosphere.

Such innovations may be used for drugs before they are developed for cosmetics. As we learn more about the functions of the epidermis and the ways chemicals react with the surface of the skin, we will learn more about transport mechanisms for various cosmetic as well as pharmaceutical ingredients.

## TOPICS FOR DISCUSSION

1. What is a vehicle?
2. Discuss the difference between a surfactant, a detergent, and an emulsifier.
3. What is a suspension? List some examples.
4. How are fatty esters formed? Why are they often used in cosmetic formulas?
5. Why are preservatives necessary in cosmetics? Name some frequently used cosmetic preservatives.
6. Why are "natural" products more likely to need more effective preservatives?
7. Discuss microencapsulation. Why is it important for some ingredients?

# CHAPTER 10

# Performance Ingredients and Active Ingredients

## OBJECTIVES. . .

It is very important to understand the difference between an active ingredient used in a drug and a performance ingredient used in a skin-care product or cosmetic. The U.S. Food and Drug Administration (FDA) defines a **drug** as "articles (other than food) intended to affect the structure or any function of the body." **Cosmetics** are defined as "articles intended to be rubbed, poured, sprinkled, or otherwise applied to the human body or any part thereof for cleansing, beautifying, promoting physical attractiveness or altering the appearance."

Ingredients within a skin-care product or cosmetic that actually cause changes to the appearance of the skin are known as **performance ingredients** or **active agents**. They are intended to affect the *appearance* of the skin. **Active ingredients** are chemicals or substances within a drug that is intended to cause *physiological changes*, meaning they are intended to affect a structure or biochemical function of the body, including the skin.

Performance ingredients are, by far, the most important ingredients in cosmetic chemistry. In this chapter, we will discuss many different performance ingredients used in cleansers, moisturizers, and treatment products for various skin types and conditions, as well as active ingredients used in over-the-counter (OTC) drugs like sunscreens and acne products.

**Drugs** are articles that are intended to affect the structure or any function of the body.

**Cosmetics** are articles intended to be applied to the human body to alter the appearance or promote attractiveness.

**Performance** agents or **ingredients** are ingredients within a skin-care product or cosmetic that actually cause changes to the appearance of the skin.

**Active agents** is another term for performance agents.

**Active ingredient** is the chemical within a drug that causes physiological changes.

**Cosmeceuticals** are products that are not drugs intended to treat disease, but they still benefit the skin in a positive way.

**Detergents** are cleansing ingredients that help break up and remove fatty residues and other impurities from the skin.

**Defatting agents** remove fats and lipids, along with dirt, makeup, and debris, from the surface of the skin.

Every skin-care product or cosmetic has at least one performance ingredient. Performance ingredients may also be functional ingredients, or vehicles. For example, an emollient that helps to spread a moisturizing cream can also serve as a barrier to keep moisture from leaving the stratum corneum. The emollient is both a functional and a performance ingredient.

## "COSMECEUTICAL" INGREDIENTS

In the past two decades, many new ingredient and technology discoveries have been made to significantly help the appearance of aging skin. Scientists understand both the aging process and the function and structure of the skin much better than ever before. We understand that although the epidermis is technically dead, it is biochemically active, which means that there are many biochemical reactions that take place in the epidermis. We also know now that there are many topical ingredients that definitely affect the appearance of the skin and the biochemical reactions that occur in the epidermis and the dermis.

Again, although we know that there are definite changes in these reactions and understand that these changes are definitely responsible for the appearance changes we see when we use certain skin-care products, we cannot tout these physiological reactions because of the legal definitions of "drugs" and "cosmetics."

**Cosmeceuticals** refer to products that are not drugs intended to treat diseases, but purportedly benefit the skin in a positive way, help to restore normal skin behavior, and enhance the health of the skin. Although not officially recognized by the FDA, this category of ingredients refers to ingredients that promote skin health and have positive effects on the appearance of the skin.

Many scientists believe that, eventually, this category of ingredients may be officially recognized by the scientific community. When and if this happens, FDA definitions will have to be re-written. In the meantime, cosmetic companies and estheticians must adhere to the laws and rules as they are currently written, discussing only the appearance effects of these ingredients.

That being said, in this chapter we will discuss what we know about the biochemical effects of certain ingredients and why they likely affect the appearance of the skin.

## CLEANSING AGENTS

Performance ingredients in cleansers may be of two types: detergents or emulsion cleansing agents. **Detergents** cause cleansers to foam, as we discuss in the functional ingredients chapter. A performance ingredient detergent is present in any foaming cleanser, rinseable cleanser, or shampoo. They are essentially **defatting agents**, which means they remove fats and lipids, along with dirt, makeup, and debris, from the surface of the skin.

Commonly used detergent ingredients used in cleansers are the following:

- Sodium lauryl sulfate
- Sodium laureth sulfate
- Ammonium lauryl sulfate
- Disodium lauryl sulfosuccinate
- Decyl polyglucoside

◆ Lauramphocarboxylglycinate

◆ Cocamidopropyl betaine

Detergents work by loosening sebum and debris from the skin surface. Individual detergents can be stronger than others. Strength of a cleanser is also related to the amount of detergent ingredients in the cleanser and how long the cleanser is left on the skin.

**Soap** also defats the skin's surface. Soaps are usually made of salts of fatty acids. There are two basic disadvantages to soap. First, many soaps have a high pH, which can irritate and dry the skin, impair the barrier function by removing too much sebum, and begin removing intercellular lipids from the corneum. Second, many soaps, because of their fatty content, leave a residue or film on the skin that is created by insoluble salts, which are formed when the soap is used.

Both fatty acid salts in soap and detergents in foaming cleansers can strip too much sebum if the soap or detergent is too strong for a certain skin type, such as dry or sensitive skin. When this happens, the skin can become dry, flaky, tight, and irritated. The cleanser can "eat" into the lipids within the intercellular cement, "the mortar," damaging the barrier function, making the skin susceptible to dehydration and irritation. Continued use of the soap or cleanser may further damage the barrier function and further dry and irritate the skin.

Because of this overdrying factor, fats and oils are often added to cleansers and soaps to prevent too much of the irritating cleansing agent from coming in contact with the skin for too long a period of time. You can think of these fats and oils as "buffer zones" set up to keep the product from stripping too much oil from a fragile, dry, or sensitive skin. When cleansers have fat added to buffer their contact with the skin, they are called **superfatted** soaps or cleansers. Of course, the fats that are added to these products can also leave a film on the skin. This can be a problem for oily skin types because the fats may cause comedone development. In dry skin, the fats may actually help retain moisture. Fats used in true bar-type soaps include the following:

Sodium tallowate
Sodium oleate
Sodium cocoate
Sodium stearate

You will notice that fatty additives in soap almost always start with the word *sodium* and end in a fatty ester of one of many fatty acids listed in the functional ingredients chapter: stearic, myristic, oleic, and so on. Sometimes potassium is used instead of sodium.

**Emulsion cleansers** are what most estheticians think of as cleansing milks. They are often used for removing makeup and are often recommended for sensitive skin because of their gentleness. Most do not have detergents, but detergents can be used in these products to help the product foam slightly, to make the product more rinseable and easier to remove, or to keep the product emulsified. Cleansing milks are made mostly of water, with an oil or fat mixed in the emulsion; therefore, they are an oil-in-water emulsion. The oil or fat is the active agent used to create a slippery surface for removal of makeup or other debris from the skin's surface. The advantage to these cleansing milks is that they are less drying and irritating to the skin and perform an efficient job of removing makeup. The disadvantage is that they generally leave a residue on the skin. This residue is usually an emollient, the same one often used as the active cleansing agent, helping to loosen the debris from the skin's surface.

The emollient film left on the skin can be good or bad. For drier skins that do not make enough oil, it can actually help condition the surface. For oily skins or acne-prone skins, it can be a problem because it leaves a residue of fat to further clog the problem skin.

**Soap** is made of salts of fatty acids. It defats the skin's surface.

**Superfatted** cleansing agents have had fat added.

**Emulsion cleansers**, better known as cleansing milks, are non-foaming cream-type cleansers.

Another type of emulsion cleanser is cold cream. Cold cream is often made primarily of mineral oil, making it a water-in-oil emulsion. It is certainly a more oily emulsion cleanser, although very effective for heavy makeup. It often leaves a significant amount of oil on the skin after use. Clients often complain about the greasy feeling after using a cold cream cleanser. These types of cleansers are slowly losing popularity. Emulsion cleansers should always be followed by using a toner.

## PERFORMANCE AGENTS IN TONERS

The main function of toners is to lower the pH of the skin after cleansing. Second, toners help remove any excess cleanser or residue left on the skin after cleansing. Performance agents in toners vary greatly, depending on the skin type.

### pH Adjusters

Most toners have a lower pH, usually around 4.0 to 5.5. This low pH helps to restore the normal pH of the skin's acid mantle after cleansing, which is normally around 5.5 to 6.2. Citric acid or lemon extract is sometimes added to toners to help lower the pH of the product.

### Toners for Oily Skin

**Astringents** have a tightening effect on the skin or pore appearance.

**Witch hazel**, or **hamamelis extract**, can be a soothing agent or, in higher concentrations, is an astringent.

**Potassium alum** is a strong astringent.

**Lemon extract**, or **citrus extracts**, have astringent effects.

**Isopropyl alcohol** is a fairly strong drying alcohol, used as a cleansing and drying agent to remove excess oil from very oily skin. Isopropyl alcohol can dehydrate and irritate if overused or used on skin that is not excessively oily.

**SD alcohol** is specially denatured ethyl alcohol, also known as **ethanol**.

**Astringents** are functional agents, but sometimes are active ingredients if used in a drug formulation, that have a tightening effect on the skin or pore appearance. Astringent ingredients include **witch hazel** or **hamamelis extract**, **potassium alum**, **lemon extract**, and other **citrus extracts**. Astringents actually work by causing a slight swelling around the pore openings, helping to tighten the skin and minimize the appearance of the pore opening. Toner products for oily skin are sometimes referred to as astringents, although to call a product an astringent is technically a drug term.

For oilier skins, alcohol is often used as a performance agent. **Isopropyl** and **SD alcohols** are drying alcohols, unlike cetyl alcohol, which is a fatty alcohol used in creams. SD alcohol is **"specially denatured" ethyl alcohol**, also known as **ethanol**. Denaturing means the alcohol is not suitable for drinking. Bittering agents are added to the ethanol to make it taste terrible to ensure safety, so that infants who might try to ingest the product will leave it alone. SD alcohol is listed on the ingredient label followed by a number. This number indicates the technique used to denature the alcohol.

SD alcohol and isopropyl alcohol are strong cleansing agents or defatting agents that help remove excess quantities of sebum from oily skin or oily areas. In larger quantities, they are antiseptics, helping to kill surface microorganisms. This, of course, is a drug claim. Isopropyl alcohol is an even stronger drying alcohol. The drying effect of these alcohols on the skin can also have an astringent effect on the oily skin and pore appearance.

## A WORD ABOUT ALCOHOL

Alcohol has an undeserved terrible reputation in the cosmetics industry. Many companies tout that their products are "alcohol-free," referring to the drying effect of certain alcohols on the skin.

Although large amounts of SD or isopropyl alcohol can be irritating or overdrying to dry or sensitive skin, they are useful in helping to control oiliness in very oily and some acne-prone skin. Do not reject a product simply because it has some SD or isopropyl alcohol. Make your decision based on the skin type you are treating. For more information on alcohol, see the chapter on functional ingredients.

# PERFORMANCE INGREDIENTS FOR DEHYDRATED SKIN

## Toners for Dry Skin

Toners for dry skin often contain humectants that help restore moisture to the dehydrated skin after cleansing. A **humectant** is an ingredient that attracts water. Toner humectants may include **butylene glycol**, **propylene glycol**, and **sorbitol**. These humectant ingredients are also known for their softening effect on the skin. More on humectants will be discussed later in this chapter. Dry skin toners also have an acidic pH.

Various other performance ingredients may be added to toners. For example, **azulene**, **chamomile**, or **bisabolol** might be added for their soothing effect in a toner for dry, sensitive skin. **Salicylic acid** might be added to an oily skin toner for its keratolytic or peeling effect on the oily, hyperkeratinized skin.

When skin is dehydrated, it is suffering from lack of water in the surface. Skin becomes dehydrated from too much sun, weather exposure, harsh cleansers, and aging. Humectants are water-binding agents. They have a strong attraction to water. Many chemically bind water to them, holding many water molecules.

We have already discussed the barrier function of the skin. Impaired barrier function can result not only in flaking and esthetic problems but also in increased skin sensitivity. Natural humectants, lipids, or hydrating agents found within the intercellular cement are known as **natural moisturizing factors** or **NMFs**. The NMFs in the skin help to preserve water or hydration within the epidermis, keeping the barrier function intact and keeping the skin soft and supple. Impaired barrier function can mean a lack of NMFs from missing lipids or other components and can cause dehydration, which is sometimes severe. It can also cause a wrinkly, unfirm appearance to the skin surface.

NMFs include **sodium PCA**, **sphingolipids** and **glycosphingolipids** (also known as **ceramides**), **phospholipids**, **fatty acids**, **glycerol**, **squalane**, and **cholesterol**. These intercellular components are produced during the cell renewal process as cells migrate from the basal layer to the stratum corneum. As we age, our cell renewal slows down and, therefore, we produce fewer NMFs. This reduces the ability of the skin to hold hydration, making the skin dry, tight, flaky, and dull-looking.

In recent years, scientists have been able to isolate and prepare special ingredients that help to "repair" or "patch" the moisture barrier. These ingredients can now be used in products for dry, dehydrated, aging, and sun-damaged skin.

**Lipid replacement** is accomplished by applying a group of lipid ingredients to the skin. These include ceramides or sphingolipids, phospholipids, cholesterol, and fatty acids. These lipid ingredients can actually be derived from plant or animal sources, although most are derived from plant materials such as **soy sterols** or **soy lecithin**. **Linoleic acid** can be derived from numerous plant sources, including **evening primrose oil**, **sunflower oil**, or **borage oil**. These lipid components are naturally in the intercellular material at a ratio of 4:1:1:1. In other words, it is four parts ceramides to one part of each of the other components. This complex of performance lipid ingredients literally patches the impaired barrier. Its function is to hold water within the intercellular matrix.

However, lipids alone are not as effective without the use of humectants or **hydrophilic ingredients**. Hydrophilic literally means water-loving. These ingredients work like "water magnets," attracting water while the lipids hold the water within the intercellular spaces between the cells. This combination of lipid complexes with hydrators is excellent for helping restore essential moisture to dry, dehydrated, and sensitive skin.

Sodium PCA is an excellent hydrator. It has a strong ability to attract water and is readily accepted by the skin. Sodium PCA is used frequently in night creams,

**Humectant** is an ingredient that attracts water.

**Butylene glycol** is a humectant often used in dry- or sensitive-skin moisturizers.

**Propylene glycol** is a humectant that penetrates the skin fairly easily, making it a good hydrating agent.

**Sorbitol** is a humectant.

**Azulene** is a hydrocarbon that is derived from the chamomile flower.

**Chamomile** is a soothing agent.

**Bisabolol** is an agent that is added to cosmetics designed for sensitive skin.

**Salicylic acid** is an antibacterial and keratolytic agent.

**Natural moisturizing factors (NMFs)** are hydrating agents found within the cells and within the intercellular cement.

**Sodium PCA** is a natural moisturizing factor ingredient.

**Sphingolipids** are lipid materials that are a natural part of the intercellular cement.

**Glycosphingolipids** are lipid materials that are a natural part of the intercellular cement.

**Ceramides** are lipid materials that are a natural part of the intercellular cement.

**Phospholipids** are naturally moisturizing humectants found within the skin.

**Fatty acids** are derived from plant or animal sources.

**Glycerol** is a humectant that is a natural part of the intercellular cement.

**Squalane** is a lipid material that is a natural part of the intercellular cement.

**Cholesterol** is a lipid material that is a natural part of the intercellular cement.

**Lipid replacement** involves using topical lipids to repair the barrier function.

**Soy sterols** are natural sources of lipid materials.

**Soy lecithin** is used as a moisture-binding material, also used for many liposomes.

**Linoleic acid** is a fatty acid that is a natural part of the intercellular cement.

**Evening primrose oil** is an excellent source of fatty acids, including linoleic acid.

**Sunflower oil** is an excellent source of fatty acids, including linoleic acid.

**Borage oil** is an excellent source of fatty acids, including linoleic acid.

**Hydrophilic ingredients**, or "water-loving" ingredients, attract and bind water.

**Glycerin** is a humectant and is a very strong water binder.

**Hyaluronic acid** or **sodium hyaluronate** is a hydrophilic agent with excellent water-binding properties.

**Mucopolysaccharides** are carbohydrate-lipid complexes that are also good water binders.

**Collagen** is a large, long-chain molecular protein that lies on the top of the skin and binds water, also helps to prevent water loss.

**Elastin** is a large, long-chain molecular protein that lies on the top of the skin and bind water, also helps to prevent water loss.

**Substantives** are ingredients that attach themselves well to the surface of the skin, sort of spreading out across the skin, to protect and hydrate the surface.

**Occlusives** are heavy, large molecules that sit on top of the skin and prevent moisture loss.

day creams, sunscreens, and other hydrating products. It can be used without lipids to hydrate oilier or combination skin. It is lightweight on the skin and does not cause clogged pores.

**Glycerin** is a humectant that has been used for many years. It is a very strong water binder. It is, in fact, so strong that it should not be used by itself. Glycerin can actually make the skin more dry over a period of time because it doesn't just pull water from cosmetics and the atmosphere when applied to the skin. In large amounts, it can pull water from the lower levels of the epidermis, causing transepidermal water loss (TEWL), which results in drier skin. Used in a moderate amount in a good hydrating cream, it is an excellent hydrating agent.

Propylene glycol is another widely used humectant. It penetrates the skin fairly easily, making it a good hydrating agent. However, because propylene glycol can increase permeability of the skin, it can cause problems for sensitive or dry skin with impaired barrier function. Butylene glycol is now being used more frequently in products for dehydrated or sensitive skin. It has less potential for sensitive skin irritation than its chemical cousin, propylene glycol. Sorbitol is another excellent hydrating agent that is frequently used in hydrating lotions.

Alphahydroxy acids, besides being surface exfoliants, are also hydrators. Lactic acid is actually used in prescription-strength moisturizers. Glycolic acid is also a hydrating agent.

## OTHER HUMECTANTS

Other water binders work very differently than the standard hydrophylic agents.

**Hyaluronic acid**, also known as **sodium hyaluronate**, is one of these agents. Hyaluronic acid can hold up to 400 times its own weight in water. The molecule is quite large. It cannot penetrate the skin to any degree. However, because of its excellent water-binding properties, it is a frequently used hydrating performance ingredient. Hyaluronic acid is an expensive hydrator. Creams and lotions containing hyaluronic acid may be more expensive than others.

**Mucopolysaccharides** are carbohydrate–lipid complexes that are also good water binders. Considered a "mother–molecule" to hyaluronic acid, it is capable of holding large amounts of water, and is an excellent hydrator. Again, it is too large to penetrate the skin.

**Collagen** and **elastin** are large, long-chain molecular proteins that lie on top of the skin and bind water, also helping to prevent water loss. Collagen and elastin have been used in creams for many years. They are too big to ever penetrate the skin, but they do a good job hydrating. Because they lie on top of the skin, they also help to "fill in" small lines and wrinkles, making skin look smoother.

All of these ingredients are known as **substantives**, which are ingredients that attach themselves well to the surface of the skin, sort of spreading out across the skin, to protect and hydrate the surface.

Some of the more recent discoveries in humectants include algae and seaweed extracts. These are quite remarkable hydrators. They are substantive, forming a surface gel. Some forms of algae are now being used as hydrating base materials for sensitive skin products without using traditional emulsifiers that can decrease the barrier function in sensitive skin with loss of lipid barrier.

## OCCLUSIVES

An **occlusive** is a heavy, large molecule that sits on top of the skin and prevents moisture loss. Occlusives are exactly what they sound like, forming a barrier on top of the skin to shield the skin from transepidermal moisture loss from the inside out, much like the barrier function, except on top instead of within the skin.

A good example of an occlusive is **petrolatum**, or **petroleum jelly**. Petrolatum can be used by itself or incorporated into a cream or lotion. The amount of occlusion created by the petrolatum depends on the amount used in the cream formulation.

The advantages of using petrolatum in formulations are many. It is extremely hypoallergenic, rarely causing a problem with allergies or irritations. Hence, it is often used in formulas, both drug and cosmetic, for sensitive or irritated skin.

Petrolatum provides an excellent occlusive barrier both to keep water in the skin and to keep allergens, antigens, and foreign bodies out of the skin. A good example of this is the application of petroleum jelly or mineral oil to a baby's bottom to avoid skin contact with urine in the baby's diaper. Petrolatum is also very inexpensive.

There are some disadvantages to using petrolatum. First, it is extremely sticky, slippery, and greasy. Most clients do not like this greasy feeling. It is also hard to accomplish any task when your hands are too slippery to handle anything. It is extremely greasy on the face, creating esthetic problems as well. Second, it is disadvantageous to use petrolatum for oily and problem skin. Although petrolatum is not comedogenic in its pure state, it is very greasy and heavy. Besides the obvious esthetic problem for oily skin, the occlusive action of petrolatum also blocks the follicles from oil dispersement, as well as from transepidermal water loss. In other words, although it keeps the water in the skin, it does not allow sebum to leave the follicle, therefore causing a "back-up" of sebaceous secretions.

Many estheticians do not like petrolatum because it is not "natural." This is simply not true. Petrolatum comes from minerals in the earth. What could be more natural? In short, petrolatum is a useful product, but it should not be used in all cases of dehydration.

## EMOLLIENTS

As the skin ages, it tends not to produce as much of the essential lipids that make up the intercellular cement, or the skin produces less sebum, which helps provide a barrier on the surface of the skin to prevent dehydration. This is when emollient ingredients are used in cosmetic systems. **Emollients** are somewhat like occlusives in that they mostly lie on the surface of the skin and prevent water loss. Emollients help to smooth the surface of wrinkled skin, filling in the cracks of dry and dehydrated skin.

Emollients are often used not only for dehydrated or water-dry skin but also for oil-dry or alipidic skin. Emollients have a second use as spreading agents, previously discussed in the chapter on functional ingredients.

**Alipidic** literally means "lack of lipids." These types of skin do not produce enough lipids. This could be true of both the intercellular lipids and the sebum produced by the sebaceous gland.

Emollients help to supplement skin that suffers from this lack of lipid production. They serve as a substitute, helping to keep the surface lubricated and protected.

These emollients are of several categories. Fatty acids have already been discussed in the chapter on functional ingredients. They are emollients. Fatty alcohols and fatty esters are also emollients. We have already discussed new types of emollients that are, again, actually a synthetic version of intercellular cement lipids. These include cholesterol, ceramides, lecithin (also a humectant), squalane, and glycosphingolipids.

Lanolin is another good emollient. Lanolin has had much bad press in the past. It was thought to cause many allergies. Although this is a problem for some people, it has recently been theorized that most of the old-fashioned lanolin formula creams were also often full of perfumes and fragrances, thought to be a major source of these allergies. Purification processes for lanolin have also improved substantially over the decades, making today's lanolin a useful and relatively harmless active agent.

Mineral oil is another emollient. Like petrolatum, it is a petroleum derivative. It has many of the same advantages and disadvantages as petrolatum. It is hypoallergenic

**Petrolatum** prevents urine and soggy diapers from irritating the baby's sensitive skin.

**Petroleum jelly** is an excellent occlusive, preventing moisture loss from the skin.

**Emollients** are somewhat like occlusives in that they mostly lie on the surface of the skin and prevent water loss. They also help to "fill in the cracks" of dry, dehydrated skin.

**Alipidic** means "lack of lipids." These skin types do not produce enough lipids.

and a good emollient, helping to soothe irritated, dry, scaly skin. But it is also greasy, particularly in its pure state. However, when formulated properly into a cream, it can be an excellent active agent emollient for dry, dehydrated skin, especially when mixed with good humectant active agents.

Silicones are often used now instead of traditional fatty-type emollients. Silicones include **cyclomethicone**, **dimethicone**, and **phenyl trimethicone**, often used in combination. Often referred to as "breathable barriers," these lightweight and unique ingredients help block water to prevent it from escaping from the surface of the skin, while keeping the skin feeling light and comfortable. Another advantage is that silicones are **biologically inert**, which means they are chemicals that are unlikely to cause reactions with the skin, making them ideal for sensitive skin formulations also. The silicones are noncomedogenic and do not irritate the pores; thus, they are ideal for oily and acne-prone formulations. They can be used in creams, lotions, cleansing milks, and foundations and are often used in concentrated lipid serums for dry and sensitive skin with impaired barrier function.

## PRODUCTS FOR DRY SKIN

Most products designed for dry skin contain a combination of humectants and emollients to help boost moisture levels and improve the skin's ability to hold the moisture. Dry skin products often contain lipid replacement ingredients to improve barrier function. Normally these products are water-based, or oil-in-water emulsions, although some may be water-in-oil emulsions designed for more severely alipidic skin.

These moisturizing products vary greatly in the amount of emollients and humectants they contain. The more oil-dry (alipidic) the skin is, the more emollient should be used.

Treatments with larger amounts of humectants and less emollients are designed for oilier and combination skin. Hydration fluids that are designed for younger or oilier skin types may contain just enough emollient to serve as a vehicle to spread the product on the skin. Because some emollients often can clog oily skin or worsen acne-prone skin, special emollient ingredients have been designed to be used in hydrating fluids for oilier skin. These special emollient complexes do not clog the follicles. For more information on these chemicals, see the chapter on comedogenicity.

## INGREDIENTS FOR AGING SKIN

The amount of information that has been discovered in the past two decades about the aging process is amazing. We are constantly discovering new ingredients and treatments that make skin look and behave like younger skin. These treatments include drug and cosmetic products and high-tech machine technology such as lasers, LED light treatments, and microcurrent technology.

### Alphahydroxy Acids

In the history of cosmetics, no other ingredient or family of ingredients has had the impact or efficacy of alphahydroxy acids. **Alphahydroxy acids (AHAs)** are a family of naturally occurring mild acids. Most AHAs are present in fruits and vegetables, but some actually occur in human cells. Most AHAs used in cosmetics have been laboratory purified or are the side product of other industrial chemical processes, such as the making of film.

AHAs have a large number of applications in skin care and can help many conditions, including oily and acne-prone skin, sun damage, dryness, and hyperpigmentation. There are several AHAs used in skin-care treatment. These include **lactic acid**; **tartaric acid**; **malic acid**; and by far the best-known AHA, **glycolic acid**.

**Silicones** help protect skin from epidermal water loss, and improve feel and spreadability of product.

**Cyclomethicone** is a type of silicone used primarily as a vehicle or emollient.

**Dimethicone** is a lightweight silicone emollient.

**Phenyl trimethicone** is a silicone emollient.

**Biologically inert** chemicals are chemicals that are unlikely to cause reactions with the skin, making them ideal for sensitive formulations.

**Alphahydroxy acids (AHAs)** are a family of naturally occurring mild acids.

**Lactic acid** is an alphahydroxy acid occurring naturally in milk, both an exfoliant and a hydrophilic.

**Tartaric acid** is an alphahydroxy acid occurring naturally in grapes and passionfruit.

**Salicylic acid** and **citric acid** are also often included when discussing hydroxy acids, but they are actually **betahydroxy acids (BHAs)**.

The chemical difference between alphahydroxy and betahydroxy acids is the location of the hydroxy group on the carbon chain of the acid. *Alpha* indicates that the group is on the first carbon atom, whereas *beta* means that the group is on the second carbon atom. Glycolic acid is the smallest, molecularly, of all the alphahydroxy acids. It has been widely researched, and, because of its size, penetrates between cells more readily than the other AHAs.

AHAs are theorized to work by loosening the bond between dead corneum cells, dissolving part of the surface intercellular cement that holds dead epidermal cells together. This makes it easy to remove dead cells from the skin surface, which has a positive effect on many conditions:

1. Removal of dead cell buildup helps to smooth the surface of dry, sun-damaged, or aging skin, improving roughness and making wrinkles appear much less deep. Results on an aging skin can become apparent in a very short period of time.

2. By removing dead surface cells, cell renewal is stimulated, bringing younger, fresher cells to the surface more quickly and increasing the production of intercellular lipids, improving barrier function and, therefore, improving hydration of the skin. Well-hydrated skin is smoother and firmer looking and is generally healthier, helping all activities of the skin proceed more efficaciously.

3. Removing dead cell buildup from the inside of follicles helps loosen clogged pores, comedones, and other impactions on an oily skin or oily area. Continued use helps keep dead cells from accumulating on the follicle wall, which prevents impactions that can lead to inflammatory acne lesions. This property of AHAs and BHAs make them good ingredients to use for acne-prone and oily skins.

4. Removal of dead cells can mean the removal of hyperpigmented cells, whereas helps to lighten discolored or splotchy skin. Used in combination with a melanin suppressant, such as hydroquinone, AHAs help remove stained cells, whereas hydroquinone helps suppress the activity of the melanocytes. A broad-spectrum sunscreen with an SPF of 15 or higher should always be used with AHA products, especially when treating hyperpigmentation.

5. AHAs can also be used on body skin, removing dead, dry cells and helping improve retention of moisture. This helps conditions such as dry, winter skin and helps dermatologists in treating medical conditions such as eczema and icthyosis. Alphahydroxy acids are also helpful in removing calluses on feet, elbows, and hands.

6. New information now indicates that routine use of alphahydroxy acids improves both barrier functions of the epidermis, and long-term studies indicate the improvement of collagen content in the dermis.

Alphahydroxy and betahydroxy acids can be used in many products, including cleansers and toners but are most effective when used in leave-on products such as treatment gels, serums, or moisturizing creams.

## Strengths and Effectiveness of AHAs

Alphahydroxy acids can vary extensively in their strengths. Products have been formulated with as little as 2 or 3 percent to as high as 20 percent in higher strength treatment preparations, which are generally available only through dermatologists and plastic surgeons. There has been a great deal of controversy over the irritation potential of various higher strengths. It is generally accepted by the esthetic industry that products contain 8 to 10 percent AHA in order to show results in helping the various conditions previously discussed, although even 5 percent can show gradual improvements to the skin conditions.

**Malic acid** is an alphahydroxy acid derived from apples.

**Glycolic acid** is the most frequently used alphahydroxy acid; it is an exfoliant and hydrophilic.

**Citric acid**, or betahydroxy acid, is most often used as a pH adjuster, but can also be used as a mild exfoliant.

**Salicylic acid** is a betahydroxy acid with exfoliating and antiseptic properties; natural sources include sweet birch, willow bark, and wintergreen.

**Betahydroxy acids (BHAs)** are a group of organic acids used in skin care products; includes salicylic acid.

The pH is also a very important factor in AHA efficacy. The lower the pH, the higher the strength of the acid and the more cells will be removed from the skin. Also, though, the lower the pH, the more potentially irritating the acid will be to the skin. AHA leave-on products of 8 percent or higher sting slightly when applied, indicating some irritancy, even though this is probably very small at this concentration.

The Cosmetic Ingredient Review (CIR) is a special panel of scientists and dermatologists who investigate cosmetic ingredient safety for the Cosmetic, Toiletries, and Fragrance Association, the largest cosmetic manufacturers association. The CIR shares its findings with the industry as well as with the Food and Drug Administration (FDA). Recently, the CIR conducted an extensive investigation of the safety of alphahydroxy acids and many derivatives of AHA. The CIR determined that home use products were generally safe, as long as they contained no more than 10 percent AHA, and had a pH no less than 3.5. Remember, the lower the pH, the stronger the acid!

Likewise, the CIR looked at salon use AHAs, and these higher strength AHAs will be discussed in Chapter 21, Chemical Peeling and Exfoliation Procedures.

## Vehicles and Other Ingredients with AHAs

The cosmetic spreading agent or vehicle for AHAs can also vary greatly. AHAs can be incorporated into leave-on gels (used frequently on oily, acne-prone, and combination skin types) and lotions or creams (which are more suitable for dry skin and body skin).

Other ingredients may also be combined with AHAs in different formulations. Hydrating ingredients or emollients may be included for dry skin, hydroquinone may be included for hyperpigmented skin, and salicylic acid may be included for acne-prone skin.

## Contraindications of Alphahydroxy Acids

AHAs should not be used on the following clients:

- ◆ Are using or have recently used Accutane®.
- ◆ Have recently had laser resurfacing, chemical peel, dermabrasion, or other peeling procedure.
- ◆ Are using tretinoin (Retin-A®, Renova®), tazarotene (Tazorac®), adapalene (Differin®), or other exfoliating prescription drugs.
- ◆ Are known to be allergic to AHA or BHA.
- ◆ Are sunburned or have visibly irritated skin.
- ◆ Have cuts; abrasions, including open acne lesions that have been scratched; or blisters.
- ◆ Are using other topical medications, unless approved by their physician.
- ◆ Are planning to deliberately expose their skin to the sun or sun beds.
- ◆ Have not had a thorough consultation and may be using products that are contraindicated.
- ◆ Are pregnant or nursing. AHA safety has not been determined for pregnant or nursing women.

In addition, AHAs should be used carefully with other peeling agents such as salicylic acid, benzoyl peroxide, sulfur, resorcinol, or products with large amounts of alcohol.

Combining peeling agents can increase irritation. Using AHA products on skin that has recently had a microdermabrasion treatment may also increase irritation potential. It is not generally advisable to combine mechanical and chemical exfoliation procedures. Be careful when using any stimulating product with AHAs, because this may increase irritation.

In general, it is best to supervise your client's entire home care program when using AHA products. This way you can determine exactly what they are using with the AHA product for best results and the least irritation.

Last, but certainly not least, the client *must* use a daily sunscreen with an SPF of at least 15 while using AHA products!

# MORE ANTI-AGING INGREDIENTS

## Sunscreens

Probably the single most important anti-aging ingredient group is sunscreens. Broad-spectrum SPF-15 or higher sunscreens that screen both ultraviolet A and B rays should be used daily on all skin types but especially on aging and sun-damaged skin. Best used by building these into day moisturizers, regular use of sunscreens will prevent sun damage, inflammation, and free radical reactions that can cause aging skin symptoms. Individual sunscreen ingredients will be discussed in the chapter on sun and sun damage.

## Antioxidants

We discuss free radicals in other chapters. Many scientists believe that free radicals, or reactive oxygen species, are responsible for not only the aging of the skin, but of the body. Free radicals cause much havoc in the skin. Free radicals occur in normal body cellular and physiological reactions. Free radicals are also caused by forms of inflammation such as sun exposure, smoking, pollution, and certain types of chemical exposure. Free radicals are essentially unstable oxygen atoms that rob electrons from the surface of skin cell membranes, creating another form of free radical called lipid peroxide and starting a domino effect of chemical reactions that lead to skin damage and even damage to DNA. The **inflammation cascade** is a series of biochemical reactions that lead to the production of self-destruct enzymes in the skin called **proteases**. **Collagenase, elastase,** and **hyaluronidase** are three of these self-destruct enzymes. As you might guess by their names, they cause destruction of collagen, elastin, and hyaluronic acid. Collagen and elastin are fibers responsible for elasticity, firmness, and smoothness of the skin, and hyaluronic acid in the lower dermis makes up the ground substance that gives the skin further cushion and support. Constant, cumulative free radical damage eventually results in the skin damage we think of as aging skin.

**Antioxidants** are free radical scavengers. Some neutralize free radicals before they attack cell membranes, beginning the inflammation cascade. Others squelch other forms of free radicals. Antioxidants work by supplying electrons to radical oxygen atoms, which need electrons to be stable. This prevents the need for the free radical to attack the cell membrane, avoiding the start of the inflammation cascade.

The routine use of topical antioxidants can help improve the visible signs of aging and help prevent the inflammation process that leads to cell and skin damage. Because there are numerous types of free radicals that form during the inflammation cascade, it is now theorized that different types of antioxidants should be combined to squelch the different types of free radicals at all levels of the reaction cascade. When different types of antioxidants are combined in a formulation, the formulation is said to be a **broad-spectrum antioxidant**.

Antioxidants are, by nature, very unstable substances. Because they are so reactive, they must be stabilized to remain effective in a skin-care product. Antioxidants have been used for many years to keep products fresh by neutralizing free radicals within the product. This helps prevents rancidity. However, the ingredient worked in the product, not on the skin! Only in the past few years have we learned how to stabilize antioxidants so they can be used as performance ingredients.

**Inflammation cascade** is a series of biochemical reactions that lead to production of self-destruct enzymes that damage the skin.

**Proteases** are enzymes that dissolve proteins.

**Collagenase** is an enzyme produced during inflammation that breaks down collagen in the skin.

**Elastase** is an enzyme produced during inflammation that breaks down elastin fibers in the skin.

**Hyalurodinase** is an enzyme produced during inflammation that breaks down hyaluronic acid in the skin.

**Antioxidants** are topical free radical scavengers that help neutralize free radicals before they can attach themselves to cell membranes, eventually destroying the cell. They are added to cosmetic formulas to prevent oxidation.

**Broad-spectrum antioxidant** is a formulation that contains several antioxidants that help to neutralize different types of free radicals.

The invention of liposomes and other forms of microencapsulation helped provide a way to keep these reactive substances stable until they could be used. Besides acting as protective "shells" to keep the antioxidants **bioavailable**, or able to be used as a performance ingredient in the skin, the lipid-based microencapsulation also improved penetration of the antioxidants.

**Bioavailable** means able to be easily used by the skin.

Common antioxidant ingredients include the following:

- **Superoxide dismutase** (an enzyme that helps prevent the start of the cascade)
- **Tocopherol** (vitamin E)
- **Tocopherol acetate** (another form of stabilized vitamin E)
- **Ascorbic acid** (vitamin C)
- **Magnesium ascorbyl phosphate** (vitamin C ester)
- **Grapeseed extract** (contains very strong antioxidants known as proanthocyanidins)
- **Green and white tea** (contain strong antioxidants called polyphenols)
- **Stearyl glycyrrhetinate** (an anti-inflammatory antioxidant derived from licorice)
- **Malachite extract**
- **Silymarin** (from milk thistle)
- **Elagic acid** (from pomegranate)
- **Hypericin** (from St. John's wort)
- **Lipoic acid**
- **Coenzyme Q-10** (naturally occurring antioxidant)
- **Idebenone** (a newly discovered powerful topical antioxidant)

## Lipid Replacement for Aging Skin

As with dry skin, lipid replacement ingredients are often used to repair and support the barrier function of aging or sun-damaged skin. These ingredients improve hydration, plumpness, and smoothness of the skin, helping make wrinkles look less apparent. Improvement of the barrier function also reduces sensitivity by making the skin more resistant to irritant penetration and therefore reducing the chances of inflammation that can lead to cascade reactions.

## Hydrating Aging Skin

Hydrators added to emollients and lipid replacement ingredients help to bind water to the skin, improving hydration. Sodium PCA, hyaluronic acid or sodium hyaluronate, seaweed or algae extracts, and glycerin are frequent hydrators used for aging skin.

## Peptides and Collagen Stimulants

**Peptides** are chains or amino acids used in skin-care products to produce different changes in the appearance.

**Palmitoyl pentapeptide-3** is a peptide also known as Matrixyl® that is used in cosmeceuticals to have a firming effect on the skin's appearance.

**Peptides** are chains of amino acids that can cause various responses when applied to aging skin. Peptides are a recent discovery for treatment of wrinkles and lack of elasticity.

**Palmitoyl pentapeptide-3** is the most commonly used peptide for aging skin. Also known as Matrixyl®, palmitoyl pentatpeptide-3 has been demonstrated to significantly increase collagen synthesis, improving the appearance of wrinkles and sagging of the aging skin. Palmitoyl pentapeptide-3 is basically a sequential piece of a collagen molecule. It is theorized to work by "tricking" the skin into "believing" that too much collagen has been broken down, curbing the production of collagenase, the enzyme that destroys collagen, and stimulating fibroblasts, the cells that produce collagen. The results of the use of palmitoyl pentapeptide-3 are remarkable, and the performance ingredient does not cause the irritation that can be caused by other anti-aging ingredients such as retinol.

**Acetyl-hexapeptide-3** is another peptide ingredient. Acetyl-hexapeptide-3 is used in "wrinkle-relaxing" creams. This ingredient is reported to prevent certain reactions in the skin that create skin folding as a result of facial expressions, softening pronounced wrinkles and expression lines.

Other peptides are being developed that help with dark circles under the eyes, eye puffiness, and eye wrinkling. These include **palmitoyl oligopeptide**, **dipeptide-2**, and **palmitoyl tetrapeptide-3**. Peptide technology is an area that is very promising, and new ingredients will surely be developed that have other appearance effects on the skin.

**Hydrocotyl (Centella asiatica)** and **coneflower (Echinacea purpurea) extracts** are a patented complex of botanical ingredients that has been demonstrated to stimulate collagen production. Often, peptides are combined with this complex in products to improve collagen content, soften wrinkles, and improve skin firmness.

## Retinol

**Retinol** is a natural form of vitamin A that seems to stimulate cell repair and regulate skin functions and is theorized to be necessary for skin cell generation. Retinol is incorporated into serums and moisturizers to stimulate collagen production. Retinol has some side effects in a significant number of people, sometimes producing redness and irritation.

## COMBINING ANTI-AGING INGREDIENTS

All of these anti-aging ingredients we have discussed definitely help the appearance of the sun-damaged and aging skin. However, the best results are achieved by combining products and performance agents. Choosing just one ingredient modality will not provide the benefit that you will see when you combine all the types of ingredients discussed here. Using a good sunscreen in a lipid-based hydrating vehicle, antioxidant/peptide collagen-stimulating serums, and AHA gels or creams provides a program approach to helping the appearance of aging or sun-damaged skin.

## PLANT EXTRACTS

Hundreds of plant extracts are used as performance ingredients in skin-care products. One-third of all prescription drugs are made from plants. Plant extracts are generally liquids that are pressed, boiled, or chemically extracted from different plants.

Most plant extracts are used for their **anecdotal** properties. Anecdotal means that the ingredient is reputed to have certain benefits for improving the appearance of the skin, but the benefits not been substantiated, or proved, by accepted scientific means. Many ingredients are studied individually for their effects on the skin, but that does not necessarily mean that it will work in a particular product, unless the finished product has also been studied.

Plant extracts are simply natural complexes of various chemicals. Many estheticians like plant extracts because they believe they are "natural." Nevertheless, they ARE chemicals! All life forms are made of chemicals. There can be literally hundreds of chemicals that make up a single plant extract.

Research is ongoing on some plant extracts to substantiate their effectiveness and understand which chemicals within the particular extract cause the appearance changes and other effects on the skin.

**Acetyl-hexapeptide-3** is a peptide used in "wrinkle-relaxing" products.

**Palmitoyl oligopeptide** is a peptide used to improve the appearance of elasticity.

**Dipeptide-2** is a peptide used to help reduce puffiness.

**Palmitoyl tetrapeptide-3** is a peptide that has both soothing effects and is also used to improve the appearance of elasticity.

**Hydrocotyl** (Centella asiatica) is part of a patented botanical complex that helps to improve the appearance of elasticity.

**Coneflower** (Echinacea purpurea) is part of a patented botanical complex that helps to improve the appearance of elasticity.

**Retinol** is a natural form of vitamin A, appears to regulate skin function, and is theorized to be necessary for skin cell generation.

**Anecdotal** means that an ingredient is supposed to provide certain benefits to the skin, but they have not yet been substantiated, or proved, by scientific means.

Plant extracts are normally used in relatively small quantities in skin-care products. Usually they are listed as extracts, but if they are in a solution of water or alcohol, which most of them are, they may be listed near the top of the ingredient label. This simply means that water is the main ingredient in the extracts and that the extracts have been prepared before the formula was actually combined.

# PERFORMANCE INGREDIENTS FOR SENSITIVE SKIN

Treating redness and sensitive skin can be tricky because there are so many ingredient factors that can influence or worsen redness-prone or sensitive skin. As we discuss in the chapters on sensitive skin and rosacea, there are many ingredients, including fragrances and some preservatives, that can cause irritation, inflammation, and allergies and overstimulate fragile, reactive skin. These known irritants and common allergens must be avoided in sensitive skin formulations.

## Protecting the Barrier Function in Sensitive Skin

Guarding and replenishing the barrier function is very important in treating sensitive skin. Not only does the barrier function need to be reinforced, we must be careful not to strip the barrier function. Strong detergents and surfactants, some emulsifiers, drying alcohols, and other ingredients can eat away at the fragile barrier function in sensitive skin. If the barrier function is stripped, the skin turns red from inflammation and exposure.

Lipid replacement ingredients such as sphingolipids, glycosphingolipids, phospholipids, cholesterol, and certain fatty acids can serve as a complex to patch and reinforce barrier function, just as it does in helping the aging skin. Use of physical emulsifiers reduces the chances of damage to the natural barrier function lipids.

## Soothing and Anti-Redness Agents

Soothing agents have an anti-reddening effect on the skin. They make the skin feel cooler and more comfortable. Many antioxidants also serve as soothing agents, probably because they interfere with the inflammation cascade that can lead to redness. They are often added to many products designed for sensitive skin, and are most effective in leave-on products.

The following ingredients are used for their soothing benefits:

◆ Stearyl glycyrrhetinate (derived from licorice)
◆ Dipotassium glycyrrhizinate (derived from licorice)
◆ Matricaria extract (a type of chamomile)
◆ Green tea extract
◆ Grapeseed extract
◆ Ginseng extract
◆ White tea extract
◆ Allantoin (derived from comfrey root)
◆ Licorice extract
◆ *Aloe barbadensis* extract (aloe vera)
◆ Chamomile
◆ Azulene (derived from chamomile)
◆ Bisabolol (derived from chamomile)
◆ Calendula extract

◆ Zinc oxide

◆ Horse chestnut extract (strengthens capillaries)

◆ Mallow extract

◆ Hamamelis extract (nonalcoholic witch hazel)

Finished products designed for sensitive skin should be independently tested to ensure their low irritancy potential. For more information, see the chapter on sensitive skin.

## OVER-THE-COUNTER DRUGS

The U.S. Food and Drug Administration (FDA) regulates both prescription and **over-the-counter (OTC) drugs**. OTC drugs have been determined to have relatively few side effects and, therefore, are deemed safe for consumers to use without a doctor's prescription. OTC drugs are sold without a doctor's prescription, are carried by stores, and are often sold by estheticians. These include acne medications, skin lightening products, and sunscreens.

**Over-the-counter (OTC) drugs** are available without a prescription.

### OTC and Drug Facts Labeling

OTC drugs are required by law to use special chart labels called **drug facts** labels (Figure 10-1). These standardized labels are designed to be uniform and clearly inform the consumer what the product is used for and how to use the product. It also includes

**Drug facts** are special charts used on the packages of over-the-counter drugs to inform the consumer about the drug's uses and possible problems.

### Drug Facts

| **Active Ingredients** | | **Purpose** |
|---|---|---|
| Octinoxate | 7.5% | Sunscreen |
| Octisalate | 5.00% | Sunscreen |
| Oxybenzone | 4.5% | Sunscreen |

**Uses**
• Sun Protection Factor 15
• Helps prevent sunburn

**Warnings**
• External use only
• Keep out of reach of children

**When using this product**
• Keep out of eyes. Rinse with water to remove

**Stop use and ask a doctor if**
• Rash or irration develops or lasts

**Directions**
• Apply generously and evenly before sun exposure and as needed.
• Children under 6 months: ask a doctor.
• Reapply after swimming, perspiring, or towel-drying.

**Inactive Ingredients:**
Water (Aqua),Butylene Glycol, Caprylic/Capric Triglycerides, Stearic Acid, Glyceryl Stearate, Propylene Glycol Dicaprylate/Dicaprate, Aloe Barbadensis Leaf Juice, Dimethicone, PEG-100 Stearate, Glycerin, Paraffin, Silk Amino Acids, Glycoproteins, Sphingolipids, Glycosphingolipids, Phospholipids, Cholesterol, Sodium Hyaluronate, Sodium PCA, Ceteth-20, Cetyl Alcohol, Carbomer, Disodium EDTA, Triethanolamine, Propylene Glycol, Diazolidinyl Urea, Methylparaben, Propylparoben.

**Figure 10-1** Drug facts label

warnings as to possible side effects and contraindications. Drug facts labels are required to be printed on the outside container of any OTC drug. For most products, this means the drug facts label is printed on the box, but if the product is not sold in a box, it must be on the actual container. For small containers, "accordion" labels may be attached.

Active ingredients are the ingredients within a drug that cause the physiological change that occurs when the drug is used. They are listed first on the drug facts label, along with their purpose. Uses for the product are listed second. Warnings are listed third. After the warnings are sections for "when using this product" advice and "stop use and ask a doctor if," instructing consumers when they should seek a physician's advice if the drug is not working or they are experiencing an adverse reaction. Directions follow this, with clear instructions on how to use the product. Last, the "inactive" ingredients are listed. The inactive ingredients are the functional ingredients in the OTC product. Ingredients that are considered to be cosmetic performance ingredients affecting skin appearance are considered to be "inactive ingredients" when listed on the label of an OTC drug.

OTC products can also be cosmetics. A sunscreen that contains moisturizing ingredients is both a drug and a cosmetic. However, it must be labeled as an OTC drug, and cosmetic claims cannot be made on the drug facts label. Any appearance claims must be made somewhere else on the package.

You may notice that products from different companies have very similar wording on their drug facts labels. This is because the FDA has very strict rules about what a company can say about an OTC drug product. There are specific words and phrases that are specifically approved for different active ingredients and for explaining how to use an OTC drug product.

## Sunscreen Ingredients

There are two types of sunscreen ingredients—absorbing sunscreens and physical sunscreens. Absorbing sunscreens work by absorbing and neutralizing ultraviolet sunrays. Physical sunscreens work by reflecting the rays. For much more on these ingredients and how they work, see the chapter on sun and sun damage.

In the past few years, the FDA has changed the official name of numerous sunscreen ingredients. The following lists are some of the new names with the old names in parentheses. Also listed is the type of UV light screened by these agents. Often these sunscreen active ingredients are used in combination to screen various parts of the spectrum of ultraviolet light from the sun.

The most widely used absorbing sunscreen active ingredients include the following:

Octinoxate (octyl methoxycinnimate) UVB screen
Octisalate (octyl salicylate) UVB Screen
Oxybenzone (benzophenone) UVB and partial UVA screen
Avobenzone (also known as Parsol 1789) UVA screen

There are only two physical sunscreens. These screen both UVA and UVB rays:

Zinc oxide
Titanium dioxide

## Sunscreens or Sunblocks?

What is the difference between a sunscreen and a sunblock? In the old FDA regulations, a sunblock claim could be made if the sunscreen product contained a physical sunscreen active: titanium dioxide or zinc oxide. The new regulations do not allow the term sunblock to be used. No sunscreen agent or product blocks 100% of the sun's rays.

## Active Ingredients for Acne Medications

There are four major OTC approved ingredients for the treatment of acne:

◆ **Benzoyl peroxide**—used in 2.5%, 5%, and 10% concentrations, depending on the acne severity. Usually these are in a gel spreading agent but can also be in a cream base or a drying paste. Benzoyl peroxide is a **keratolytic**, which means "keratin-dissolving," and works by loosening dead cells stuck in the follicles. It also releases oxygen in the follicle. Because acne bacteria are anaerobic, they cannot survive in the presence of oxygen. Benzoyl peroxide essentially works both as an interfollicular exfoliant and as an antibacterial.

◆ **Salicylic acid**—a betahydroxy acid that also sloughs dead cell buildup within the follicle, acts as a mild antibacterial, and has soothing properties. Salicylic acid is regarded to be less irritating than benzoyl peroxide, and has less allergy potential, but is also less aggressive in treating acne. It is often used for treating milder forms of acne. The concentration in OTC drugs is limited to a 2% concentration. Salicylic acid is also used as a performance ingredient exfoliant in smaller concentrations, without making a drug claim.

◆ **Sulfur**—is both a follicular exfoliant and a mild antibacterial. Sulfur also tends to be less aggressive than benzoyl peroxide, and it often is marketed for adult acne conditions. It is used in up to 10% concentration in OTC products.

◆ **Sulfur mixed with resorcinol**—Resorcinol is a peeling agent, and when combined with sulfur, it seems to enhance its anti-acne activity. Resorcinol can be toxic and should not be used on large areas or on broken skin. Sulfur–resorcinol lotions are often marketed as "spot-drying" products.

It should be noted here that salicylic acid, sulfur, and resorcinol are all keratolytic agents and are also often used as performance agent exfoliating and drying agents, without making anti-acne drug claims.

## Skin Lightening

There is only one FDA-approved OTC drug ingredient for lightening of skin hyperpigmentation. **Hydroquinone** is used at up to 2% concentration in OTC products, but it is used at higher concentrations in prescription lightening products. Hydroquinone works by interfering with the physiological processes that cause pigment to form.

It is sometimes combined with performance ingredient exfoliants such as salicylic or glycolic acids to exfoliate dead cells for better absorption of the hydroquinone.

## Skin "Brightening"

There are many performance ingredients that have a lightening effect on hyperpigmentation. Because they are not approved OTC active ingredients, they cannot be marketed with "lightening" claims. Therefore, many of these are marketed as "brighteners" or "whiteners." These agents include **magnesium ascorbyl phosphate**, **arbutin**, **kojic acid**, **bearberry and mulberry extracts**, and others.

## PERFORMANCE INGREDIENTS FOR OILY AND ACNE-PRONE SKIN

The goal in treating oily and acne-prone skin is to clear the follicles of dead cell buildup and to control the excessive sebum produced by these skin types. Use of foaming cleansers with higher concentrations of the rinseable, foaming detergent

**Keratolytic** is a keratin-dissolving ingredient type used in exfoliators and acne drugs.

**Hydroquinone** is an active topical ingredient that inhibits the production of melanin.

**Magnesium ascorbyl phosphate** is an ester of vitamin C that is a fat-soluble antioxidant, often considered to be a stable form of topical vitamin C; also used for skin brightening.

**Arbutin** is an ingredient used for skin brightening.

**Kojic** is an ingredient used for skin brightening.

**Bearberry and mulberry extracts** are ingredients used for skin brightening.

cleansing agents already discussed is helpful in controlling the excessive oil. Sometimes **oil absorbers** such as **nylon** (actually made from nylon fibers) and **silica** are used in "oil-control" lotions or gels that are worn under makeup.

Use of follicular exfoliants like **glycolic acid** help to slough dead cells from the inside of the follicle that clog the pores. Additionally, the previously listed OTC drug exfoliants are used.

Even oily skin needs to be properly hydrated. Because of the excess sebum produced by these skin types, little emollient is required in products for oily skin. Use of hydrating agents such as sodium PCA and glycerin help to bind water without adding oily emollients to an already oily skin. Special nonclogging lightweight emollient spreading agents have been developed so that these products may be applied without making the skin feel oily or heavy.

## Exfoliants

An **exfoliant** is a performance ingredient that helps to remove dead cells from the skin surface. Exfoliants help the appearance of the skin by removing dead cells, making the surface look smoother and more refined, and actually help to stimulate the skin to replace these old cells with fresher cells. **Mechanical exfoliants** are usually granular particles that bump or scratch the skin surface to remove cells. Polyethylene, ground shells or nuts, and hydrogenated jojoba oil beads are example of these types of particles. Sometimes these ingredients are mixed into cleansers to increase their rinseability. Applied with the fingertips and gently massaged, these agents bump off surface excess dead cells.

**Chemical exfoliants** include alphahydroxy acids, such as glycolic and lactic acids, and the betahydroxy salicylic acid. They help improve the appearance of wrinkles, fine lines, rough textures, and clogged pores, and they improve cell renewal and the lipid content in the barrier function. They also can shed off discolored cells, helping with hyperpigmentation. On oily skin they can loosen clogged pores and remove dead cell buildup within the follicles. They are best used when applied to the skin in a gel, serum, or cream and worn under a moisturizer or sunscreen. These acids work by dissolving surface intercellular lipids in the top of the corneum, loosening the cells so they can shed. Sometimes these acids are added to cleansers or rinseable scrubs, but they work best when left on the skin. Benzoyl peroxide, sulfur, and resorcinol are stronger exfoliants and are used in OTC acne products, as discussed earlier.

**Enzymes** such as **papain** (derived from papaya), **bromelain** (derived from pineapple), and **pancreatin** (a pancreatic enzyme derived from beef or pork processing) work by dissolving protein in dead cells. They are keratolytics known as **proteolytic enzymes**. Proteolytic literally means "protein dissolving." Enzymes are often used in professional salon skin-care treatments. Enzymes can be used in "vegetal" peels or **gommages**, roll-off surface exfoliation treatments, or they can also be in powder form and mixed with water to activate them.

## Other Ingredients

Clays such as **bentonite**, **kaolin**, **hectorite**, and **silica** are used for their tightening and oil-absorbing benefits. They are also sometimes used in drying lotions for acne blemishes. They have drawing effects on clogged pores, helping to remove impactions and tighten the appearance of pores.

## CONCLUSION

Hundreds of chemicals are used as performance ingredients in cosmetics. Some active agents, as you have seen, are also vehicles and have more than one function in a cosmetic.

---

**Oil absorbers** are agents used to absorb excess sebum.

**Nylon** is a synthetic molecule used in oil-control products to absorb excess sebum and reduce shininess.

**Glycolic acid** is an alphahydroxy acid used primarily as a cellular exfoliant. It has many beneficial effects on the skin's appearance.

**Exfoliants** usually come in the form of scrubs. They are water-based products with a humectant mixed with some sort of abrasive agent such as almond meal or polyethylene granules.

**Mechanical exfoliants** are ingredients used to bump off dead cells from the skin's surface. Some examples include granules, jojoba oil beads, or ground nut shells.

**Chemical exfoliants** are ingredients used to remove dead cells from the skin's surface by chemically dissolving the bond between dead cells or dissolving the dead cell itself.

**Enzymes** are naturally occurring chemicals used in cosmetics primarily as chemical exfoliants.

**Papain** is a keratolytic enzyme derived from papaya fruit.

**Bromelain** is keratolytic enzyme derived from pineapple.

**Pancreatin** is a keratolytic enzyme derived from bovine (cow) or porcine (pig) pancreas extract.

**Keratolytic** or **proteolytic** means "protein dissolving," and these agents work by dissolving keratin protein within dead surface cells, helping to remove these cells and making the skin look clearer and smoother.

**Gommages** are roll-off exfoliation treatments.

**Bentonite** is a clay often used in cleansing masks.

**Kaolin** is a clay used in oil-absorbing and cleansing mask products.

**Hectorite** is a clay used in cleansing masks.

**Silica** is an oil absorber.

We have touched on only a few performance ingredients, but you will be able to use this knowledge to understand ingredient labels and their functions. With additional study, you should eventually be able to pick up a product and, simply by reading the ingredient label, know what kind of product it is and for what skin problem it is intended.

## TOPICS FOR DISCUSSION

1. What is a performance ingredient? How does it differ from an active ingredient?
2. What are the two basic types of cleansing ingredients? Discuss the products in which each is used.
3. What are natural moisturizing factors? Name some that are used in cosmetics.
4. Discuss some ingredients used to help aging skin.
5. What are free radicals?
6. Discuss some ingredients used to treat oily skin and problem acne skin.

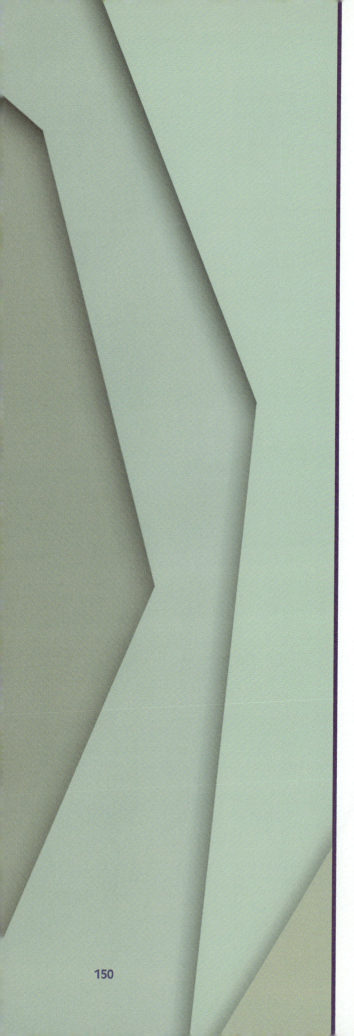

# CHAPTER 11

# Skin-Care Products

## OBJECTIVES. . .

After the esthetician graduates from school, he or she will be amazed at the variety of skin-care products available. This chapter discusses various types of skin-care products available, products for different skin types and problems, and the chemical makeup of products for different skin types.

Although this chapter provides only an overview of the products available, it will teach the esthetician about factors involved in choosing products for various skin problems and clients' needs.

In the chapters on cosmetic chemistry and functional ingredients and performance ingredients and active ingredients you learned about various ingredients used in manufacturing cosmetics. Now you will learn about practical application of various formulas of cleansers, toners, creams, and other products.

There are literally hundreds and hundreds of different products available to estheticians. These are products that you will use in the treatment room and recommend that your clients use at home. It is important to carry a variety of products to sell to your clients for home use. There are many good esthetic product manufacturers, and the most successful skin-care salons carry lines made by at least two or three of them. There is no one line that is the answer to every problem you will see. What your client is doing to their skin at home is actually more important than your in-room treatments. Your client is treating his or her skin with something twice a day—that's 60 times a month! What could be more important than what products are used on your client's skin 24 hours a day? It is essential to the success of any skin-care program that the client participates at home by using the correct products you recommend (Figure 11-1).

## A VISIT TO THE PRODUCT STOCKROOM

Let's take a trip to the stockroom of a successful skin-care salon. We will not talk about name brands, but we will talk about various products available in chemical terms. You will be able to use what you have learned. Remember, a primary objective is for you to be able to read ingredient labels and tell what kind of product you are examining and for what skin type it is intended. As we look into this imaginary stockroom, we will look at various types of products. There are enough types of products in this stockroom to handle most esthetic problems (Figure 11-2).

The most important factor in prescribing the right home care for your clients is your education and knowledge of skin analysis. Make sure you receive good training in analysis. It is one of the biggest keys to success in esthetics.

Before we enter the imaginary stockroom, it must be understood that many products are available to the esthetician, and new products are developed every year. We will cover only a portion of the products available, but this will be a representative sampling of what is frequently used in skin-care salons.

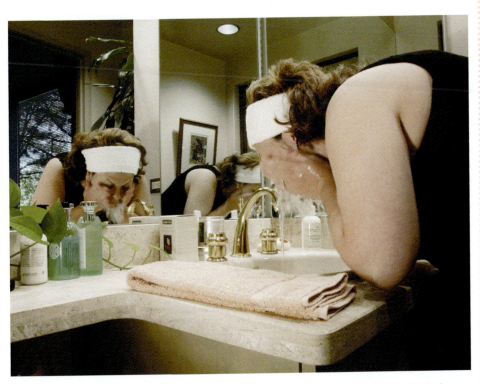

**Figure 11-1** It is essential to the success of any skin-care program that the client participates at home

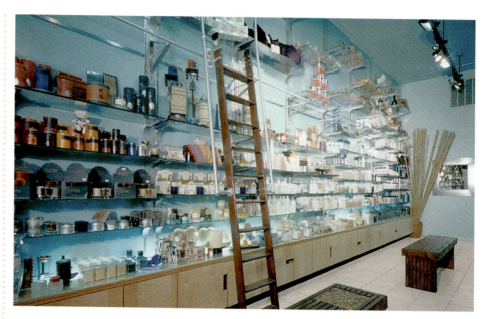

**Figure 11-2** A well-organized retail area is important to the esthetics practice

## CLEANSERS

As we enter the stockroom, the first thing you notice is the wide assortment of cleansers. There are milk-type cleansers and rinseable detergent-type foaming cleansers, and there are some specialty cleansers for acne- and clog-prone skin.

Let's talk about rinseable cleansers first. Rinseable cleansers usually come in a tube, sometimes in a bottle. They vary in strength and texture. Rinseable cleansers are important to carry because you will find that many clients are used to washing their faces with bar soap, like the foaming action, and do not "feel clean" unless they have "washed" their faces.

### Product Profile: Rinseable Cleanser for Oily and Combination Skin

**Client and Skin Type:** The first rinseable cleanser we will look at is a rinseable cleanser for oily and combination skin. Clients with oily and combination skin are especially fond of rinseable cleansers because these clients need some detergent to help cut excess amounts of oil. However, we don't want our cleanser to overdry them or strip the acid mantle.

**Product Characteristics:** This particular cleanser is in a tube. The product consistency feels almost like soap. When the client adds water, it begins to foam moderately. It rinses completely, leaving the skin feeling fresh and clean, but not too tight. This clean but not tight feeling is a good sign that the product is pH balanced correctly for the skin type.

**Chemical Action and Design:** Chemically this product uses disodium lauryl sulfosuccinate as a detergent-surfactant. It also contains smaller amounts of avocado oil and cetyl alcohol, emollient ingredients added to cut the detergent action on the skin's surface so that it will not be stripping. This cleanser is also fragrance-free, a helpful characteristic when treating sensitive skin. This cleanser is a good recommendation for adult oily and combination skin or for clients who are used to heavier moisturizers but really need to switch to a lighter program for oily or combination skin (Figure 11-3A).

**INGREDIENTS:** Deionized Water, Mineral Oil, Cetyl Alcohol, Sodium Lauryl Sulfate, Cetearyl Alcohol, Ceteth-20, Imidazolidinyl Urea, Methyl Paraben.

A

**INGREDIENTS:** Deionized Water, Disodium Lauryl Sulfosuccinate, Cetyl Alcohol, Ceteth-20, Propylene Glycol, Avocado Oil, Methylparaben, DMDM Hydantoin.

B

Which cleanser is stronger? The first one is weaker. The surfactant (sodium lauryl sulfate) is buffered by dominating ingredients cetyl alcohol and mineral oil, which help to prevent too much contact with the surfactant. In the second formulation, the surfactant (disodium lauryl sulfosuccinate) is diluted only by water as a larger percentage ingredient. The further the surfactant is down the list, the weaker the cleansing action. The first product is designed for dry-combination skin, and the second is for oily-combination skin.

**Figure 11-3** Sample ingredient labels for cleansers

## Product Profile: Rinseable Cleanser for Dry and Combination Skin

**Client and Skin Type:** This cleanser is designed for clients who have dry skin but still want the action of a detergent cleanser. This cleanser will be good for an older client with dry skin who prefers soap over milk cleanser.

**Product Characteristics:** This rinseable cleanser is also packaged in a tube. It foams very slightly. It rinses well but leaves the skin feeling very soft. This cleanser will not be aggressive enough for oily-combination skin. However, for more alipidic skin it is excellent.

**Chemical Action and Design:** If you look at the ingredient label of this product you will notice that its detergent agent, sodium lauryl sulfate, is listed about halfway down the list of ingredients. This means that the product is not nearly as strong a cleanser as the first cleanser listed on the label. The ingredients listed after water are different types of emollients, fatty alcohols, and esters. This cleanser contains lots of emollients because it is designed for dry skin. The large amounts of emollients will keep the detergents from stripping too much lipid from the skin's surface. This product is superfatted (Figure 11-3B).

## Product Profile: Rinseable Cleanser for Very Oily Skin

**Client and Skin Type:** This stronger rinseable cleanser is designed for clients who have very oily skin. Their skin is covered with enlarged pores, and they almost never have any dryness or dehydration. This type of client's skin is extremely oily by 10 or 11 o'clock in the morning.

**Product Characteristics:** This cleanser is a liquid in a bottle. It has almost the consistency of shampoo. It foams quite strongly and rinses thoroughly, leaving the skin feeling very clean. It is much too strong for any skin type except extremely oily skin.

**Chemical Action and Design:** The active detergent in this rinseable cleanser is an anionic surfactant called ammonium laureth sulfate. This cleanser contains some glycolic acid, which, in a cleanser, is helpful in loosening surface cells. Glycolic and other alphahydroxy acids can be used in cleansers but, of course, are rinsed off and do not have the same long-term conditioning effects as AHAs that are used in leave-on products. This cleanser is mixed with gelling agents to form shampoo-like consistency. The surfactant concentration in a cleanser such as this is somewhat higher than other rinseable detergent cleansers that are designed for less oily skins. There are no emollients in this product, and therefore the product has no buffer against stripping oil from the skin's surface. However, this is appropriate for a cleanser that is designed for very oily skin.

## Product Profile: Rinseable Medicated Cleanser for Acne

**Client and Skin Type:** This cleanser is made for mild to moderate acne, excessively oily, and chronic acne-prone skin. This type of skin is not sensitive and is fairly thick, due to the accumulation of corneocytes on the surface of the skin. This client may have a currently active acne condition or may tend to develop moderate acne frequently. This product may also be excellent for teenage acne.

**Product Characteristics:** This cleanser is very similar to the one designed for chronically oily skin, except that it contains an antimicrobial agent to kill bacteria. Medicated cleansers such as this are usually registered as over-the-counter drugs. (See Chapter 12, Claims in Cosmetics.) It is a strong foaming cleanser. It may also be made to be an exfoliant, depending on the ingredients.

**Chemical Action and Design:** Benzoyl peroxide may serve as the antimicrobial in a product like this, or another antimicrobial such as salicylic acid, sulfur, or hexetidine may be used. Benzoyl peroxide (see Chapter 15, Acne and the Esthetician) is also a keratolytic agent, as is salicylic acid, which serves to lightly peel away dead corneocytes from the surface of the skin as well as flush the follicular canal. Some products like this cleanser may also contain a mechanical exfoliant such as polyethylene granules. These small, bead-like granules are used in the cleanser because they are gritty and literally "bump off" dead cell buildup.

As you move across the shelf from the rinseable cleanser, you may notice a variety of milk cleansers in several different colors. As you look closer, you notice that these cleansers are designed for a variety of skin types.

## Product Profile: Milk Cleanser for Oily and Combination Skin

**Client and Skin Type:** This cleanser is an emulsion to be used for makeup removal on oily and combination skin. Milk cleanser for acne and extremely oily skin is rarely used, at least not by itself. For acne, a milk cleanser may be used strictly as a makeup remover, followed by a rinseable detergent cleanser for extra cleansing action. This cleansing milk is a good choice for the older person with oily or combination skin who has a tendency toward oiliness and minor but persistent breakout problems. This type of client may find twice daily cleansings with detergents to be too dehydrating. Older skin tends to dehydrate much more easily than younger skin. This skin type may use a rinseable cleanser in the morning and then a gentler milk for nightly makeup removal.

**Product Characteristics:** This milk is a water-based fluid. It is slightly slippery to the touch and leaves the skin feeling fairly clean when removed. This product should be applied and removed with a room temperature damp sponge cloth or cleansing sponge. It is necessary with all cleansing milks to use a very soft cloth to apply and remove these cleansers, because they do not contain much detergent, if any, and do not rinse as easily as detergent cleansers. This cleanser, however, rinses well when used with a sponge or sponge cloth. Makeup is removed very easily with this product. This product should not be used on the eyes, because it is designed for oily and combination skin and is not chemically appropriate for the eye area.

**Chemical Action and Design:** The emollients used in this cleanser are tridecyl stearate, neopentylglycol dicaprate/dicaprylate, and tridecyl trimellitate, which are a complex of emollients designed to be a noncomedogenic oil replacement. They do not clog the skin and are easily removed from the skin. The emollients mix with the dirt, makeup, and oils and work to dissolve these foreign materials so they may be removed from the skin's surface. This product has a pH of about 7.0, typical of a cleanser designed for oily and combination skin. The slightly higher pH helps the cleanser be a more aggressive solvent. The cleansing process should be followed by a lower pH toner to lower the pH and remove any film left from the emollient.

## Product Profile: Cleansing Milk for Combination Skin

**Client and Skin Type:** This thicker cleansing emulsion is made for clients who wear heavier makeup and therefore need a more oily cleanser to dissolve the thicker, oilier makeup. This cleanser is often prescribed for older clients with combination skin. It is considerably heavier than many other cleansing milks. This cleanser may also be used frequently by actors and other performers who wear heavier stage makeup routinely.

**Product Characteristics:** This cleanser is a thicker liquid in a bottle. It absolutely must be used with a sponge or a soft cloth. Otherwise, it would leave a residue on the skin. Its emollients dissolve makeup very readily, making it an excellent product for heavy makeup wearers. This product should be followed by a toner designed for combination skin. The toner needs to be strong enough to remove any residue left from this cleanser.

**Chemical Action and Design:** Petrolatum and mineral oil are the secrets of the slipperiness of this cleanser. There is enough emulsifier in this product to make it relatively thick. The petrolatum makes the product physically heavy. Mineral oil mixed with petrolatum is an excellent makeup dissolver. Plant extracts have been added to this product for soothing.

## Product Profile: Cleansing Milk for Sensitive Skin

**Client and Skin Type:** This lightweight milk cleanser is designed for sensitive skin. It is designed for the client with thin, fragile skin that reddens easily. It is not specifically designed for oily skin; its emollient content is meant more for dry, irritated skin. The client who has sensitive, thin skin can use this product.

**Product Characteristics:** This is a lightweight cleansing milk designed to be used with a soft cloth or sponge. It does not leave much residue when rinsed and has very little fragrance. It will remove liquid makeup well.

**Chemical Action and Design:** This water-based cleanser combines a relatively large amount of water with a mixture of emollients to dissolve makeup. It does not contain a traditional emulsifier. It is a physical emulsion, blended by homogenization. As we have discussed in the chapter on cosmetic chemistry and functional ingredients, traditional emulsifiers can impair barrier function when used on sensitive skin, increasing reactivity. Using cleansers that are physically emulsified will not further damage an already thin barrier. This cleanser contains azulene, bisabolol, and chamomile extract, which are included for their soothing properties. No fragrance is used because of allergy potentials. The only fragrance is from the plant extract used.

## Product Profile: Cleansing Milk for Dry Skin

**Client and Skin Type:** Dry, mature skin will benefit from the use of this fairly lightweight milk for dry skin.

**Product Characteristics:** Again, this product should be applied and removed with a damp, soft cloth. This cleanser is slightly richer to the touch than our other milk cleansers. It does leave a residue if not carefully removed and should be used with a toner designed for dry skin.

**Chemical Action and Design:** The ultra-rich emollient oils in this cleanser are added to help condition the surface of the skin while cleansing, helping to avoid overstripping of the natural oils. It contains no detergents, which can strip older alipidic skin.

Some skin-care companies add expensive conditioners to cleansing product. These conditioning ingredients are normally used in creams, lotions, and fluids that are in the form of day or night treatments. In other words, they stay on the face for long periods of time. Many cosmetic scientists believe that it is useless to include expensive conditioning ingredients in cleansers, because they simply do not stay on the face long enough to do any good. Soothing agents and agents that are meant to strengthen or weaken the action of the cleanser are the only type of these agents that should be added.

## TONERS

Toners, clarifying lotions, fresheners, and astringents are all basically the same type of product. Products that are titled "astringents" are considered to be OTC (over-the-counter) drugs. Toners vary in strength, drying ability, and alcohol content. They are made for three specific reasons:

1. They remove excess cleanser and residue from liquid cleansers.

2. They have a relatively low pH, helping to adjust the pH of the acid mantle after cleansing so it is not overstripped.

3. It provides a temporary tightening effect to both the skin and the individual follicle openings, helping to temporarily shrink "pores."

## Product Profile: Toner for Oily and Combination Skin

**Client and Skin Type:** This toner is designed for oily and combination skin. It is good for the client who develops clogs easily but still needs a hydrating moisturizer. Adult oily-combination skin will benefit from this toner.

**Product Characteristics:** This toner is a clear, water-based liquid. It should be applied with a predampened cotton pad, a sponge, or a soft cloth after using a rinseable cleanser or cleansing milk, or it can be atomized onto the skin with a fine-mist sprayer. Sprayers have become popular in nonalcoholic toners because they are so convenient to use. Sprayers cannot be used in toners containing alcohol because of possible accidental contact with the eyes. This toner has a lemon fragrance. After use, the skin feels clean and toned but not dry. Pores do seem to shrink after using this product. Men can also use this product as an aftershave. It is a good product for men, because it is not femininely fragranced and has enough astringent action for after shaving. This will help constrict the follicles, helping to keep the hair pointed in an outward direction so it does not become an **ingrown hair** by growing into the side of the follicle wall.

> **Ingrown hair** is an infected follicle caused by a hair that grows into the side of the follicle wall.

**Chemical Action and Design:** The low pH in this toner is due to a combination of citric acid and lemon extract, which has an astringent action. It is blended into a liquid with mostly water, but it also contains a glycerin derivative, which is a humectant that helps to restore water to dehydrated skin.

## Product Profile: Toner for Extremely Oily Skin

**Client and Skin Type:** This toner is made for skin that becomes very oily after only a short period of time and has very large pores that clog very easily. This client never gets dehydrated because the skin is so oily. The client uses a strong, rinseable cleanser for very oily skin, which we discussed earlier. This toner should be applied on a predampened cotton pad or damp sponge.

**Product Characteristics:** This toner is a water-based liquid that is used after cleansing milk or rinseable cleanser. It has a strong astringent action. It leaves the skin feeling very clean and tight. Application to dry skin would be too drying.

**Chemical Action and Design:** This oily skin astringent contains plant extracts for oily skin as well as sulfur, a keratolytic peeling agent, and potassium alum, a strong astringent agent. They are in a base vehicle of water and propylene glycol, a hydrating agent.

## Product Profile: Astringent for Acne-Prone Skin

**Client and Skin Type:** This very strong astringent is made for inflamed acne and extremely oily skin. It is a good product for teenage acne, grades II and III. (See Chapter 15, Acne and the Esthetician.)

**Product Characteristics:** This astringent is a light-colored liquid and has a strong medicinal (alcohol) odor. It is applied with a damp cotton ball after cleansing. It is very stripping, removes lots of sebum, and is very drying to the skin. It may burn or tingle slightly when applied, especially if applied to open acne lesions. Some extremely oily skin needs this much oil removal.

**Chemical Action and Design:** This product is actually an over-the-counter drug. Isopropyl alcohol is the active ingredient for its astringent properties and also for its oil-stripping action. Isopropyl alcohol and water are the main ingredients in this liquid astringent. Witch hazel distillate provides astringent properties and temporary pore "tightening." Camphor is included as a soothing agent.

## Product Profile: Toner for Normal Skin

**Client and Skin Type:** This toner is a medium-strength tonic designed for normal and sensitive skin. It is for adult skin that basically needs moderate hydrating and has no particular problems.

**Product Characteristics:** This toner is a liquid and has a very mild astringent action. It does not pull on the skin. It has a moist feeling when applied. It has a slight soothing effect on the skin. It is applied with cool, wet, cotton pads after cleansing.

**Chemical Action and Design:** This is a very simple formula made with water, rosewater, propylene glycol (as a humectant), cucumber extract for soothing, and allantoin. It contains a smaller amount of witch hazel extract than toners for oily skin.

## Product Profile: Toner for Extra-Dry Skin

**Client and Skin Type:** Dry, mature skin is the type of skin that this toner will help. It has moisturizing properties and helps gently remove traces of cleanser from dry, sensitive skin. This type of dry skin can become so dehydrated that the face becomes very tight even after a very gentle cleanser. This toner is designed for dry skin that becomes tender after cleansing. This toner should be used after cleansing and applied with a cool, damp cotton pad.

**Product Characteristics:** This a very moist toner, almost soft to the touch. It has practically no astringent action. It is designed to moisturize the skin with humectants that provide a buffer so that the skin will not become stripped if the toner is used after cleansing.

**Chemical Action and Design:** A large amount of butylene glycol provides humectant effects for the skin in this water-based, fluid toner. Glycerin also has hydrating action on the surface of the dry skin. Extracts of chamomile, mallow, and cornflower are included for their softening and soothing properties. This is an unusually moisturizing toner.

## DAY CREAMS AND TREATMENTS

Day creams are made for various skin types. Treatments for everything from acne to extremely dry and aging skin are available. These products vary greatly in texture and thickness, depending on the amount of fats or emollients that are added.

Sunscreen is probably the biggest health benefit that can be contained in a day cream. Besides preventing premature aging of the skin, using sunscreen is one of the best ways to help prevent skin cancer. Many day creams are also sunscreens, making them OTC drugs. Because sunscreen is such an important feature and benefit, it is becoming traditional to combine broad-spectrum UVA-UVB protection in day treatment products. Sunscreen product ingredient labels will be drug facts labels, as discussed in the performance and active ingredients chapter. They will list the sunscreen ingredients as the active ingredients. Other ingredients will be listed in the "inactive ingredients" section of the drug facts label. It is illegal to claim sunscreen protection and not list the active ingredients in a drug facts label.

Day creams almost always contain either an occlusive agent or some sort of protective ingredient that helps hold moisture in the surface layers of the skin. They may also contain various hydrating ingredients, emollients, or other performance ingredients, depending on the skin type for which they are included.

There are companies who market day creams that are basically moisturizers with hydrating and protective inclusive ingredients and do not have sunscreen ingredients. If these day creams are used, it is necessary to apply sunscreen over the moisturizer. Again, most companies now have sunscreen built into their day creams, which also include hydrating and protective ingredients. This is much more convenient for the client, who will only have to apply one product.

## Product Profile: Day Sunscreen Protection Fluid for Oily and Combination Skin

**Client and Skin Type:** This product is designed for oily and combination skin. Clients who have oily skin appreciate this product because it does not feel oily or greasy and is noncomedogenic. It is a good choice for 20- to 50-year-old clients who develop clogged pores easily. This product is a good choice for people who need hydrating but become oily easily. These clients generally have trouble with their makeup not staying on well and becoming oily during the day. The lack of many emollients in this cream will benefit the client who prefers a light-textured, nonheavy day product. This will also serve well as a daytime moisturizer-protectant for oily skins during the winter months.

**Product Characteristics:** This lightweight day protection fluid comes in a tube. It is not a thick product and feels very light and nongreasy when touched. It absorbs quickly, helping to hydrate the skin and protect against daytime water loss, and it contains SPF-15 sunscreen to shield against routine daily sun exposure during daily activities. It is applied with the fingertips in the morning before makeup, or alone. It is noncomedogenic, which means that it has been tested and found not to clog pores. This product is unusual because it hydrates, protects, conditions, contains two sunscreens, and is noncomedogenic.

**Chemical Action and Design:** This fluid is water-based, with small amounts of noncomedogenic emollients added. These emollients are tridecyl stearate, tridecyl trimellitate, neopentylglycol dicaprate/dicaprylate, and glyceryl stearate. The active humectants that help to bind water in this fluid are glycerin and sodium PCA. Other conditioning agents include allantoin, cornflower extract, tocopherol, and retinyl palmitate. Octinoxate (formerly called methoxycinnimate) and titanium dioxide are the sunscreen ingredients, and dimethicone is used as a water-loss shielding agent because of its lightweight characteristics.

## Product Profile: Day Cream for Dry and Dehydrated Skin

**Client and Skin Type:** Designed for oil-dry (alipidic), dehydrated, or mature skin, this cream will help the client who becomes dry very easily due to lack of oil production. It is for clients who have a slight amount of oiliness through the T-zone, but the large part of the outer perimeter of the face is dry and dehydrated.

**Product Characteristics:** This cream is packaged in a tube. It is definitely cream, containing a substantial amount of emollient. It contains a broad-spectrum SPF-15 sunscreen and a protective agent. It is not extremely greasy or heavy, so it may be worn by clients who prefer a lighter weight day cream. It is blue due to the azulene content. It should be applied under makeup or alone during the day.

**Chemical Action and Design:** This cream contains propylene glycol and aloe as hydrating agents. It contains dimethicone as a shielding protective agent, a broad-spectrum sunscreen combining UVA-UVB sunscreen active oxybenzone (formerly called benzophenone), and UVB actives octinoxate (formerly called methoxycinnimate) and octisalate (formerly called octyl salicylate). These active ingredients are mixed into a water-based blend of emollients, including sphingolipids, cholesterol, cetyl palmitate, and beeswax. Azulene provides soothing benefits.

## Product Profile: Sunscreen Day Lotion for Sensitive Skin

**Client and Skin Type:** The client with sensitive, dehydrated, redness-prone skin will appreciate this product. This product is designed for skin that turns red easily. It helps reduce the appearance of redness, and provides SPF-15 sunscreen protection.

**Product Characteristics:** This is a medium-weight fluid in a tube. It can be applied under makeup or alone.

**Chemical Action and Design:** This lotion contains performance soothing ingredients such as aloe barbadensis gel, matricaria extract, green tea extract, and licorice extract. Its sunscreen active ingredients are octinoxate and zinc oxide, with glycerin as a hydrator. Protective emollients include sunflower oil and caprylic/capric triglycerides. It does not contain fragrance or color agents, which is important for sensitive skin; has been dermatologist-tested for irritancy potential; and has been determined to be noncomedogenic.

## NIGHT CREAMS AND TREATMENTS

Night treatment creams are normally extraintensive treatment products designed to help hydrate and condition skin during the night, a time when normal tissue repair is taking place all over the body, including the skin. Night treatments are often heavier in consistency and texture than day products. They normally contain more emollient than day cream and are not made for use under makeup. Night creams should be applied all over the skin, according to manufacturer's instructions. It is important that the skin be thoroughly cleansed before night treatment is applied.

### Product Profile: Night Treatment Fluid for Oily-Combination, Dehydrated Skin

**Client and Skin Type:** This fluid is made to provide hydration to adult oily skin that is also dehydrated. It can be used on oily and combination skin. These clients are normally adults who need to use a hydrating agent but develop clogged pores and break out easily. This fluid has been laboratory tested and found to be noncomedogenic. It is also ideal for the client who prefers a lighter weight night treatment.

**Product Characteristics:** Due to its low emollient content, this fluid is very light in texture and feel. It does not feel oily at all because it contains mostly humectants to attract water to the skin, rather than oils and fats that will clog this type of skin. This fluid comes in a tube and should be applied in moderate amounts to the entire skin before bedtime.

**Chemical Action and Design:** This fluid contains sodium PCA, a natural moisturizing factor (NMF), and glycerin as hydrating agents. It also includes allantoin, retinyl palmitate, and tocopherol in its formula for their conditioning properties. This fluid has been carefully designed without comedogenic ingredients (see the chapter on comedogenicity) to avoid clogging the oily and combination skin for which it is intended. The emollients added are tridecyl stearate, tridecyl trimellitate, and neopentylglycol dicaprate/dicaprylate. This fluid adds hydration to the skin without adding excess emollients that cause buildup of cells, which cause clogs to form.

### Product Profile: Night Treatment for Oily, Clogged Adult Skin

**Client and Skin Type:** This product is designed for oily skin or oily, clogged areas. It is for clients who have a tendency to break out but find that most drying agents overdry. Adult acne can benefit from this type of product because it incorporates both a peeling agent and a hydrating agent as well as a protectant. This product is also ideal for an adult oily skin client who is used to using heavy moisturizers that are clogging the skin. It feels like a moisturizer but is actually a very light peeling agent.

**Product Characteristics:** This lightweight product has an unusual texture somewhere between a gel and a cream. It is very light and dries quickly when applied. It has a matte dry feeling when used. It should be applied in the evening after cleansing and toning. It takes the place of moisturizer and can be used under makeup or alone.

**Chemical Action and Design:** Salicylic acid, a betahydroxy acid, is used in a very small quantity in this product to promote some exfoliation. This product contains glycerin and propylene glycol as humectants, and dimethicone provides protection against excess water loss.

## Product Profile: Night Hydrating Cream for Combination Mature Skin

**Client and Skin Type:** Designed for older oily and combination skins that need hydration but do not need extra oils, this lightweight cream is good for older clients who still have a tendency to break out. It provides hydration without oiliness. This cream could also be used as a night treatment for younger, extra-dehydrated skin types. The cream is laboratory tested to be noncomedogenic.

**Product Characteristics:** The cream is extremely lightweight and is absorbed by the skin easily. After use the skin feels smooth and "plumped up." It is contained in a tube and should be applied to clean skin before bedtime. It contains no color or fragrance, which is helpful for sensitive and allergy-prone skin.

**Chemical Action and Design:** A mixture of lipids, including fatty acids, sphingolipids, phospholipids, and cholesterol, help to reinforce the barrier function of the mature combination skin. Hydrating agents include sodium hyaluronate, glycerin, and butylene glycol. Protective emollients that help prevent dehydration include caprylic/capric triglycerides and dimethicone.

## Product Profile: Night Moisturizing Lotion for Dehydrated Combination Dry Skin

**Client and Skin Type:** This lotion is formulated to help skin that is both oil- and water-dry. This type of skin has a very narrow T-zone with little oil production or visible pore structure. Most clients will be mature women.

**Product Characteristics:** This treatment is a lotion and is packaged in a bottle. It is slightly oily to the touch, leaving a slight film on the surface of the skin. This characteristic is helpful for drier skin types. It is a light blue color, due to its azulene content. It should be applied before bedtime.

**Chemical Action and Design:** The lotion contains a mixture of oils, emollients, and humectants, providing both hydration and oils for the oil-dry skin. It contains the humectants urea, propylene glycol, and butylene glycol and is mixed with sesame oil, peanut oil, and various emollient esters and fats. Because it contains a good amount of both hydrator and oils, it contains sodium lauryl sulfate, used as an emulsifier to keep the oils in the water-based emulsion.

## Product Profile: Night Cream for Dry, Dehydrated Skin

**Client and Skin Type:** Alipidic (oil-dry), dehydrated, mature skin is the target for this heavier cream. This type of client is very dry for most of the year and needs a richer cream.

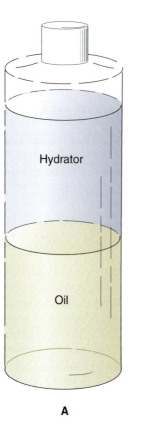
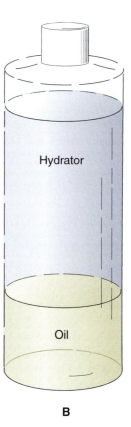

**A**　　　　　　　　　　　　**B**

**Figure 11-4** Bottle A has more oil and emollient for dry skin. Bottle B has less oil and more hydration for dehydrated, oilier skin

**Product Characteristics:** This cream comes in a jar. It is rich in texture and leaves an emollient residue on the skin when applied and stays on the skin all night. The product is nonfragranced.

**Chemical Action and Design:** This cream is a mixture of humectants and emollients containing large amounts of the latter. The chief humectant in this cream is sorbitol, with emollients caprylic/capric triglycerides, jojoba oil, and squalane, which help to prevent moisture loss. It is nonfragranced and has been tested to be noncomedogenic, although it is intended for skin that does not tend to develop comedones (Figure 11-4).

## Product Profile: Firming Night Cream for Mature Skin with Lack of Elasticity

**Client and Skin Type:** This is for clients with combination to dry, dehydrated, sun-damaged skin that needs more elasticity.

**Product Characteristics:** This cream comes in a jar. It has a fluffy, light texture and absorbs easily. It has no color or fragrance, which are helpful features for sensitive skin. The product has been tested for irritancy potential and comedogenicity.

**Chemical Action and Design:** This high-tech cream is a mixture of humectants and emollients with a complex of botanical performance ingredients, hydrocotyl and coneflower extracts, that are helpful in firming the appearance of skin with poor elasticity. The chief humectants in this cream are sodium hyaluronate, glycerin, and butylene glycol, with protective cyclomethicone, a silicone derivative, which helps to prevent moisture loss.

# ABOUT AMPOULES AND SERUMS

**Ampoules** are sealed vials of concentrated ingredients. They are designed to give ultra-intensive treatment to the skin. They often contain larger amounts of performance ingredients in a water base, although occasionally they are in an oil base. Ampoules must be applied under a night cream or fluid.

Ampoules are available for a wide variety of skin types and problems. Ampoules are often designed to be used in a series once a month or several times a year. Others are designed to be used nightly. Ampoules are frequently found in European skin-care lines. The disadvantages of ampoules are that they are more trouble to use and are often very expensive. Clients who are extremely conscientious about their home care will often take the time to use ampoules and will not mind paying extra for them.

In the past decade, **serums** have replaced ampoules, at least in many American lines. Like ampoules, serums contain concentrated ingredients, often in liposomes or other advanced delivery systems, but they are easier to use. Many serums are designed to be used daily, sometimes twice a day.

Serums are usually in pump bottles or tincture bottles. Many contain antioxidants, peptides, lipids, or other intensive ingredients. Like ampoules, they are applied under a day or night cream or fluid.

## Product Profile: Firming Serum for Mature Skin with Lack of Elasticity

**Client and Skin Type:** This product is for dehydrated, sun-damaged skin of any skin type that needs more elasticity.

**Product Characteristics:** This water-based serum is in a pump bottle. It has a liquid-gel consistency. Because it contains no fats or oils, it can be used on any skin type. It has no color or fragrance, which are helpful features for sensitive skin. The product has been tested for irritancy potential and comedogenicity.

**Chemical Action and Design:** This advanced serum combines palmitoyl pentapeptide-3, a peptide known for firming skin and improving the appearance of mature, sun damage and wrinkles. The base of the serum contains hyaluronic acid, boosting water levels; the peptides improve elasticity. Additionally, this serum contains four different liposomed antioxidants and a botanical complex of coneflower and hydrocotyl extracts, known for their firming effects.

## Product Profile: Lipid Serum for Wrinkles and Dry Skin

**Client and Skin Type:** This product is for dry, dehydrated, mature skin and wrinkle areas.

**Product Characteristics:** This serum is in a pump bottle. It has a slippery feel, but when applied to the skin it seems to absorb quickly, leaving a velvety feel to the skin. Applying this serum to wrinkled areas shows almost immediate smoothing effects. The serum does not contain color or fragrance, which are helpful features for sensitive skin. The product has been tested for irritancy potential and comedogenicity.

**Chemical Action and Design:** This serum for very dry skin is **anhydrous**, which means it contains no water. Because it contains no water, no preservatives are needed. The vehicle of this serum is a complex of three silicone derivatives: cyclomethicone, dimethicone, and phenyl trimethicone. A specific lipid complex has been added to mimic the natural proportions of lipids identical to the lipid complex in the normal barrier function.

**Ampoules** are sealed vials of concentrated ingredients designed to give intensive treatment to a skin condition.

**Serums** are products containing concentrated ingredients that are usually in pump or tincture bottles.

**Anhydrous** means that a product does not contain water.

# SPECIAL CREAMS AND TREATMENTS

Many treatment creams are available for special problems or special areas. These treatments should be used in conjunction with other day and night treatments. These include performance-oriented products like alphahydroxy acid formulations, antioxidant serums, melanin suppressant OTC formulations, and acne care treatment products.

## Product Profile: Alphahydroxy Treatment for Dry, Sun-Damaged Skin

**Client and Skin Type:** This product is designed for dry, dehydrated mature skin that is wrinkled or sun damaged.

**Product Characteristics:** This is a very emollient, thicker cream that contains multiple alphahydroxy acids. It is in a jar and should be applied after cleansing and toning and before sunscreen or night hydration cream. SPF-15 sunscreen should be used daily with this product.

**Chemical Action and Design:** Alphahydroxy acids—glycolic and lactic—and betahydroxy—citric acid—combined with fruit-derived hydroxy acids from sugarcane, orange, and apple extracts work to exfoliate dead cells and smooth surface wrinkles and lines. Long-term use helps with barrier function and moisture retention. Emollients include hydrogenated polyisobutene, cetyl alcohol, dimethicone, and polyacrylamide, an appropriate combination for a drier skin type. Green tea extract is present in a fairly large concentration to soothe potential irritation caused by this 10 percent acid blend. Even with a large emollient base, this product has tested noncomedogenic and has been dermatologist tested for irritancy. These results may be helpful when deciding which client is best suited for this product. The pH of this product is 3.5, in compliance with the Cosmetic Ingredient Review (CIR) recommendations discussed in the chapter on performance and active ingredients, Active Agents and Performance Ingredients.

## Product Profile: Alphahydroxy Treatment Gel for Oily-Combination, Clogged Skin

**Client and Skin Type:** This product is designed for any skin with clogged pores and oily or oily-combination skin. This product is appropriate for patients with acne and acne-prone skin.

**Product Characteristics:** A liquid gel in a bottle, this 10 percent alphahydroxy and betahydroxy blend should be used on oily to combination skin once or twice a day to help improve clogged pores and impacted areas. SPF-15 sunscreen should be used daily with this product.

**Chemical Action and Design:** A 10 percent mixture of alphahydroxy acids—glycolic, lactic, tartaric, and malic—with betahydroxy acids—salicylic and citric—help to exfoliate the surface as well as the follicle, removing dead cell buildup and loosening pore accumulations. The gel base contains SD alcohol 40, aloe vera gel, and hydroxycellulose, which gives the product its gel-like feel. The pH of this product is 3.5 in compliance with the CIR recommendations discussed in the chapter on performance and active ingredients.

## Product Profile: Lightening Treatment Gel for Hyperpigmented Skin

**Client and Skin Type:** This treatment gel is intended for clients who have splotchy hyperpigmentation, melasma, or chloasma on the face or hands.

**Product Characteristics:** A liquid gel in an amber bottle, this product should be applied every day for best results. Clients using this product must always wear an SPF-15 or -30 sunscreen, because the symptoms being treated are caused by sun exposure. This product oxidizes very quickly, easily turning brown, indicating decreased effectiveness.

**Chemical Action and Design:** An OTC drug, the active ingredient in this product is 2 percent hydroquinone, which suppresses production of melanin by the melanocytes in the basal layer of the epidermis. The gel also contains 10 percent glycolic acid, which helps remove stained surface cells, as well as magnesium ascorbyl phosphate, a vitamin C derivative antioxidant known for its melanin suppressive activity. Hydroquinone is a frequent allergen, and the product should be patch-tested before using on larger areas.

## Product Profile: Benzoyl Peroxide Gel for Acneic Skin

**Client and Skin Type:** This product is designed for acneic skin, grades I and II. Both adults and teenagers can use this product.

**Product Characteristics:** A lotion in a tube-bottle, this 5 percent benzoyl peroxide lotion is used at night only on active acne papules and pustules. A light application to all areas should be followed by dabbing a small amount on any raised lesions. Do not use in the eye area.

**Chemical Action and Design:** This is an OTC drug. A 5 percent concentration of benzoyl peroxide is the active ingredient, which helps flush and exfoliate debris from the follicle. The oxygen released from the benzoyl peroxide kills anaerobic *Propionibacterium acnes* bacteria. The lightweight, glycerin-based lotion is a simple emulsion that serves as a spreading agent for the benzoyl peroxide. Benzoyl peroxide acts as a bleach to fabric and hair. It can be irritating if overused, and some clients are allergic to it.

**Eye creams** are specially designed for the skin around the eye area. This area of the skin is usually more oil-dry and more sensitive than other areas of the skin. Therefore, creams designed for these areas are generally higher in emollient and lower in humectant content. Because the skin around the eyes is very thin, if you "plump it up" by using lots of hydrating agents, you end up making the eyelid look puffy. More emollient is added to these creams to help supplement the lack of oil production associated with the eye area. Because this area is very sensitive, eye creams must be carefully designed not to irritate. Nevertheless, eye creams often do cause irritation and allergic reactions. Eye creams should be used twice daily.

**Eye creams** are designed for the skin around the eye area.

**Neck creams** are also made with more emollients and less humectant. The neck area has thinner skin that dries easily. Neck creams should be massaged into the skin twice daily. They are available in a variety of formulations.

**Neck creams** are made with more emollients and less humectant, because the neck area has thinner skin that dries easily.

**Masks** are designed to treat a variety of skin problems, from oil-dryness to acne. They are formulated with less water than creams, lotions, and fluids and are considerably heavier than any of these products.

**Masks** are designed to treat a variety of skin problems, from oil-dryness to acne.

Masks for oily skin generally contain bentonite and kaolin; these clays are helpful in absorbing excess oil and drying the skin. These clays cause the drying of masks designed for cleansing oilier and combination skin types. These masks may contain other conditioning ingredients. For example, for acne-prone skin the mask might contain sulfur, salicylic acid, or benzoyl peroxide. For oily and combination skin it might contain camphor for soothing and antiseptic action or cornstarch for soothing action.

Dry skin masks often do not dry tightly and contain large amounts of emollients. To give substance to the mask, the chemist may use titanium dioxide or may use a gelling agent or thickener to give the mask a thicker texture. These dry skin masks may contain a variety of plant extracts, conditioning agents, emollients, and humectants. They work by adding water to surface layers as well as emollients, helping to temporarily fill in or plump up small lines and wrinkles. They can have a lasting effect on the skin, particularly if preceded by the use of a good humectant or other active agent. The effects may last up to several days.

Mechanical **exfoliants** usually come in the form of scrubs. They are usually water-based products with a humectant, mixed with some sort of abrasive agent such as almond meal or polyethylene granules or hydrogenated jojoba oil beads. They are applied after cleansing and massaged over the skin. The granules literally "bump off" dead cells from the skin's surface. The humectant keeps the product from overdrying the skin. Exfoliants should be used several times a week for best results. They should be followed by a toner and a night or day cream. New treatments are constantly being developed. Improvements in both active agents and vehicle and delivery transport systems for active ingredients constantly help improve the quality of cosmetics and their positive effect on the appearance of the skin.

## HOW PRODUCTS ARE DEVELOPED

There are many steps in developing new skin-care and cosmetic products. Let's go through the steps involved in developing a new skin-care product.

### Step One—The Idea

The first step is, of course, recognizing the need for a new product. It must be determined that a product is needed and will sell. What is the appearance change that is desired? What type and condition of skin will benefit from this product?

Let's suppose that we want a new cleanser for combination skin. We want a product that will be strong enough to remove some oil from the oily areas of the skin but not so strong that it will strip areas of the facial skin that is more alipidic and prone to dehydration.

### Step 2—Product Characteristics and Client Type

What characteristics do we want this product to have? Will it be a foaming or non-foaming cleanser? Will it be a gel or lotion? How easily will it rinse? Will it have fragrance? How sensitive is the skin we want it to cleanse?

Let's think about the lifestyle of the client that will likely buy this product. We need to know the client type, which is best determined from day-to-day client interaction. What age is the client that is most likely to buy this product? Are they asking for a particular type of product? Have they asked for a particular characteristic?

Let's suppose that we are aiming this product toward a 30–40-year-old client, who is likely to have combination skin. This typical client has a family, and ease of use is important because they do not have a lot of free time. We have determined that the best product for this client will be an easy-to-rinse, lightly foaming cleansing lotion.

### Step 3—Choosing Ingredients and Budgeting

We need to choose the individual ingredients for the product. We talk this over with our chemist, making sure the chemist understands the product idea, the product characteristics, and the client type.

Budgeting is an important part of product development. We need to determine how much we want to charge for this product. What type of packaging will we use? A cheap container will not necessarily support a higher price for the product. Attractive packaging is important, but it is more important here to be practical. Is the packaging type acceptable with the specific chemicals being used in the products? Sometimes packaging materials can cross-react with the chemicals in the product. This must be

**Exfoliants** usually come in the form of scrubs. They are water-based products with a humectant mixed with some sort of abrasive agent such as almond meal or polyethylene granules.

determined. The use of exotic or expensive ingredients may be prohibited to keep the cost and price of the product reasonable.

If this product will foam, we need a detergent foaming cleansing agent. There are many to choose from. We choose a classic detergent, ammonium lauryl sulfate. Ammonium lauryl sulfate is not the strongest detergent, and we can vary the strength of the cleanser by carefully deciding how much detergent we use in the formula. The more we use, the more aggressive the cleanser will be. Ammonium lauryl sulfate might not be the best choice for ultra-sensitive or delicate skin, but this is not the target client or skin type.

With the chemist, we need to decide what type of preservative, emulsifier, thickener, and fragrance to use with this product, based on the type and condition of the skin and the client's lifestyle desires.

## Step 4—The Prototype and Use Testing

A **prototype** product is a product sample that has been developed by the chemist and is ready to try. The sample cleanser will be tried by actual people, and we will gather their opinions about the use of the product. Is the smell of the product nice? Does it rinse well? How does the skin feel after its use? Did it cleanse enough, or did the skin feel stripped? How did other products feel after the skin was cleansed? Did the packaging work well during use?

Of course, we want the client to love the product, but it is important that we get unbiased, honest opinions. If the majority of test participants like all the characteristics of the product, we have an acceptable product. If most of the participants dislike a characteristic of the product, we need to change this characteristic and re-test until we have a product well liked by all participants. This phase of development can take a substantial amount of time.

> A **prototype** is a product sample that has been developed by the chemist and is ready to try.

## Step 5—Independent Testing

If we are making specific claims about the product, we need to arrange claims substantiation testing, performed by an outside lab. Let's say we want to make an irritancy-tested claim. We contract with an independent testing lab to perform irritancy testing on the cleanser. We need to send the lab enough cleanser for testing on 200 people. This testing can take a few months to perform, depending on the type of testing, the product, the claims, and other factors.

## Step 6—Production

All the tests have come back with acceptable results. We have budgeted and chosen our packaging. We need to have artwork made to silkscreen the bottle and make sure that all the labeling complies with FDA regulations. We need to decide on the size of the batch and how many bottles will be produced. The finished product must be tested in microbiology to make sure the product is not contaminated and that the preservative system is working properly.

## Step 7—Marketing

Marketing of a product actually begins with the initial idea. We have to get the word out that the product is great and why people need to use it. Marketing involves every step of the development. Without proper marketing, no one will know how great the product is, and it will not sell well.

As you can see, there is a lot involved in developing a new product. The more claims and more specific the skin condition, the more complicated the development.

## TOPICS FOR DISCUSSION

1. What are the differences between rinseable cleansers and emulsion cleansers?
2. What determines the difference between types of rinseable cleansers?
3. Describe some different types of toners.
4. Describe a good day cream for oily or combination skin.
5. Describe some of the various types of day creams you may find in a salon.
6. What is the difference between a day treatment and a night treatment?
7. Describe some of the different types of products that use AHAs and how they might differ for oily and dry skin types.

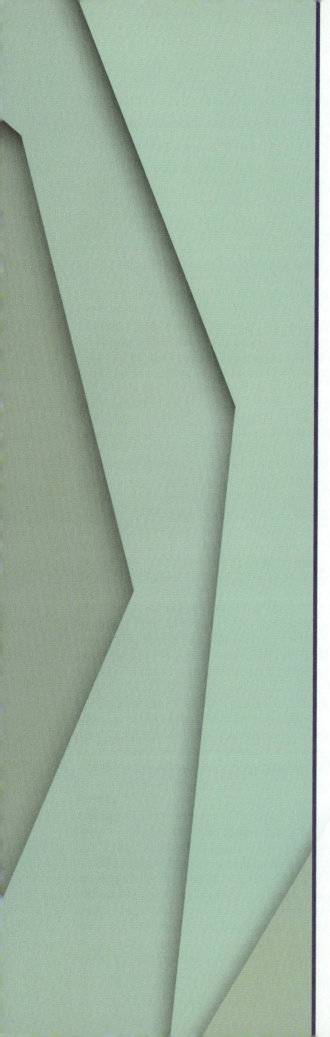

# Claims in Cosmetics

## OBJECTIVES. . .

The Food and Drug Administration (FDA) is a federal agency that regulates the cosmetics industry. In this chapter you will learn about the FDA and how it functions. You will also learn about various claims made about cosmetics and what the difference is between a drug claim and a cosmetic claim.

You will learn what kind of questions to think about when evaluating claims made by cosmetics companies about their products, which you may be using in your salon.

In 1938 the Food, Drug and Cosmetic Act was passed by the United States Congress. The act called for certain definitions of cosmetics and drugs.

The FDA is a federal government agency designed to ensure safety of consumer products, namely food, drugs, and cosmetics. They regulate the cosmetics industry. Unlike the regulation of the drug industry, where approval of drugs is necessary before they are marketed, the FDA only controls cosmetics from a disapproving perspective. The FDA does not "approve" cosmetics.

This means, essentially, that the FDA only regulates the cosmetic industry when the agency disapproves of a claim or product. This also means that cosmetic companies are not required to list their products or formulas with the FDA. They are required to register only on a voluntary basis.

When a "bad" cosmetic is found by the FDA, the agency begins investigating the cosmetic or claim. If the cosmetic is found to be unsafe, or to be making untrue claims, or to be making drug claims, the FDA will move to warn the company or remove the product from the market.

## DRUG VERSUS COSMETIC

The Food and Drug Act of 1938 defines cosmetics and drugs as follows:

◆ "Drug—Articles (other than food) intended to affect the structure or any function of the body."

◆ "Cosmetics—Articles intended to be rubbed, poured, sprinkled, or otherwise applied to the human body or any part thereof for cleansing, beautifying, promoting attractiveness or altering the appearance."

Now, we have discussed how functional or performance agents work on the skin in the last few chapters. But even if these performance agents do affect the function of the skin, we cannot make this claim if the product is a cosmetic. We can, however, say that the product "improves the skin's appearance."

Does this sound silly? Many cosmetic scientists agree, but this is the law as it exists. Cosmetics affect the appearance. If it is claimed that they affect the body or the skin's physiological function, they are considered drugs.

The key words here are *claims* and *intention*. If your product does affect the skin's function, and you do not mention it while selling the product as a cosmetic, you have not broken the law. You are selling the product and claiming that it only improves the appearance.

In other words, what you *intend* for the product to do makes it a cosmetic or a drug. Let's look at a few examples. A toner for oily skin contains an antiseptic ingredient. Killing bacteria is a drug claim because it affects the skin's function and rids the body of possible disease-causing microorganisms. But if the toner contains the antiseptic ingredient and no claim about the antiseptic action is made, then it is not a drug claim. You can say that the toner "helps reduce the appearance of enlarged pores" or "helps remove excess oil" or "improves the appearance of oily areas." These are all claims about the appearance. The fact that the toner also probably kills bacteria is just not mentioned.

Now, if you register the same product as a drug, you can say, "This product helps kill bacteria" or "Kills germs that can cause infection." You are permitted to make these physiological claims if the product is registered with the FDA as a drug. Over-the-counter (OTC) drugs are drug products for which a physician's prescription is not needed. Prescription drugs require a written prescription from a licensed physician. Dentists and veterinarians are also permitted to write prescriptions. Estheticians only use OTC drugs unless they are working directly under the supervision of a licensed physician. OTC drugs that are used by or sold by estheticians may include sunscreens, melanin suppressants for hyperpigmentation, acne medications, and hydrocortisone creams.

Let's explore another possibility. A cream is made with good vehicle ingredients that are very acceptable to the intercellular cement, making the probability of deeper penetration of the product higher. The cream includes the free radical scavengers tocopherol and grapeseed extract that help reduce irritation and redness. It also contains alphahydroxy acids, shown to stimulate new collagen production when used routinely.

Now these theories may be true, but if the claim is made that "this cream makes cells healthier by reducing free radicals with vitamins A and E and stimulates the production of new collagen," a drug claim has been made. You are saying that the product (1) contains vitamins, which are known to affect body functions; (2) "makes cells healthier," which is a physiological claim; and (3) "stimulates the production of new collagen," another physiological claim.

So you have three drug claims in just one descriptive phrase. In order to make these claims, the product would have to be registered as a drug. If you claim that the cream makes skin look healthier and helps to smooth the appearance of rough textures, you have made a cosmetic claim. You have simply made the claim that the product improves appearance and have not said anything regarding physiological function.

Registering a product as a drug means that the product must have had substantial testing to support its ingredient claims, efficacy, and safety. It takes years to have new ingredients approved.

Drug ingredients that have been used for long periods of time safely and effectively are permitted for the uses for which they are approved. Salicylic acid, for example, has long been approved for use in OTC acne products. It is recognized as safe and effective for treating minor acne. Because of its long history of safety, manufacturers may use it in acne products and must register the product if they are making a drug claim. They do not need to file for "new ingredient" testing, though.

## VERBAL CLAIMS

As a licensed esthetician or cosmetologist, you must be careful of what you say to clients regarding claims for products. If you say that a product affects the physiology of the skin, then you intend for that product to have drug effects, and you are therefore making drug claims.

You must be careful never to make a claim about a cosmetic that is a drug claim. Always describe products as "improving the appearance," "reducing the visible signs of wrinkles" (intention: you are reducing the appearance of the wrinkle, not the wrinkle itself), "lessening the appearance of puffy eyes" (you are treating the appearance of puffiness, not the physiological factors that caused the puffiness). Good key words include the following:

- ◆ "helps to . . ."
- ◆ "reduces the appearance of . . ."
- ◆ "diminishes the visual signs of . . ."
- ◆ "improves the appearance of the skin . . ."

Any words that imply that the skin looks better are usually appropriate. Remember, a cosmetic cleanses, beautifies, promotes attractiveness, and alters the appearance.

But what about how cosmetics really affect the skin? It is the opinion of this author and many other cosmetic and health scientists that we need a new product classification with the FDA. It has been proposed that a "cosmeceutical" category be established. A **cosmeceutical** would be defined as a product that is designed for appearance improvement but may have positive physiological effects on the skin on a cellular level. Because cosmetic scientists, as well as scientists from the medical community, do have evidence that many cosmetic ingredients affect the behavior and function of the skin, it is felt by many that this new category is needed. Cosmetologists and estheticians cannot legally explain the actual chemical reactions that occur in products.

**Cosmeceutical** is a product that is designed for appearance improvement, but may have positive physiological effects on the skin, on a cellular level.

# THE LABELING LAW

In 1977 the Federal Packaging and Labeling Act was instated by the FDA. This package of regulations required all cosmetic manufacturers to list ingredients used in their products. The initial reasoning for this package of regulations was to protect consumers who suffered from allergic reactions to particular ingredients.

In theory, the consumer could check the ingredient label for allergen ingredients and thus, theoretically, avoid a potential allergic reaction.

The ingredients are required to be listed on the outermost part of the packaging. If the product is in a box, the ingredients must be listed on the box. Products that are marketed in jars or containers without using a box or other outer packaging must list ingredients on the container itself. The reason for the requirement for the ingredients to be on the outermost surface of the packaging is so the consumer can easily find the list.

Again, in this author's opinion, this is both helpful and hurtful. It is true that a consumer can check for ingredients to which he or she is allergic. But the consumer often reads other chemical names that he or she does not understand or knows nothing about. As an example, a consumer once said that she did not want to use a particular moisturizer because it contained methylparaben, and she did not like to use products with oils in them! The consumer had mistaken the preservative *paraben* for the oil *paraffin*. An easy mistake, perhaps, but nevertheless this illustrates the fact that consumers do not, in general, know enough about chemistry to read an ingredient label, much less know what it means.

The names of the chemical listed must be registered in the CTFA (Cosmetics, Toiletries, and Fragrance Association) compendium, which is essentially a directory of generic chemical names agreed on by the CTFA (which is the largest association of cosmetic manufacturers), the FDA, and other interested consumer and manufacturing groups. These names are used so that any two companies who use a particular ingredient will list it in the same way on their ingredient labels. These names are the industry standard. It is not acceptable by the FDA to list chemicals by their trade names or functions.

The ingredients listed on the label must be in the order of concentration that they are present in the product. In other words, a cream that is a mixture of 70 percent water, 10 percent mineral oil, and 5 percent sodium lauryl sulfate must list the ingredients in descending order of concentration such as, "water, mineral oil, sodium lauryl sulfate. . . ."

The exception to the concentration listing rule is that any ingredient that is less than 1 percent concentration in the product can be listed in any order. In other words, toward the end of the list, after ingredients with 1 percent concentration are listed, any ingredient (at less than 1 percent concentration presence in the product) may be listed in any order.

The sources of the ingredients are also illegal to use on the ingredient label. Some "natural" cosmetics manufacturers will list cetyl alcohol, for example, and then afterwards list in parentheses *(coconut oil)*, indicating that cetyl alcohol is derived from a "natural" source. This is an illegal listing, because it may be confusing to the consumer. Second, just because a chemical is naturally derived does not necessarily mean that the quality is better.

Extracts from plants are usually listed by the plant name and the word *extract*. Plant extracts or derivatives must include the Latin genus and species of the particular extract. For example, lemon extract must be listed as "*Citrus medica limonum* (Lemon) extract." This rule is intended to designate exactly what specific type of plant was extracted. For example, there are numerous types of seaweed. Different types may have very different functions. The extract may or may not contain a solvent such as oil, propylene glycol, water, or alcohol. The term *extract* implies, according to the industry rules, that there may be solvent ingredients in this plant extract constituent. It is generally accepted that this is an acceptable labeling practice. Sometimes extracts will be

listed as "essence of . . ." or "infusion of. . . ." This means that the extract is in a suspension of water or that extracts have been added to water used in the formulation.

# DRUG LABELING

On OTC products, the manufacturer must print an OTC drugs facts label, as discussed previously in the chapter on performance and active ingredients (Figure 12-1). The active ingredients are listed first, with their purpose, and all other ingredients must be listed in the inactive ingredients section of the drug facts label. All OTC products, regardless of type, must have a drug facts label. For example, an eye cream that is also a sunscreen must have a drug facts label. The active ingredients section might read:

| **Active Ingredients:** | **Purpose** |
| --- | --- |
| Octinoxate 4% | Sunscreen |
| Zinc Oxide 4% | Sunscreen |

The inactive ingredients section will list the other ingredients, even if they are performance ingredients with cosmetic benefits:

*Inactive Ingredients:*

Water (aqua), butylene glycol, caprylic/capric triglycerides, stearic acid, glyceryl stearate, propylene glycol dicaprylate/dicaprate, *Aloe barbadensis* (aloe) extract, PEG-100 stearate, cetyl alcohol, glycerin, dimethicone, paraffin, disodium EDTA, sodium PCA, carbomer, sodium hyaluronate, ceteth-20, triethanolamine, silk amino acids, phospholipids, sphingolipids, fatty acids, glycoproteins, glycosphingolipids, cholesterol, propylene glycol, diazolidinyl urea, methylparaben, propylparaben.

There are other rules regarding claims for OTC drugs. Often, there are standard phrases that must be used for usage instructions or to describe functions of the drug, along with warnings. These are mandated by the FDA.

Once again, the FDA is a disapproving agency, meaning that they only investigate a cosmetic if it is believed that a fraudulent or medical claim is being made or if

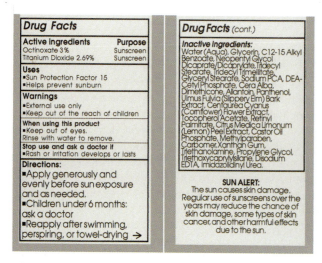

**Figure 12-1** Drug facts label

the product is unsafe or contaminated. The FDA does not approve cosmetics. Claims that a particular cosmetic is "FDA approved" are false, misleading, and illegal.

## OTHER COSMETIC CLAIMS

### Hypoallergenic

**Hypoallergenic** cosmetics are cosmetics that have generally been manufactured without the use of certain ingredients that are known to frequently cause allergic reactions.

A cosmetic that is claimed to be **hypoallergenic** has generally been manufactured without the use of certain ingredients that are known to frequently cause allergic reactions. Fragrance is generally left out of the hypoallergenic cosmetics, because fragrance is one of the main causes of allergic skin reactions.

The term *hypoallergenic* does not mean nonallergenic. There is no such thing as a nonallergenic cosmetic. Someone could be allergic to any one (or more) ingredients in any product in the cosmetic industry. Although there is no way to guarantee a product as nonallergenic, hypoallergenic cosmetics statistically cause fewer allergic reactions.

Some companies run sophisticated allergy tests on their products to demonstrate their hypoallergenic status. This unfortunately still does not guarantee nonallergenicity; it simply shows that the company cares and believes in their product enough to have it tested.

The truth is that most cosmetics today are hypoallergenic and are designed that way. Most companies take great care to make sure their products can be used by most people. It is in their financial interest to do so as well.

### Fragrance-Free Cosmetics

As discussed earlier, many cosmetic manufacturers purposely do not use fragrances in their products to reduce the chances of allergic reaction. Such products may still have an odor or smell. This is the odor of the actual ingredients used in the product formulation. However, not adding fragrance to a cosmetic is a generally good idea, when possible.

### Preservative-Free Cosmetics

**Anhydrous** products are treatment products that do not contain water.

Recently, thanks largely to the advancement in silicone technology, some preservative-free cosmetics have been developed. These treatment products are **anhydrous**, which means they do not contain water. Water is an essential element to sustain life of pathological bacteria. Most of these products are serums, based with silicone mixtures or petrolatum. Most cosmetics and skin-care products do contain preservatives, which are necessary to inhibit growth of harmful bacteria.

### Noncomedogenic

This means that certain ingredients that are known to cause comedone development and acne flareups have not been used in these cosmetic formulations. Fats and emollients are the principal agents that cause these reactions.

Unfortunately, there is no standard industry definition of the word *noncomedogenic*, and the FDA does not require that testing be performed to make such a claim. Unfortunately, certain companies take advantage of lack of rules and make claims that their products are noncomedogenic without performing the proper testing. For much more information on noncomedogenic testing, see the chapter on comedogenicity.

### Nonacnegenic

Often this term is used interchangeably with noncomedogenic, but *nonacnegenic* means that the product has been designed not to cause comedones to develop or

follicle irritancy that can cause immediate acne flareups. It can take as long as six months for comedones to form, whereas follicle irritancy potentially can cause an acne flareup much more quickly.

Again, a variety of tests for follicle irritancy can be run, but some companies make the claim without proper testing.

## Dermatologist Tested

Once again, this can be a very confusing term. Generally, ethical companies mean that the product has been tested for irritancy under the supervision of a dermatologist. One writer asks the question, "Dermatologist tested—for what?". That's a good question. This can be a misleading term.

## Natural Cosmetics

One of the latest rages in cosmetic development is so-called "natural" cosmetics. Naturally derived ingredients in cosmetics have been used for decades. Although nature has some wonderful chemicals to contribute to the cosmetics industry, they are not sufficient by themselves, nor are they always superior to synthetic chemicals.

The fact is that in one form or another everything comes from the earth. Think about it. Even the ingredients used to make plastic come from Mother Nature.

Natural products can also cause allergic reactions. For more on this, see the chapter on sensitive skin. Do not choose a cosmetic solely on the basis of its "naturalness."

## Organic Cosmetics

The term "organic cosmetics" is probably also supposed to mean that the cosmetic ingredients used are derived from "natural" sources. The term *organic* actually means that the chemistry of a substance involves the element carbon.

## Puffing

*Puffing* is a term used to describe the way some companies make their products sound better. This is actually an insulting term, because it usually used to mean that the cosmetic company is making the product sound better than it actually is.

Most companies want their products to sound good. Companies that use outrageous claims to promote their products, like "face-lift in-a-jar," make the entire industry suffer. Companies that promote their cosmetics for their real benefits are fortunately in the majority. However, there is always one unscrupulous company that will make outrageous claims in order to make money. Fortunately, consumers soon find that their claims aren't true.

## Animal Testing

Some companies claim that they do not perform testing on animals. Although many companies do not believe in excessive animal testing, certain tests must be performed to ensure a safe product.

Formulas often are not tested on animals, but almost all ingredients used in cosmetics have, at one time or another, been tested on animals. This is the only way to make sure that the individual ingredients are safe for human use.

In general, cosmetics companies have made a legitimate effort to reduce animal testing, eliminating excessive and unnecessary testing. However, some important tests cannot be performed without using animals.

Some estheticians are single-mindedly against animal testing. Many of these estheticians do not understand that it is vital to ensure ingredient safety. Some of these safety tests cannot be run without the use of animals.

**In vitro** refers to scientific testing that occurs outside of a living organism. It has not been tested on a live specimen.

Rapidly developing technology may eventually eliminate animal testing. Laboratory-produced skin, and other **in vitro** tests not performed on live organisms, are being discovered. Progress is being made, but as of this writing there are still a few very important safety tests that cannot be run without the use of animals. We all hope that eventually this will no longer be an issue, but we also must be scientific enough to understand the need for nontoxic products that are safe for human use.

## International Companies

Some products are imported from other countries where laws regarding cosmetics may be different than those of the United States. Because of this, some companies make claims that are legitimate by their country's standards but are illegal or misleading by U.S. standards. Importers of these products should be aware of these differences and change claims that are not permitted in the United States. Although many companies are extremely conscientious about this, a few companies, out of ignorance, do not make the proper changes.

Today's consumer is generally better informed than consumers of years past and knows better than to believe unrealistic claims. Unfortunately, enough "bad guy" companies have "cried wolf" often enough that the consumer is often wary when buying cosmetics.

## Discussing Claims with Clients

Always try to be honest with clients about a product's true benefits. Hard selling only offends clients. Estheticians should educate their clients about proper products for their skin. The client is only interested in making the skin look the best it can look. Do not make promises you can't keep. Each client has unique problems and conditions, and clients will not always react to products in the same way. There is no way an esthetician can absolutely be sure any product will work. All an esthetician can do is give the best advice possible.

## BUYING PRODUCTS FOR YOUR SALON

You will, no doubt, attend many trade shows throughout your career where cosmetics companies display their products for you to purchase. You should do your homework before you purchase products from any company.

You should ask many questions before buying a product line. Some of these questions are as follows:

1. Are the theories used by the company's products rational?
2. Do they make legitimate claims? If the product sounds too good to be true, it probably is too good to be true!
3. How much care do they take in developing cosmetics?
4. Are their products formulated with allergies and comedogenicity in mind?
5. If they make claims about hypoallergenic or noncomedogenic products, do they test their products?
6. Are these tests run by the company or by an independent testing company? (It is better if they are performed by an outside company—they are less likely to be biased.)
7. Are they willing to explain their testing procedure and results?
8. Are their prices competitive with similar products?

9. Do they use ingredients that you have never heard of? If you are current on your skin-care journal reading, you should be aware of new and innovative ingredients that are legitimate.

10. What is the company's history? Who is its founder, and what are the founder's credentials?

The more education you have, the better you will be at selecting the best reputable companies. Be careful not to be pressured. Good, solid companies don't mind if you think about a purchase before making it.

Many more questions should be asked of companies before you choose a line. You should investigate their reputation with colleagues you respect. You should look into their marketing programs and find out if they are accessible if you have questions and how fast their service is.

The bottom line is are they honest, and do they have a quality, legitimate product?

## TOPICS FOR DISCUSSION

1. What does the FDA regulate?
2. Why is the FDA called a "disapproving" agency?
3. Discuss the Food and Drug Act's definitions of cosmetics and drugs. How do these definitions differ?
4. What is the reason for listing ingredients on a cosmetic label?
5. What are the labeling laws for drug products?
6. Discuss the terms *noncomedogenic* and *nonacnegenic*. What tests should be run to legitimately make these claims?

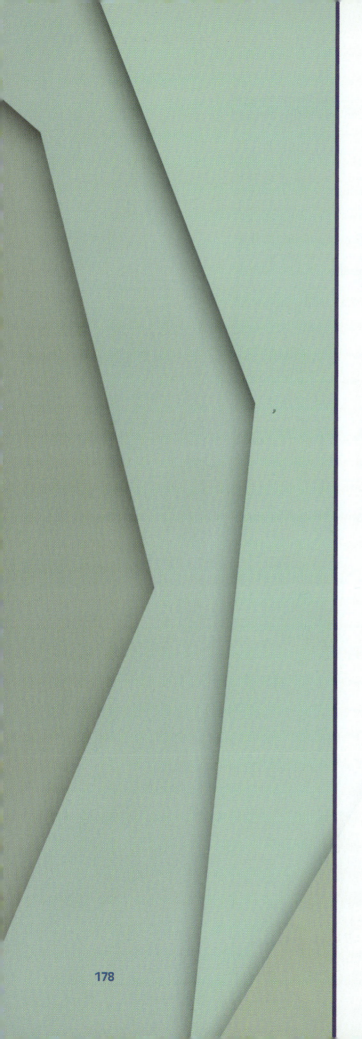

# CHAPTER 13

# Sensitive Skin, Allergies, and Irritants

## OBJECTIVES. . .

Sensitive skin is a common condition frequently seen by estheticians. More and more women seem to have sensitive skin. Skin sensitivities can be attributed to a variety of causes, from hereditarily sensitive skin, to irritant and allergic reactions, to skin that has been overexposed to peeling agents.

In this chapter, we will discuss analysis of sensitive skin, treatment and management of skin that is chronically sensitive, and identifing ingredients and procedures that should be avoided on sensitive skin.

## SENSITIVE SKIN

Sensitive skin is very thin, fragile-looking, pink-colored skin. People with red hair and blue eyes or of Celtic, Irish, Scottish, or British decent are more likely to have sensitive skin than other ethnic groups with darker-colored skin, hair, or eyes. Because of the skin's thinness, the blood vessels and nerve endings are much closer to the surface of the skin. This explains why this type of skin tends to be more easily irritated by skin-care and cosmetic products.

Sensitive skin is becoming more and more common. In some studies, 40–90% of women surveyed report that they believe their skin is sensitive. Some of these clients actually do have sensitive or reactive skin, and some have "perceived sensitive skin," meaning that they simply believe their skin is sensitive. These clients have often had one bad experience with a topical reaction to a skin-care or makeup product or have experienced clogged pores or breakouts from products that were too oily or fatty for their skin. It is important to understand as much as possible about sensitive skin and know that all reactions are not fully understood by medical science.

## ANALYSIS OF SENSITIVE SKIN

Sensitive skin is often obvious on examination. It is most often Fitzpatrick Type I, which always burns when exposed to the sun. It is often thin in appearance, bruises easily, and blanches (or turns white) easily when touched. **Blanching** is caused by pressing on the thin skin, which actually pushes the blood away from the surface tissues, thus causing a temporary white, or lighter, appearance (Figure 13-1).

Clients with sensitive skin often report frequent inflammation during their first visit to the esthetician, including histories of **erythema** (redness), **urticaria** (the medical term for **hives** (Figure 13-2), **wheals**, or **welts**), and sometimes **edema** (swelling). All three of these symptoms are **objective symptoms**, which means they can be physically observed or measured. Symptoms like **pruritus** (itching), stinging, tingling, or burning are **subjective symptoms**. Subjective symptoms are felt by the client but cannot be seen by the esthetician. Sometimes, clients will have both types of symptoms, and sometimes only one. The most difficult situation is when the client

**Blanching** refers to the skin turning white when touched firmly with the fingers.

**Erythema** refers to any area of redness associated with a lesion.

**Urticaria**, or hives, is due to allergies.

**Hives** are a localized swelling, usually caused by allergies.

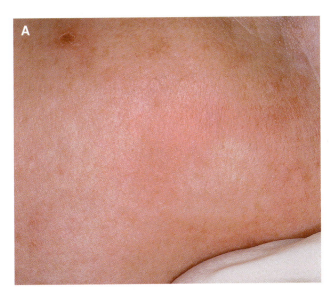

**Figure 13-1A** In sensitive skin, the area appears whiter than the surrounding skin after pressure has been applied and first removed

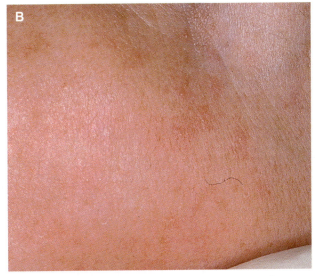

**Figure 13-1B** The skin quickly regains its pink tone, sometimes becoming darker after pressure

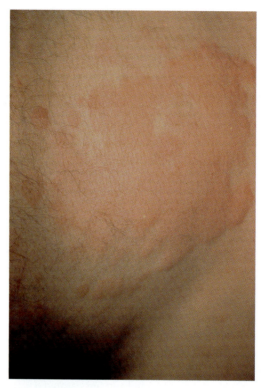

**Figure 13-2** Urticaria (hives) (Courtesy Rube J. Pardo, M.D., Ph.D.)

**Wheals,** or **welts,** are raised, swollen, red lesions, usually caused by allergies.

**Edema** is swelling.

**Objective symptoms,** such as redness or swelling, are physically observable.

**Pruritus** is the technical term for itching.

**Subjective symptoms** include itching or burning.

has only subjective symptoms because the esthetician cannot observe any indications and must rely solely on the feelings experienced by the client. Most scientists now believe that chronic subjective symptoms are neurological (caused by irritated nerve endings) or may be caused by an over-reactive immune system.

The client with sensitive skin will often be very vocal about sensitivity. They have experienced problems before, and they don't want to experience them again! It is important to listen carefully to your client's past experiences to help determine the exact cause of the sensitivity. Even if they don't know the exact cause of the sensitivity, they may be able to give you clues about what to avoid using or what might be appropriate treatment. It is important to ask about previous allergies or irritant reactions to cosmetics, skin-care products and topical medications, drugs, and foods. Some clients may have already had dermatological testing to determine exact causes of allergic reactions.

## SENSITIVE SKIN AND BARRIER FUNCTION

**Permeable** means easily penetrated.

It is extremely important to protect the barrier function of sensitive skin, which, in general, does not have a natural barrier function that is as effective as that of normal, nonsensitive skin. Impaired barrier function means that there are holes in the lipid barrier between the epidermal cells, resulting in a more **permeable** (more easily penetrated) epidermis. Irritants are more likely to cause inflammation because it easier for them to penetrate the skin's surface, where they come in contact with poorly protected nerve endings and blood vessels. Impaired barrier function also results in **transepidermal water loss**, also known as **TEWL**, meaning that water is escaping from the layers of the epidermis, causing severe dehydration and inflammation. If skin is inflamed due to a diminished barrier function, it is more likely to react to skin-care products and cosmetics.

**Transepidermal water loss (TEWL)** is the evaporation of excess intercellular water.

Sensitive skin may be hereditary or transient. **Hereditary** sensitive skin is chronically sensitive for life. **Transient** sensitivity is usually caused by an injury to the barrier function, such as overuse of exfoliants, sunburn, or windburn. These sensitivities usually resolve themselves when the cause is determined and avoided or removed. As an example, an acne client overusing drying agents may have stripped the barrier function and may have redness and burning. When the barrier is restored by reducing the exposure to the drying products, the redness and burning are no longer a problem.

## RESPECTING THE BARRIER FUNCTION

In sensitive skin, avoid exposure to strong detergents and surfactants and other solvents that can decrease barrier function by stripping important lipids. Heavily foaming washes contain large amounts of surfactants, which are chemicals that remove oils form the skin. They are designed to remove excessive oil from the skin surface but often also remove lipids within the intercellular cement. They tend to damage barrier function in fragile, sensitive skin. Propylene glycol is a solvent that can be used on oilier skin but should be avoided on sensitive skin. Products containing **drying alcohols** such as isopropyl or SD alcohol should be avoided on sensitive skin. It is important to note that not all alcohols are drying. Cetyl alcohol, for example, is a wax-like ingredient that acts as an emollient to smooth the skin surface.

Desincrustation products, if used, should be used for a shorter time and only if necessary. Chemicals used for exfoliation, such as alphahydroxy acids and other peeling and exfoliation agents, can damage the barrier function if overused and should never be used if the skin is inflamed. Scrubs, microdermabrasion, brushing, and other mechanical exfoliation techniques must also be avoided.

Oils and water are often mixed to make a moisturizer or skin-care product. **Chemical emulsifiers** are used in products to keep oil-in-water emulsion products properly mixed. They work by dispersing oils from water to keep the product in a uniform blended state. Unfortunately, these normally harmless chemicals can also dissolve lipids within the lipid barrier, damaging barrier function in sensitive skin. State-of-the-art sensitive skin products are now being produced with special **physical emulsifiers** that separate oil particles, keeping the product blended without damaging the barrier function. The process of making these products is known as physical emulsification, which sometimes involves using high-pressure manufacturing techniques. Inclusion of special barrier-protective agents, such as lipids or silicones, helps protect the barrier function from contact with emulsifying agents.

## THE INFLAMMATION CASCADE

The **inflammation cascade** is a series of chemical reactions that occurs when the skin is irritated. When a cell is irritated, it releases special chemicals called **inflammatory mediators**, which alert the immune system to the irritation. The immune system then sends **leukocytes**, or white blood cells, to the site of irritation. Because the leukocytes are mixed with red blood cells, if the inflammation is severe enough, the site of irritation becomes red.

The leukocytes release another special chemical called a **cytokine**. The cytokine signals cells to produce "self destruct" enzymes called **proteases**. Proteases break down substances in the skin including collagen, elastin, and hyaluronic acid, which are responsible for skin firmness, elasticity, and moisture content.

Chronic skin inflammation has a cumulative effect on skin aging and deterioration due to the constant cascade of reactions. Although many of these reactions are **subclinical**, which means that they are not visibly detectable, they produce a slow, gradual deterioration of the skin. Therefore, it is extremely important to avoid

**Hereditary** describes a trait or condition inherited from parents; genetic.

**Transient** means temporary.

**Drying alcohols** are alcohols used in cosmetics that have a drying effect, such as isopropyl or SD alcohol

**Chemical emulsifiers** are agents that cause an even blending of water and oil in a lotion or cream.

**Physical emulsifiers** are used in skin products to separate oil particles, which keeps the product blended without damaging the barrier function.

**Inflammation cascade** is a series of chemical reactions that occurs when the skin is irritated.

**Inflammatory mediators** are chemicals released by irritated cells that alert the immune system to the irritation.

**Leukocytes** are white blood cells.

**Cytokine** is a chemical released by cells that signal other chemical immune responses.

**Proteases** are enzymes that dissolve proteins.

**Subclinical** symptoms, such as stinging or tingling, have no visible appearance.

**Dermatographic** literally means "skin writing." Skin turns red and swells at the slightest scrape.

**Telangiectasias** are small, red enlarged capillaries of the face and other areas of the body.

**Couperose** are small, red enlarged capillaries of the face and other areas of the body.

chronically inflaming or irritating the skin, whether the inflammation is from sun exposure or constantly stripping the skin with harsh chemicals.

## ANALYSIS TECHNIQUE

1. Begin by cleansing the skin with a very mild, nonfoaming, fragrance-free cleanser using cool, wet cotton pads. Using sponges or other implements may cause a friction reaction in extremely sensitive skin. Redness during the very beginning of treatment is a surefire symptom of sensitive skin. Skin that turns red from friction or the slightest touch or scrape is called **dermatographic**, which literally means "skin writing." Persons with dermatographic skin experience hive-like swelling from slight scratches from an activity as simple as carrying a cardboard box if the edges of the box lightly scrape the arms. These same people will be likely to experience swelling and redness from common skin-care practices such as mechanical exfoliation (brushing or scrubs), microdermabrasion, extraction, waxing, hardening masks, and other physical or mechanical skin treatment techniques. All physical treatments previously listed should be avoided as much as possible on these clients.

2. Remove all traces of makeup and cleanser. Do not tone the skin. Toning before analysis may distort the true appearance of the skin and lead to an error in the analysis procedure.

3. Using your magnifying lamp, look carefully at all areas of the skin. Sensitive skin will generally have a pink tone and may have red areas or red or pink splotches or blotchiness. It may have **telangiectasias**, or distended red capillaries, also known as **couperose** (Figure 13-3). Not all clients with telangiectases are sensitive because telangiectases can also be caused by sun damage, injuries, and high blood pressure. However, if the client has both telangiectases and red–pink splotchiness, the client probably has sensitive skin that will likely be reactive to some treatments and products.

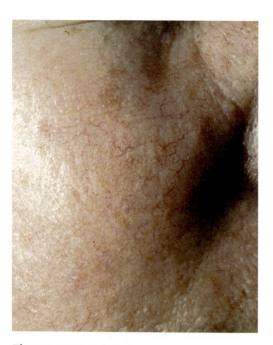

**Figure 13-3** Telangiectasias

4. Press gently on different areas of the face, especially the forehead and cheeks. If these areas turn lighter in color when pressed, this indicates blood close to the surface of the skin, another sensitive skin trait. Remember from our chapter of the immune system that the immune system is largely within the blood and uses the blood as a vehicle to react to invaders. Hence, the sensitive skin may be more likely to have immune responses and reactions because of the close proximity of the blood to the skin surface.

5. Make careful notes of your observations, and write down points of your discussion with the client, along with any pertinent information obtained from the client's health history form.

## ALLERGIES, IRRITANTS, AND CONTACT DERMATITIS

**Dermatitis** is a term used by dermatologists to describe general skin inflammation. There are many types of dermatitis. **Contact dermatitis** means skin inflammation resulting from physical contact with a particular substance (Figure 13-4). **Allergic contact dermatitis (ACD)** means inflammation resulting from an allergy to a particular chemical or substance. **Irritant contact dermatitis (ICD)** is inflammation due to a substance that is irritating the skin. There are many differences between allergies and irritants. An **allergy** is, clinically, the body's immune system rejection of a particular agent or substance. The immune system has identified that substance (or cosmetic ingredient) as a foreign invader. It reacts by sending out T cells to fight off the **allergen**, the offending substance. The immune response is what causes the redness and inflammation associated with an allergic reaction on the skin. This is a true allergy.

**Dermatitis** means inflammation of the skin.

**Contact dermatitis** is an irritation caused by either an allergic reaction or irritation to something or some substance touching the skin or coming in contact with the skin's surface.

**Allergic contact dermatitis (ACD)** is inflammation resulting from an allergy to a particular substance.

**Irritant contact dermatitis (ICD)** is inflammation resulting from a substance that is irritating the skin.

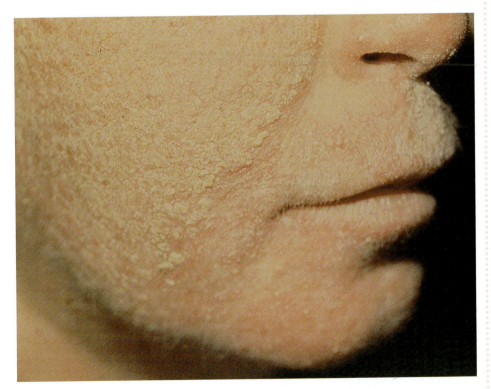

**Figure 13-4** Severe contact dermatitis as a reaction to cosmetics (Courtesy Rube J. Pardo, M.D., Ph.D.)

**Allergy** is the body's immune system rejection of a particular substance.

**Allergen** is a substance that provokes an allergic reaction.

**Irritant** is a substance that can inflame the skin.

As an example, many people are allergic to peanuts. If you had a room full of 1,000 people and gave all of them peanuts to eat, a few would have an allergic reaction. Allergies only affect a small number of individuals.

If you took the same room full of people and gave each person three microdermabrasion treatments followed by five glycolic peels in one session, all would have inflamed skin! This is an **irritant** reaction. An irritant reaction can happen to anyone, whereas an allergic reaction only affects certain individuals.

## IRRITANT REACTIONS

Irritant reactions are usually caused from overexfoliating the skin and are often transient reactions. They are frequently caused by overuse of a product or using too many products that exfoliate. Often this skin is referred to by estheticians as **overprocessed** skin. Irritant reactions are characterized by red, flaking, and uncomfortable skin. It often stings from almost any product applied.

**Overprocessed** describes irritation resulting from overuse of a product or use of too many products that exfoliate.

Irritant reactions can happen to any client. Irritant reactions can be frequency or dose-related. In other words, treatments that are used too frequently and in too high a concentration can be culprits. A 10 percent glycolic acid product may be tolerated, but a 15 percent product may overexfoliate. A client may be able to tolerate a glycolic acid gel once a day but not twice a day. Irritant reactions are usually caused by damaging the barrier function from overwashing, stripping the skin of oils to the point that the barrier lipids are damaged. Detergents, heavy foaming washes, extreme high or low pH products, and clients washing their face too frequently are all examples of treatment that can strip the barrier lipids.

Mechanical irritations are caused by substances rubbing against the skin. They, too, can cause skin reactions such as urticaria. Clothing, bras, belts that are too tight, helmets, chinstraps, poorly fitting eyeglasses, and even playing the violin can cause skin reactions and dermatitis.

Mechanical exfoliants, including scrubs, brushes, microdermabrasion, roll-off (gommage) products, should all be avoided or used sparingly on sensitive skin, and should NEVER be used on obviously inflamed skin.

Drying chemicals such as isopropyl or SD alcohols, drying clay masks (particularly if left on too long or used too often), and peeling/exfoliation agents such as alphahydroxy acids (glycolic, lactic, etc.), benzoyl peroxide, sulfur, resorcinol, and salicylic acids can all cause an irritant reaction if overused or used in too high a concentration. Hereditarily sensitive skin is especially vulnerable to this type of irritant reaction.

Stimulating treatments that increase circulation can also cause irritant reaction. Overuse of hot steam, aggressive and stimulating massage, too much extraction, and some essential oils and aromatherapy treatments can all set off irritant reactions, especially in known sensitive skin.

The main goal in treating irritant reactions is to remove the source of the irritation.

Clients who are overprocessed tend to try to many products at once and may be a little obsessive about anti-aging and having perfect skin. Clients may need education about the overuse of certain products or attempting to exfoliate too often. Using products that help to repair barrier function may be helpful in resolving the reaction. A thorough consultation and education session with the client may help her understand the stripping of the barrier function and subsequent irritation. Set a very specific program for the client using simple, fragrance-free, nonstripping products that have been tested for irritancy potential. Make sure she understands that she is not to use ANY products not in the program.

# ALLERGIC REACTIONS

When a person develops a routine allergic response to a substance, the person has become **sensitized** to that substance. The substance or chemical is known as a **sensitizer**. The immune system has identified this particular substance as a foreign invader. **Sensitization** to a particular product may take place after many exposures or uses of that product or ingredient. This can even take place after *years* of using a product! **Late onset allergies** are allergies developed to a product after years of use.

Signs of an allergic reaction usually involve edema (swelling) and erythema (redness) and may involve neurological symptoms (pain, stinging, burning, itching). Other symptoms include the following:

**Rash**—a splotchy, red, usually flat area, sometimes associated with itching. The area is seldom raised.

**Wheal** (also called a **welt**)—a raised lesion associated with allergy.

**Hives** (also known as **urticaria**)—a group of wheals with surrounding erythema. They often itch and sting. Hives are caused by the release of a hormone-like chemical called **histamine**.

Histamine causes dilation of blood vessels to the area. **Antihistamines** are drugs that combat the formation of histamines. Often associated with nasal allergies to decrease swelling of the nasal tissues, antihistamines are also used to treat skin allergies. In severe allergic reactions, dermatologists may inject antihistamines.

**Sensitized** is having developed an allergic reaction to a substance.

**Sensitizer** is the substance or product a person has developed an allergic reaction to.

**Sensitization** refers to the process of becoming allergic to a substance and the establishment of antibodies that will always react to exposure to that substance.

**Late onset allergy** is the development of an allergy to a cosmetic after years of use.

**Histamine** is a hormone-like chemical released during allergic reactions.

**Antihistamines** are drugs that are produced to combat the formation of histamines.

# COMMON ALLERGENS

Clients who have allergies are frequently allergic to similar ingredients. It is important to know these ingredients and avoid them when treating sensitive skin with allergy histories and tendencies.

**Hypoallergenic cosmetics** are skin-care or cosmetic products that have had many well-known allergens removed. These ingredients have a history of causing allergic reactions in many people. Hypoallergenic does not mean nonallergenic. There is no such thing as a nonallergenic cosmetic! More and more companies now claim that their products are designed for sensitive skin. Unfortunately, no one really governs this claim. Skin-care and cosmetic products intended for sensitive skin should be tested by an independent testing laboratory for potential irritancy and allergies.

**Hypoallergenic cosmetics** are cosmetics that have generally been manufactured without the use of certain ingredients that are known to frequently cause allergic reactions.

## Fragrance Allergies

Many different fragrances, derived from various sources, are used in skin-care and cosmetic products. Some are natural, having been derived from plants, such as essential oils. Turpenes extracted from trees are another variety. Some musks are derived from animal by-products, and synthetic fragrances are developed.

The beauty and esthetics industries frequently use fragrances in many products for their psychological effects; they also use them during aromatherapy treatments. These agents certainly can be pleasant for the client who has nonallergy–prone and nonsensitive skin.

**Fragrances, however, are the number one cause of cosmetic allergies.** It does not matter if the fragrance is natural or synthetic. Frequent fragrance allergens include eugenol, hydroxycitronellal, cinnamic alcohol, geraniol, and ylang ylang. One of the basic rules in treating sensitive skin is to use as few ingredients and as few products as possible. Fragrances, including essential oils, can contain as many as 600 individual chemicals. Combining these chemicals with vehicles and delivery systems can increase the potential for skin penetration and, therefore, increase the potential for skin reaction.

There are approximately 400 essential oils, which are also fragrances or groups of fragrances. Many essential oils have had very little scientific testing and may present a major problem for sensitive skin.

Another interesting fact is that so-called natural products that contain a lot of botanical ingredients actually require more preservatives to be added because of the breakdown of the plant ingredients and the presence of fungi in the plant extracts. Many people think of natural ingredients as being less irritating, but they actually can be more irritating because of the presence of so many chemicals in each extract and the need to use larger quantities of preservatives to inhibit the growth of unwanted organisms in the product.

Essential oils, although naturally derived and widely used in esthetics, can be a problem for sensitive skin. Although they are natural, one extract may contain a large variety of chemical components, including proteins, a major biochemical cause of allergic reactions. They are fragrances, and many are stimulating to the immune and circulatory systems, which can cause redness and inflame sensitive skin. It is best to avoid these ingredients and treatments when dealing with sensitive or redness-prone skin.

Fragranced products should be avoided when treating any reactive, sensitive, or allergy-prone skin. There are products available to the esthetician that are fragrance-free. Some products are labeled "no added fragrance," "no artificial fragrance," or "perfume-free." This is not the same as fragrance-free. Fragrance-free products have no obvious fragrance whatsoever.

## Color Agents

Color agents are used in skin-care products strictly for marketing appeal and generally have nothing to do with the function of the product. There are clients sensitive to various color agents. Because they serve no purpose besides making the product visually attractive, they can easily be omitted from formulations designed for sensitive skin.

Color agents used in makeup products are a different story. They are obviously used for their visual appeal on the skin. However, many clients with very sensitive skin have difficulties finding makeup products that do not cause problems. Color agent allergies are often associated with lipstick and eyeshadow allergies. Swollen, peeling lips characterize lipstick allergy after using a particular lipstick. Eyeshadow allergy shows up as red, flaking upper lids and sometimes lower lids. Although it is possible to be allergic to any color agents, many people are allergic to the D & C yellow colors and the D & C red colors.

## Preservatives

Preservatives are necessary ingredients in almost every skin-care or cosmetic product and in many foods and drugs. The function of a preservative is to keep harmful bacteria form contaminating these products.

Although preservatives must be used in almost all cosmetic and skin-care products, they are, unfortunately, a very frequent allergy-producer. There is no strict rule to determine allergies and sensitivities to preservative ingredients.

The most frequently used preservative complex in the cosmetic industry is paraben. Methylparaben, propylparaben, butylparaben, and ethylparaben are used in literally thousands of cosmetic formulations. It has been estimated that 1 percent of the U.S. population is allergic to these preservatives.

Imidazolidinyl urea is the next most commonly used preservative. It is often used with methylparaben and propylparaben because these three agents work well together against a large number of microorganisms.

Many preservatives work by emitting minute quantities of formaldehyde. Unfortunately, formaldehyde is a well-known skin irritant. Preservative ingredients that emit formaldehyde are known as **formalin donors**. Commonly used formalin donors include imidazolidinyl urea, diazolidinyl urea, 2-bromo-2-nitropropane-1, 3-diol, DMDM hydantoin, and quaternium compounds. These important ingredients do not cause problems for most people, but they may be problem ingredients for people with sensitive or allergy-prone skin and skin with impaired barrier function.

The parabens make up, again, the most common preservative system and are not formalin donors. Phenoxyethanol is another nonformaldehyde–releasing preservative, often used with the parabens. Methylisothiazolinone is another preservative that does not release formaldehyde. Methylisothiazolinone is often coupled with its chemical cousin methylchloroisothiazolinine, and both are primarily used in rinse-off cleansers and products because they have caused some allergies in leave-on products such as lotions and creams when used together.

Although these ingredients are not formalin donors and generally are considered the safest preservatives for allergy-prone skin, they still may cause problems in some individuals.

If you are treating clients who have known preservative allergies, in addition to checking labels for documented allergens, you should also patch-test each individual product on the client before using in larger areas. Second, it is best to have a variety of products with different preservative systems on hand. For more information on preservatives, see the chapter on cosmetic chemistry and functional ingredients.

**Formalin donors** are preservatives or chemicals that release small amounts of formaldehyde.

## Sunscreen Allergies and Sensitivity

Sunscreen ingredients are another potential source of skin allergy. Para-amino benzoic acid, better known as PABA, is not commonly used anymore in sunscreens because of its allergen potential. PABA is an excellent UVB (ultraviolet B) sunscreen agent, but unfortunately it caused many allergic reactions. Padimate-O and Padimate-A are chemical cousins of PABA. Oxybenzone, also known as benzophenone-3 is another good sunscreen ingredient with occasional allergic reactions.

The two sunscreen ingredients that are the least likely to cause allergies are zinc oxide and titanium dioxide. Zinc oxide is the white cream that surfers use on their noses to prevent sunburn. Both these agents are **physical sunscreens** that work by reflecting the sun rather than absorbing it. In the past few years, new technology has been developed to micronize these normally white, opaque ingredients so that they can be easily mixed into a product without looking white and powdery on the skin. The downside to these ingredients is that, when used alone, they must be placed in rather thick formulations to suspend the sunscreen agents evenly throughout the product. To make a more user-friendly product that is not thick and uncomfortable to wear, companies often mix zinc oxide or titanium dioxide with a different sunscreen such as octinoxate (also known as methoxycinnimate) or octisalate (also known as octyl salicylate). Mixing some of the physical sunscreen with an absorbing sunscreen such as octinoxate produces a product that is lighter weight, is easy to use, and does not look white on the skin. In addition, a mix of these ingredients provides excellent broad-spectrum protection against UVA and UVB sunrays.

**Physical sunscreens** work by reflecting rather than absorbing UV rays. Examples are zinc oxide or titanium dioxide.

## Salicylate Allergies

Many people are allergic to the salicylates, a group of chemicals related to salicylic acid. Salicylic acid in its oral form is aspirin. Be careful to screen products carefully if your client tells you she has an aspirin allergy or salicylate allergy.

Salicylic acid is a betahydroxy acid, frequently used for treating acne and oily skin. It is also used in exfoliating products, and some chemical peels. Although it is an excellent ingredient for these skin conditions, salicylic acid should never be used on clients with aspirin or documented salicylate allergies. Octisalate (octyl salicylate) and phenyl salicylate are excellent sunscreen ingredients and likewise should be avoided in clients with salicylate allergies.

## Other Sunscreen Irritations

Many people complain that sunscreen burns their eyes. This often occurs when the client gets hot and perspires when wearing the sunscreen. Often the client has applied too much product or has gotten the product too close to the eyes.

Advise your client to apply the sunscreen 30 minutes before going out into the sun. This will allow the sunscreen to absorb better into the skin and avoid running into the eyes. Using a cream-based sunscreen rather than a gel seems to work better for many of these clients.

Another helpful tip for clients is not to apply sunscreen on hot skin. Many clients will wait until they are already outside to apply sunscreen. Any irritating factor will be more pronounced when applied on skin that is at an elevated temperature. Again, advise the client to apply the sunscreen before going outside.

Gel screens are lighter weight products and are in general more comfortable for oily and acne-prone skin. They are, however, not very water-resistant. They often have a base that is SD alcohol, which may irritate some sensitive skin when applied.

## Nail Products

Many nail products contain formaldehyde or a formaldehyde derivative. Many people are allergic to nail products. Nail polish, hardeners, conditioners, top and base coats, and other nail chemicals often contain these allergens.

Eyelid allergic reactions and irritations are often caused by nail products. People rub or touch thin, delicate eyelids with painted or treated nails.

## Acne Product Allergies and Irritations

Because many acne products are also exfoliants or peeling agents, they tend to irritate the skin. Some irritation caused by acne products is often necessary for the products to work. Slight redness, minor inflammation, and flaking or peeling skin is a fairly normal occurrence, especially when first using peeling agents to treat acne and oily skin. Although allergies to acne products are certainly possible, most of these are irritant reactions and can be resolved by applying the product less often, applying a smaller amount of product, or using a decreased strength of the product. Clients frequently misinterpret irritant reaction as allergies. However, severe peeling, redness, or swelling is NOT normal and may indicate an allergic reaction or more severe irritant reaction.

Treating acne on sensitive skin can be tricky. You may find that your client cannot tolerate nightly use of an acne medication or exfoliating agent. For these clients, recommend that they apply the product lightly every other night. On the alternate night, suggest that they use a noncomedogenic, fragrance-free, hydrating fluid. Alternating these two products seems to work well for many clients with sensitive-oily or sensitive-acne skin. The theory is that you are peeling one night and hydrating the next. Therefore, you are reducing the amount of irritation and soothing the skin on alternate nights.

Another helpful solution for clients sensitive to acne peeling agents is to have the client use them daily, but only for short periods, slowly building up to a longer exposure. For example, a sensitive skin client may only use benzoyl peroxide for 10–15 minutes the first night of treatment. If this short treatment is tolerated, on the next night the client can leave the product on for 30 minutes, and so on. This will slowly build the client's tolerance for the treatment. Your client will learn or establish her own tolerance level.

Benzoyl peroxide, an excellent acne treatment, is available in several strengths. The standard strengths are 2½%, 5%, and 10%. Sensitive clients often tolerate 2½% much better than the higher strengths.

There are some clients who are truly allergic to benzoyl peroxide. These clients experience much more severe redness and possibly edema. They should completely discontinue the use of benzoyl peroxide.

There are several alternatives for clients who are allergic to benzoyl peroxide. They are alphahydroxy acids, sulfur, sulfur combined with resorcinol, and salicylic acid.

Salicylic acid is generally a milder treatment for acne than benzoyl peroxide, but it cannot be used by clients with salicylate allergies. Salicylic acid has already been discussed as a possible allergen. Salicylic acid, however, is a good alternative for sensitive acne clients who are not allergic to salicylates.

Sulfur or sulfur combined with resorcinol are standard alternatives to benzoyl peroxide and are some of the oldest acne treatments. Unfortunately, again, some clients are allergic to sulfur, resorcinol, or both. Some clients will tell you they are allergic to sulfur, when they are actually allergic to sulfa, an oral antibiotic. It is important to clarify with the client what type of reaction she experienced. Most people allergic to oral sulfa are not allergic to topical sulfur.

Alphahydroxy acids, in particular glycolic acid, are not OTC-approved acne ingredients. However, they are excellent and generally gentle exfoliants that help remove dead cell buildup that can cause comedones and therefore are very helpful ingredients for clogged and acne-prone skin. Sometimes they are mixed with salicylic acid. Alphahydroxy acids seem to cause very few allergies, but they can cause stinging and if overused can cause irritant reactions resulting in redness and flaking. Also, some alphahydroxy products have pHs that are very low and acidic and cause barrier function problems. Look for home care products that have a pH of at least 3.5. They are safer and less irritating than lower pH products.

In general, when treating oily or acne-prone sensitive skin, the key rule is to be slow and less aggressive with treatments and products. Avoid harsh washes, astringents, and scrubs, and stick to one gentle product for exfoliation. Routine use of a gentle, noncomedogenic, fragrance-free hydrator helps to balance moisture that can be lost from exfoliating products.

## Common Allergens

The following list of common cosmetic allergens may help you pinpoint possible allergic or irritant ingredients when helping your client with sensitive or allergy-prone skin. Remember, no ingredient is nonallergenic! All of these ingredients have important functions in cosmetics, and listing it here does **not** mean they are bad ingredients. Many can be used successfully on sensitive skin. These ingredients, listed by type, are simply some of the more common allergens and irritants that may affect sensitive skin.

## Fragrances

Clove oil
Eucalyptus
Jasmine
Sandalwood oil
Cinnamics
Essential oils
Geraniol
Musk ambrette
Other plant oils

## Preservatives

Methyl-, propyl-, ethyl-, or butylparaben
Imidazolidinyl urea
Diazolidinyl urea
Quaternium-15
Benzalkonium chloride
Triclosan
Methylchloroisothiazolinone/methylisothiazolinone
2-Bromo-2-nitropropane-1, 3-diol
DMDM hydantoin
Phenoxyethanol

## Sunscreens

PABA
Padimate-O
Padimate-A
Octinoxate (methoxycinnimate)
Octisalate (octyl salicylate)
Oxybenzone (benzophenone)
Methyl Salicylate
Avobenzone

## Other Ingredients

Hydroquinone
Propylene glycol
Salicylic acid
Alphahydroxy acids (glycolic, lactic, malic, tartaric)
Benzoyl peroxide
Sulfur
Resorcinol
Tocopherol
Triethanolamine
Formaldehyde
Hydrolyzed animal protein
Lanolin

## NONCOSMETIC ALLERGIES

**Hard water** is water that contains a lot of minerals and lime.

Frequently, you will have clients who are allergic to products other than cosmetics, but these allergies will result in skin symptoms. Many clients are allergic to nickel, which is frequently used in powder laundry detergents and jewelry. Dryer sheets or fabric softeners cause problems for some individuals. Clients with nasal allergies will sometimes have skin reactions related to their nasal allergies. Clients with obvious and chronic allergies should be referred to an allergist. **Hard water** is water that contains a lot of minerals and lime. Hard water can contribute to dry and irritated skin, especially on the body and especially in the winter months. If your client lives in an area with hard water, suggest to the client that they consider installing a water softening system that removes minerals from the water. This may be particularly advisable for clients who suffer from atopic eczema (see chapter on medical conditions).

# EYELID DERMATITIS

A frequent problem seen by the esthetician is **eyelid dermatitis** (Figure 13-5). The eyelid skin is the thinnest skin on the human body and is also the most sensitive to allergies and irritants. Red, flaky, swollen upper and/or lower eyelids are signs of eyelid dermatitis. If you see a client with eyelid dermatitis, you need to check the following:

1. Has the client started any new eye treatment, eyeshadow, liner, mascara, false eyelashes, or any other new eye products?

2. Is the client wearing nail polish? If so, is it a new color or brand?

3. Has the client had a nail service recently?

4. If yes is the answer to question 3, did the nail technician use any new treatment?

5. Does the client have a new hand cream?

6. Does the client have a history of nasal allergies?

7. Has the client had an eyebrow waxing recently?

8. Is the client taking any new prescription drugs?

9. Does the client wear contact lenses and therefore use contact lens solution?

10. Does the client use eye drops or have any new eye drops?

All or any of these factors can cause eyelid irritation and dermatitis (Figure 13-6). If the reaction is severe or chronic, the client should be referred to a dermatologist, ophthalmologist, or allergist.

Frosted eye shadow, and those containing **mica**, can be a source of irritation on the lid. Besides products used directly on the affected eye skin, nail and hand products cause many of these eye skin irritations. Clients touch their eyes, or wipe their eyes, and the skin comes in contact with the nail or hand product.

Suggest that they remove all products from the eyes and hands until the inflammation clears completely. Then, they can add one product at a time, waiting a few

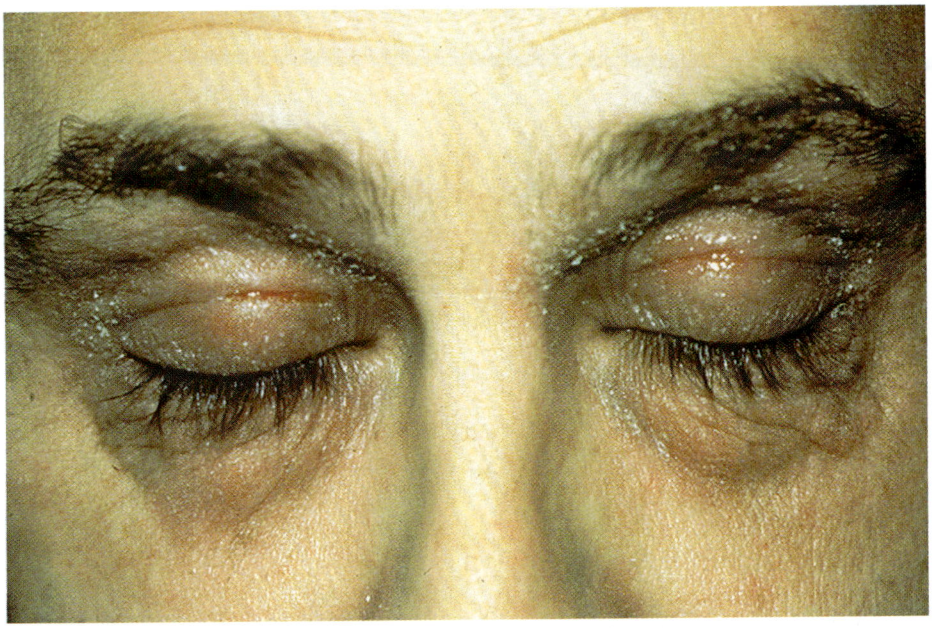

**Eyelid dermatitis** is a lid irritation resulting in swelling and redness of the eyelids.

**Mica** is a coloring agent used in makeup to cause a shiny effect.

**Figure 13-5** Eyelid contact dermatitis from cosmetics (Courtesy Rube J. Pardo, M.D., Ph.D.)

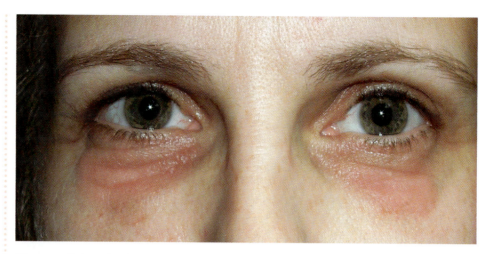

**Figure 13-6** Irritant eye reaction after using a new eye product (Courtesy Mark Lees Skin Care, Inc.)

days between adding each product. If the irritation re-occurs, often the offending product can be determined.

Clients using systemic steroids for treatment of autoimmune diseases, such as lupus, frequently have lid dermatitis. These clients should be referred to their doctor for treatment.

Clients with a history of eyelid dermatitis should avoid waxing the eye area should avoid using frosted or excessive use of eyeshadow, fragranced eye creams, or other products for the eye. Simple products with few ingredients are the best ones for these clients.

## TREATMENT CONCEPTS FOR SENSITIVE SKIN

There are several basic concepts that are widely accepted when treating sensitive skin:

1. Be very careful about protecting the barrier function of the skin. Use products that support the barrier function, and avoid any product or procedure that might strip or impair it, including strong foaming soaps and cleansers.

2. Avoid known irritating and sensitizing materials, products, and procedures. This includes fragrances; certain preservatives; many "natural" ingredients (many of which have little or no irritancy research data); stimulating products; or products that can injure the barrier function such as strong soaps, surfactants, solvents, and emulsifiers. Avoid any ingredient to which the client has had a previous allergic or irritant reaction.

3. Use products that have been shown through independent testing to have low **irritancy potential**. This means that the product has been determined to be unlikely to cause irritation or allergy. It does NOT mean that the product will be appropriate for every single client. Remember, somewhere in the world, there is someone allergic to every single ingredient.

4. Certain ingredients added to skin-care products have been shown to decrease sensitivity. These include **chamomile extract, cornflower extract, licorice extract, bisabolol, stearyl glycyrrhetinate, dipotassium glycyrrhizinate, matricaria extract,** and **azulene.** Also, the inclusion of ingredients that protect or enhance the barrier function, such as lipid complexes, are helpful in a sensitive skin product.

**Irritancy potential** is the tendency of a substance to cause skin irritation.

**Chamomile extract** is a soothing agent.

**Cornflower extract** is a soothing agent.

**Licorice extract** is a soothing agent.

# IRRITANCY AND ALLERGY TESTING

Products developed for sensitive skin should be tested by an independent laboratory to determine their irritancy potential (Figure 13-7). There are several types of irritancy testing:

1. Primary irritation testing, also known as a 48-hour patch test, involves the simple procedure of applying a small amount of the product (or ingredient) to be tested to the back skin of test participants, occluded with a bandage (hence the term patch testing), and checking the area for any irritation 48 hours later. This is a very simple, basic, inexpensive test and should be administered and interpreted by a board-certified dermatologist. This test, to be truly reflective of irritation potential, should be run on at least 50 people. The more people tested, the more reliable the results of the test.

2. A repeated insult patch test (RIPT) is similar to the primary irritation test but considered by physicians and scientists to be much more reliable and indicative of potential sensitivities or allergy potential. The human patch is tested over and over again on the same participants. Breaks of a few days are taken between test applications, allowing the body's immune system time to develop antibodies to the material being tested. Repeat testing will likely reveal any delayed allergy.

**Bisabolol** is an agent that is added to cosmetics designed for sensitive skin.

**Stearyl glycyrrhetinate** is a soothing agent derived from licorice extract.

**Dipotassium glycyrrhizinate** is a soothing agent derived from licorice extract.

**Matricaria extract** is a soothing agent.

**Azulene** is a hydrocarbon that is derived from the chamomile flower.

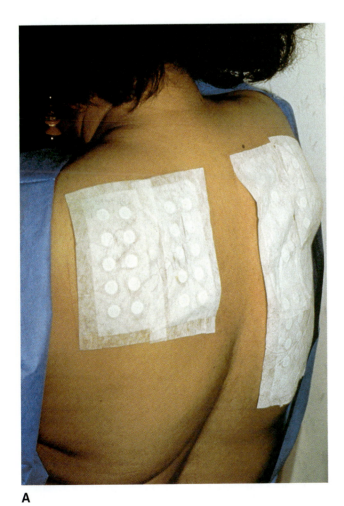

A

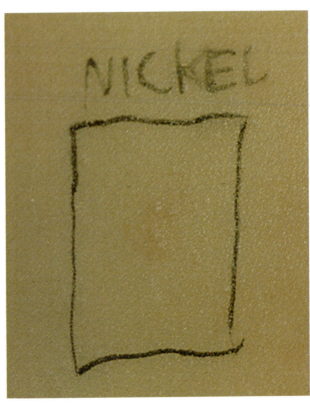

B

**Figure 13-7** *A*, Dermatologist-administered patch tests for various contact allergies. *B*, Positive patch test indicating allergy to nickel (Courtesy Rube J. Pardo, M.D., Ph.D.)

Again, to be reliable and be considered scientifically sound, this test should be run on 50 to 200 test participants.

3. Tape strip irritation testing is a relatively new test in which the skin is purposely irritated by repeated pulling tape off the area to be tested. Once the skin is irritated, the test product is applied and observations are made. Irritating products will increase the irritation in the stripped area.

4. Sensitive skin actual-use testing involves using participants who are known to have sensitive skin. These individuals actually use the product for several weeks, and the results are observed at the end of the time allotted. This is a good method of testing but involves many variables. This test should be run in addition to one of the more controlled procedures, such as the RIPT.

## TREATMENT CONTRAINDICATIONS FOR TREATING SENSITIVE SKIN

In the treatment room, it is advisable to avoid the following procedures when treating clients with sensitive or redness-prone skin:

1. Avoid heat exposure, including close or prolonged exposure to steam. There are cool ultrasonic steamers now available, and these may be helpful in providing the hydration of steam without the heat.

2. Avoid paraffin, electric heat masks, or exothermic mineral-type heating masks. Extremely cold compresses should also be avoided.

3. Use nonfragranced products. Fragrances are the number one cause of cosmetic skin allergies and may also be irritants.

4. Microdermabrasion, brushing machines, enzyme treatments, gommages (roll-off treatment products), and granular scrubs may be too aggressive.

5. Waxing should be avoided on sensitive skin.

6. Use of extremely low pH exfoliation chemicals, such as low pH alphahydroxy (AHA or glycolic) acid or enzymes. AHA exfoliants with pHs of 3.5 or greater are usually acceptable as long has the skin is not already inflamed. When in doubt, don't use it! Avoid using exfoliation too often on sensitive skin.

7. Avoid prolonged or vigorous massage, such as petrissage or any deep or rapid manipulation, which may be too stimulating and increase redness. Effleurage, shiatsu, gentle tapotement, and manual lymph drainage (if you are trained on it) are usually acceptable for use on sensitive skin.

8. Avoid overdrying masks or leaving clay masks on too long. Drying clay masks are often not appropriate for sensitive skin.

9. Many essential oils or aromatherapy products may be too stimulating for sensitive skin.

10. Extraction must be gentle and limited to a brief period to avoid redness. As you become better acquainted with an individual client's skin, this can be adapted.

11. Avoid heavily mentholated or alcohol-based treatment.

12. Avoid using isopropyl or SD alcohol-containing products on sensitive skin.

## SUGGESTED TREATMENT FOR SENSITIVE SKIN

1. Dampen the skin using cool (not cold), wet cotton compresses. Apply a gentle, nonfragranced cleanser with your gloved hands. Gently massage the cleanser and remove the cleanser using cool, wet cotton pads. Sponges and other cleansing implements are often too rough-textured for sensitive skin.

2. Apply a lightweight, nonfragranced hydrating fluid designed for sensitive skin to the face. Carefully focus steam on the skin. If warm steam is used, it should be used at a distance of 18–20 inches from the face and should be used for only a few minutes. Cool steam, if available, is preferable. Cool steamers use ultrasonic vibration to create a mist that is not hot. They help hydrate the skin without exposing the sensitive skin to heat. Cool steam can be used for a longer period of time.

3. Brushing and suction should be avoided on sensitive skin.

4. Most sensitive skin should not be exfoliated during treatment. If you do use a bead-type exfoliant, it should be nonfragranced, very gentle, and easily removed from the skin. Enzymes and peels of any type should be avoided.

5. Gentle extraction may be performed using the cotton swab technique discussed in the extraction chapter. Avoid using comedone extractors on sensitive skin. If skin begins to welt, redden severely, or swell, stop extraction immediately. Extraction should be limited to 3–4 minutes only, particularly during the first visit.

6. Spray the skin with a mild, nonfragranced, nonalcoholic toner designed for sensitive skin.

7. If the skin is still very red after extraction, apply cool, wet compresses for about five minutes. Do NOT apply any product, just cool water compresses. This will help calm the skin.

8. After the skin has cooled down, apply a nonfragranced hydrating fluid designed for sensitive skin. Using very gentle movements such as effleurage, massage the face for a short period of time, using the fluid as the treatment product for massage. If redness increases, discontinue the massage immediately and remove the product with cool, wet cotton compresses.

9. Assuming the skin is not inflamed, apply some more of the same hydrating fluid. Unfold a 4 × 4 piece of gauze and place across the face. Move cool "globes" over the gauze to help the hydrating fluid penetrate. These globes contain refrigerant, much like the type used in freezer packs. It is important NOT to apply the globes without the gauze buffering the contact. Remember, any treatment should be cool but not cold. High frequency or ionization treatments at low settings can be used on most sensitive skin; however, the cool globes are a better choice, at least during the first treatment.

10. Apply a nonsetting, nondrying, nonfragranced gel mask designed specifically for sensitive skin. It should contain soothing agents such as matricaria, chamomile, or licorice extract. Allow the mask to sit on the face for 10 minutes. Check frequently with the client to make sure the treatment is not stinging or burning.

11. Wet the mask with a cool spray, and remove the mask with cool, wet cotton pads. Pre-wetting the mask allows less pressure to be used during the physical removal of the mask.

12. Apply a gentle, nonfragranced hydrating fluid or sunscreen designed for sensitive skin.

14. It is best to avoid immediate makeup application after a treatment on sensitive skin. Wait at least two hours before makeup application.

## IF A CLIENT HAS A REACTION IN THE TREATMENT ROOM

Occasionally, a client will experience a reaction in the treatment room. Most of these reactions are irritant reactions and are mild. They are not true allergies. A client may complain of a particular product stinging or burning. Some products such as alphahydroxy acids are supposed to cause a mild tingling sensation. Most of the time these minor sensations quickly dissipate.

Red, rashy, and swollen skin, however, is not normal. Severe burning and stinging are not normal. If a client experiences extreme burning, redness, or swelling, remove whatever is on the face immediately by using cool cotton pads. Apply cool, wet compresses or spray atomized water on the skin to soothe it. Many times simply removing the irritant greatly reduces the inflammation. It is always best to end the treatment if a client has a reaction. Applying further products, even if you are trying to help, may only aggravate the reaction. Wait several days until the reaction has completely subsided for before trying a different plan. As always, severe reactions should be immediately referred to dermatologist.

## HOME CARE CONCEPTS FOR SENSITIVE SKIN

You should spend some time educating your clients about treating their skin at home. Emphasis should be placed on avoiding activities and procedures that can increase redness or the chance of reactions and damage to the barrier function. The following should be stressed to the client. Many of these concepts are similar to the previously mentioned treatment room concepts.

1. Avoid heat, including sun exposure, sitting directly in front of fireplaces, and hot water in the shower or when cleansing the skin.
2. Avoid sun exposure, and always wear a sunscreen during daylight hours.
3. Avoid scrubs and strong exfoliants.
4. Avoid fragranced products.
5. Avoid any product that feels stimulating or overdrying.
6. Avoid overcleansing or cleansing the skin too often.
7. Avoid alcohol-based products.

Some clients with sensitive skin who also have rosacea may experience more redness during the following:

Drinking alcoholic beverages, especially red wine.
Eating spicy foods.
Drinking hot beverages.
Exercising, especially in the heat or sun.
Getting into a hot car.
Sitting in saunas and steambaths.
Experiencing extreme temperature changes of any type.

## HOME SKIN-CARE PROGRAMS FOR SENSITIVE SKIN

Choosing the right products for sensitive skin can be tricky. Products that can be used on most skin types may be too irritating for sensitive skin. You must also keep in mind the client's skin type (oily, dry, etc.) and address other skin conditions the client may have.

Always choose products that are nonfragranced; free of formalin-releasing preservatives; and most importantly, have been tested for potential skin irritation (Figure 13-8). Check with your supplier to make sure the products have been independently tested.

Unfortunately, there are many products that claim to be appropriate for sensitive skin but have never been tested for irritant potential. Even if the product has been tested, remember that there is no such thing as a nonallergenic product.

The following is a model home care program for sensitive skin with information on precautions:

**Cleansers.** Cleansers should be very mild and should not foam much. As with all products for sensitive skin, cleansers should be nonfragranced. Cleansers for sensitive skin should be easy to remove without applying much pressure to the skin. Mild surfactants, such as decyl glucoside or disodium lauryl sulfosuccinate, may provide slight foaming and are generally acceptable. Nonfragranced cleansing milks are appropriate for makeup removal. If the client has oily-sensitive skin, a slight-foaming cleanser may be a better choice.

Cleansers should be applied with fingertips with cool (not cold) water. Clients should be told to avoid any hot water exposure. Cleansers should be removed with extremely soft cloths or cotton pads.

**Toners.** Toners should be fragrance-free and alcohol-free. They should contain soothing agents and should be free of solvents such as propylene glycol. (Butylene glycol is acceptable.) Spray-type toners are convenient and often used for sensitive skin.

**Antioxidants.** Antioxidants can be very helpful for soothing sensitive skin. They are theorized to work by interrupting the cascade of chemical reactions that lead to inflammation. These are most often in serum form. Green tea, white tea, and grapeseed

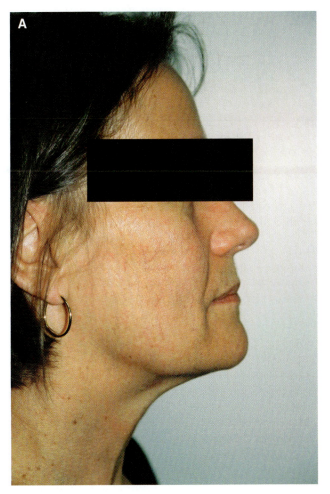
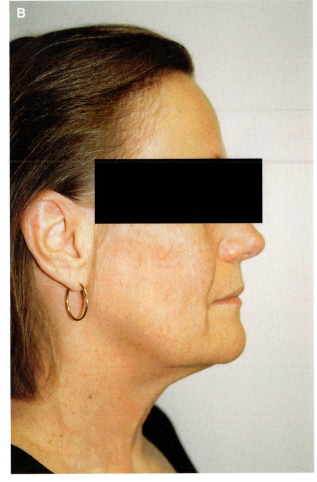

**Figure 13-8** Using a home skin-care regimen that is specifically designed and tested for sensitve skin can show reduction in the appearance of facial redness and telangiectasias (Courtesy Mark Lees Skin Care, Inc.)

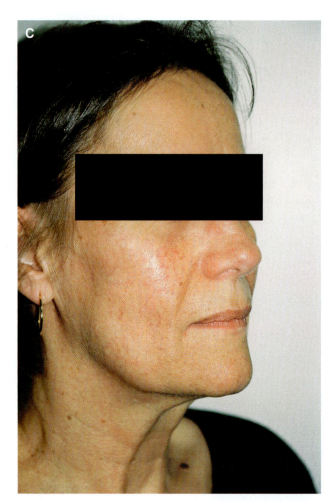

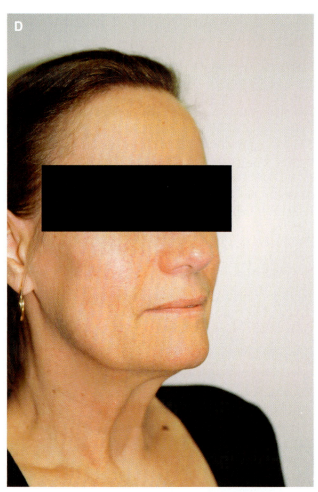

**Figure 13-8** *(Continued)*

extract are examples of soothing antioxidants. Be careful with some serums that have a very low pH. If it burns when applied, the pH is probably too low for sensitive skin use.

**Sunscreens.** This is a tricky one. Sunscreen ingredients can cause both allergic and irritant reactions. Look for a product that contains zinc oxide or titanium dioxide. These physical sunscreen ingredients are much less likely to cause irritation. They are sometimes blended with an absorbing sunscreen, such as octinoxate, so they don't appear white and pasty. Look for a product that has been tested for irritancy potential.

**Hydrators and Moisturizers.** These should be formulated carefully so that they are not only formulated without fragrance and other well-known allergens and irritants, but they also do not contain large amounts of emulsifier that can damage the barrier function. As previously discussed, emulsifiers are used in skin-care products to help keep ingredients evenly mixed in the product. They work by polarizing oil throughout the water in a lotion or cream. Unfortunately, when used on skin with impaired barrier function, they can damage the lipids in the barrier function, making the skin even more sensitive and reactive. New technology has developed, allowing products to be formulated without these irritating emulsifiers or with very low levels of the emulsifiers. These are commonly known as physical emulsions and are very helpful when treating sensitive skin. Physically emulsified products are usually in a fluid or lotion form, rather than a thicker cream.

# CONSULTATION WITH THE CLIENT WITH SENSITIVE SKIN

Clients who have sensitive, reactive, or allergy-prone skin tend to be cosmetically "gun shy." Clients with sensitive skin have had reactions before and are skeptical and self-protective because they do not want another reaction.

There are two ways to help calm the client's concerns. First, you must know what you are doing with sensitive and allergy-prone skin, and second, you must convince the client you know what you are doing.

It is important to be honest with the client. Discussing past problems with sensitivity will give you clues on what has and has not worked. Knowing that most clients with sensitive skin should avoid fragrances, formalin-releasing preservatives, stimulants, and other well-known irritants and allergens, add information you obtain from the client to choose the products for her individual skin.

Sometimes clients have had reactions to common irritants, or their skin has become overprocessed through the use of too many exfoliants. Sometimes they have had an **acnegenic** or **comedogenic** reaction, resulting in an acne breakout. This is not the same thing as an allergy, although the client knows they reacted! It is important to try to pinpoint what type of reaction the client has had in the past. This will help you establish if the reaction was transient and simply related to overprocessing, or if the client truly has a reoccurring allergy.

# MEDICAL TREATMENT OF ALLERGIES AND CONTACT DERMATITIS

Estheticians are not qualified to treat allergic reactions. Clients who have extremely sensitive skin and seem to react to many products should be referred to a dermatologist or an allergist for allergy testing. The doctor will apply small amounts of products or ingredients on the client's back and will cover each product with a small bandage. About 24 or 48 hours later, the doctor will remove the bandages and check each site for any form of inflammation. Any area that is red or swollen indicates an allergy or irritant for that client.

Standard treatment for cosmetic allergies is to remove the offending ingredient or product from use by the client. The doctor will tell the client which products or ingredients seem to cause problems and advise the client to not use those products or ingredients.

Clients having severe allergic reactions may need hydrocortisone cream prescribed by the doctor. Hydrocortisone helps to eliminate symptoms of the reaction, but it is not a cure for the problem. The client must avoid using the offending product or ingredient. In severe cases, sometimes the dermatologist will prescribe oral steroids or antihistamines.

## Salon Patch Testing

A simpler type of patch test for allergens or irritancy potential can be performed by the esthetician. If your client has extremely sensitive or a history of routine skin inflammation, it is a good idea to patch test new products on the client's back or forearm before trying them on the face. The procedure is simple:

1. Check the client's past allergy history. Does the client have any known ingredient, drug, or cosmetic allergies? If she does, you can eliminate using any products that contain those known allergenic ingredients.

2. Type and analyze the client's skin as you normally would.

3. Select the proper home care program based on your analysis, taking special precaution to avoid fragranced products or any product with long ingredient lists.

**Acnegenic** is the tendency of a product or ingredient to irritate the follicle, which can cause sudden flares of pimples

**Comedogenic** is the tendency of a topical substance to cause a buildup of dead cells resulting in the development of comedones.

The simpler the product's ingredients, the better. Also avoid essential oils and other stimulating ingredients.

4. Apply a small amount of each product on the client's back or inner forearm. Each application should be about the size of a coin. Cover each with a hypoallergenic bandage strip. Many sensitive clients are also sensitive to some bandage adhesives. Assign a number to each product tested, and write the number on the bandage. Record each number and corresponding product on the client's record. For example, the test cleanser is #1, the toner is #2, and so forth.

5. Instruct the client not to wash the area for the test period, usually 24 or 48 hours.

6. After 24 or 48 hours has elapsed, remove the bandages, and check each area for irritation, redness, swelling, itching, urticaria, or flaking. If you see any of these signs, avoid using that product.

7. Notice what ingredients are in the offending products and compare the ingredients with the ingredient list of a product to which the client did not react. What do the two lists have in common, or more importantly, what is different about the two lists? For example, if the client reacted to her day cream, which contained a certain preservative, but did not react to her night cream, which contained a different preservative, you can deduce that the client may be allergic to the preservative in the day cream.

It takes time and experience to be good at isolating allergens. An essential knowledge of cosmetic chemistry and ingredients is also important. If you do not feel comfortable with these procedures, refer the client to a dermatologist for patch testing.

Unfortunately, sometimes what occurs on the back does not occur on the face! The facial skin tends to be more sensitive than the body skin on most people, and, occasionally, a product that did not react on the back will react on the face. Again, it is important that both the esthetician and the client realize that allergic reactions are seldom predictable, unless it is known what specific ingredients are the allergens.

## EXTERNAL FACTORS THAT INFLUENCE SENSITIVITIES

Besides general product allergies and irritants, other factors can influence reactions and possibly worsen their severity. Climate is one of these factors. Hot, humid weather or extremely cold weather can play a part in sensitivity. Hot, humid weather is often accompanied by a high pollen or mold count in the air, which can make people who are allergic to pollen or mold more susceptible to nasal and skin reactions. Heat alone can aggravate sensitive skin, enlarging capillaries and making the skin more reactive than normal. Extreme cold can have similar effects. Cold weather and wind tend to impair the barrier function, reducing intercellular lipids, increasing chances of dehydration, and making the skin dry and flaky. Dry, flaky skin is always indicative of impaired barrier function and more likely to have reactions. Severely dehydrated skin may burn or tingle when moisturizers are applied. Sunburned skin can also react to cosmetics or other topicals more easily.

The general rule with all these climatic effects is to strictly adhere to all the concepts we have already discussed. Avoid stripping cleansers; avoid strong exfoliants or overuse of exfoliants, washing the skin too frequently, or any product or treatment that is fragranced or stimulating. As seasons change, you may need to adapt the proper products for the client.

## Drug Influences on the Skin

Certain drugs make the skin more sensitive to sun exposure and can cause **photoallergic** reactions. Tetracycline and other antibiotics, as well as systemic

**Photoallergic** describes drugs that can cause allergic reactions if the patient has sun exposure while using the drug.

steroids and other drugs, can increase sun sensitivity or cause allergic reactions when the client has sun exposure during their use.

Clients using prescription topical keratolytics such as the retinoids (i.e., Retin-A®, Tazorac®, Differin®, etc.) should avoid sun exposure. These drugs can also make the skin more sensitive to products the client may have used for a long time. Make sure you have carefully looked at all the client's medications to help determine if these may be factors in the sensitive skin.

If the client has started using a prescription peeling agent, you must eliminate the use of any other peeling agent or exfoliant, including home exfoliants such as alphahydroxy acids or benzoyl peroxide. Too much exfoliation impairs barrier function and causes sensitivity. The client may also need to consult with her doctor concerning proper use of the prescription exfoliant. Often, the client is unintentionally misusing the drug.

## Sudden Reactions

A client will sometimes come into the salon complaining of a sudden rash or other allergic or irritant reaction. See if you can specify any recent changes in the client's skin-care program or if the client is taking any new medications. Always check for new cosmetics or skin-care products, nail products (which can affect the face because the clients touches or scratches her face), or other possible topical contact allergens or irritants. If the client has not changed any home care products, you must look further to see if the client is taking any new medications. There is a possibility that the client has suddenly developed an allergy to a product she has used for a long time.

Have the client discontinue all products, including makeup, until the redness and sensitivity clears completely. Then, one by one, have the client use the products again, adding an additional product every couple of days. When and if the reactive product is added, the client will notice problem symptoms again, and you will know the client has a problem with that specific product.

As always, when in doubt, refer the client to a dermatologist for allergy testing.

## SUMMARY

There are many clients with sensitive skin and allergies. Most symptoms of sensitivity seen by an esthetician are caused by irritants rather than allergies.

Be very careful to help your client not strip the barrier function because this is the bottom-line problem in irritant reactions. Avoid overuse or extremely strong exfoliants and other well-established irritants. Avoid using too many treatments on clients with sensitive skin or products with many ingredients. Look for products that you know have been thoroughly tested for irritancy potential.

When you help resolve the problems for your clients with sensitive skin, you will be their hero!

## TOPICS FOR DISCUSSION

1. What is an allergy?
2. What is the difference between an allergic and irritant reaction?
3. Describe a sensitive skin.
4. Why is barrier function so important in sensitive skin?
5. What are some common allergens that should be avoided for sensitive skin?
6. Why does irritated skin turn red?
7. What are some basic concepts to follow when treating sensitive skin?
8. Why is the client's health history important when treating sensitive skin?

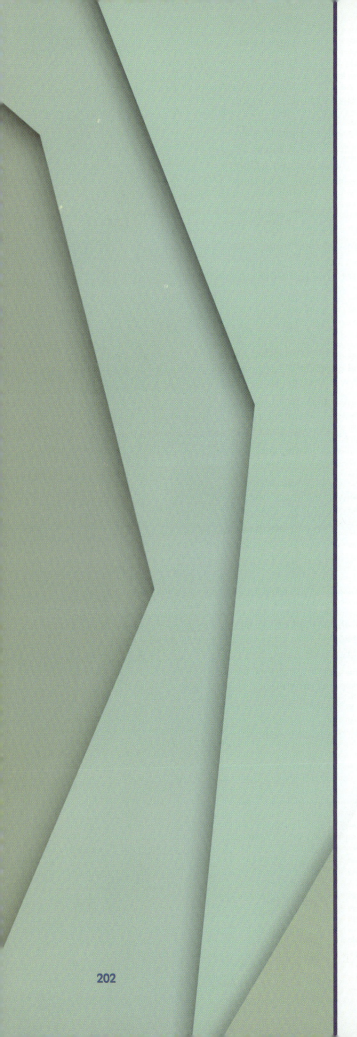

# Rosacea

## OBJECTIVES. . .

Rosacea is a common disorder of the skin associated with diffuse redness, acne-like papules and pustules, dilated capillaries, and other symptoms. Although rosacea is a medical condition and must be diagnosed by a physician, clients with rosacea can be significantly helped by proper skin care.

In this chapter we will discuss the different sub-types of rosacea and what the esthetician can do to help with the esthetic problems associated with rosacea. We will also discuss what causes flares of rosacea and how you can help your client with rosacea avoid flares and worsening of the symptoms of this disorder.

Rosacea, formerly known as acne rosacea, and sometimes referred to as **adult acne**, is a disorder of the skin characterized by redness (erythema), **flushing** (sudden dilation of capillaries causing sudden diffuse redness, often accompanied with a feeling of heat) and turning red very easily, **telangiectases** (dilated or distended capillaries) (Figure 14-1), and sometimes acne-like papules and pustules. A single distended capillary is known as a **telangiectasia**. Areas of telangiectases are also known by the European term **couperose**.

It is important to note that not all clients with telangiectases have rosacea, but almost all clients with rosacea have telangiectases. Telangiectases can also be seen in clients with sun damage and injuries to the skin and can be more apparent in clients with high blood pressure.

Rosacea is a **vascular** disorder, meaning that it is related to blood vessels and circulation of the blood. Rosacea normally affects persons older than 30 years of age, but it can appear as early as 20 or as late as 70- or 80-years-old. The sudden rushing of the blood to the facial skin can stimulate sebaceous glands and irritate follicles, causing large red papules and pustules in the nose, cheeks, and chin areas. When patients with rosacea have sudden redness or breakouts due to their condition, this is known as a rosacea **flare** (Figure 14-2). Rosacea is most prominent in light-skinned persons of Irish, Celtic, or Western European origin.

The sudden flushing of blood to the face triggers the release of a biochemical within the skin called **vascular growth factor (VGF)**. Vascular growth factor, as its name implies, triggers the growth or expansion of new blood vessels, specifically arterial capillaries in the skin. The addition of these new capillaries further increases the chances of flushing. Therefore, the disorder is self-perpetuating, or it continually progresses because of the formation of new blood vessels.

Rosacea may first appear as chronically red cheeks or a chronically red nose (Figure 14-3). Clients may notice flushing, which also produces a warming of the facial skin. Flushing can occur when the client becomes hot, drinks alcohol or wine (especially red wine), or eats spicy foods. Clients with rosacea are very likely to redden whenever they get physically hot, and some may notice flushing during or just

**Rosacea** is a condition of the skin in which the skin turns red very easily.

**Flushing** refers to the reddening of the skin due to stimulation.

**Telangiectases** are dilated or distended capillaries.

**Telangiectasia** is a single distended capillary.

**Couperose** are small, red enlarged capillaries of the face and other areas of the body.

**Vascular** means blood vessel related.

**Flare** is when pimples and redness occur in a person who has rosacea.

**Vascular growth factor (VGF)** is a biochemical within the skin that triggers the growth of capillaries.

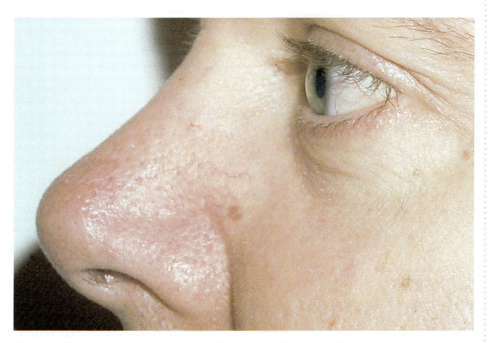

**Figure 14-1** Nose telangectasias. Dilated capillaries, called telangectasias, and a coarse textured appearance of nose ostia are typical of the rosacea client

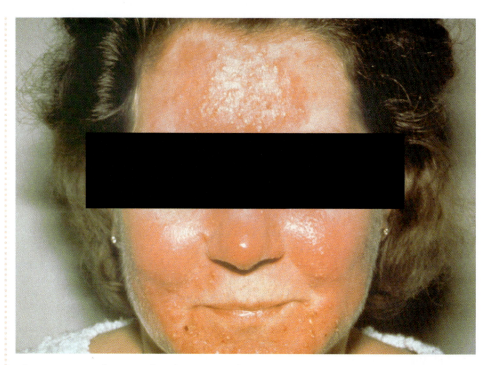

**Figure 14-2** An example of a severe flare of rosacea, which can affect the whole face

**Vasodilation** is the dilation of the blood vessels resulting in flushing.

after exercising. All these activities cause **vasodilation**, or increased blood flow due to dilated blood vessels, resulting in flushing or a rosacea flare.

## CAUSES OF ROSACEA

No one is completely sure of the exact cause or causes of rosacea, but it appears to be hereditary and strongly related to how easily a person blushes. Theories for the cause of rosacea have included the presence of a mite called ***Demodex folliculorum***. It has also been theorized that the presence of excessive yeast on the skin might be a factor. The topical drug used to treat rosacea is an anti-yeast medication, although the reason it works is thought to be because of anti-inflammatory action. An intestinal bacterium found in patients with ulcers, ***Helicobacter pylori***, has also thought to be involved. None of these theories alone have ever been confirmed to be a cause of rosacea because the presence of mites, yeast, and bacteria vary among patients with rosacea. The search for real causes and a cure continues. As of the time of this writing, there is no confirmed cause or cure for rosacea. There are, however, many known successful ways to control and manage rosacea and to keep its symptoms under control for long periods through the use of medical treatment and lifestyle and skin-care changes. When the flares of rosacea are under control for a long time, this is referred to as rosacea **remission**.

*Demodex folliculorum* is a type of skin mite that has been sometimes associated with rosacea.

*Helicobacter pylori* is a type of intestinal bacterium that has been sometimes associated with rosacea.

**Remission** is a phase of disease where the disease is dormant and no symptoms are present.

## LIFESTYLE TRIGGERS FOR ROSACEA FLUSHING AND FLARES

It is evident that constant flushing of the face makes rosacea worse and is responsible for flares. We know that there are certain triggers for flares, and all of these triggers cause flushing of the facial skin. Remember, flares and flushing cause the release of

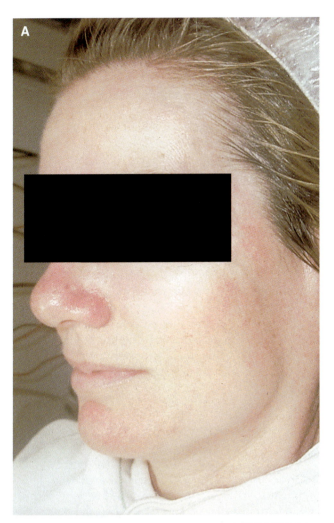

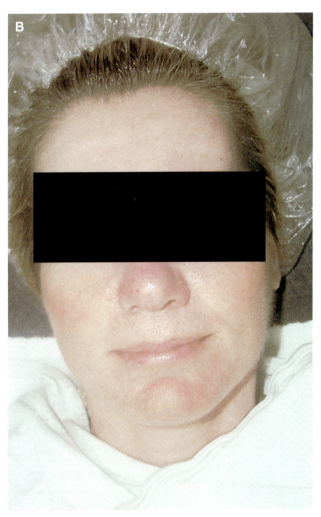

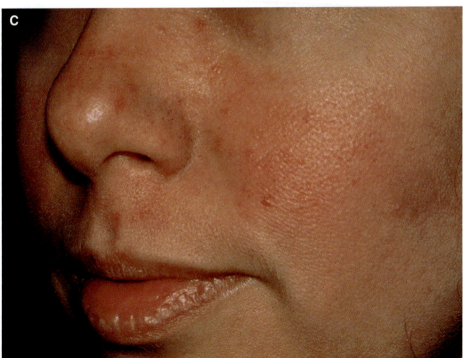

**Figure 14-3A–C** The beginning stages of rosacea. The first symptoms of rosacea may be just a redness pattern across the nose and cheeks or a red, slightly swollen nose (Courtesy Mark Lees Skin Care, Inc. and National Rosacea Society)

biochemicals that grow and expand capillaries, which further increase flushing during subsequent flares.

Flushing triggers, which should be strictly avoided by patients with rosacea, include the following:

- Sun exposure of any type—the worst culprit in rosacea flares. Sun must be avoided at all times. Besides ultraviolet rays, sun also radiates heat, a known cause of flushing and flares. Patients with rosacea should wear sunscreen every day.
- Heat exposure to the face of any type—including exposure when opening ovens, sitting in front of fireplaces, or experiencing indoor heating that is too warm. Allow hot cars to air out before getting in.
- Hot or cold weather.
- Extreme temperatures of any type—including saunas, steambaths, and hot water on the skin. Cold water should also be avoided.
- Ingestion of alcohol, especially red wine.
- Exercise that raises body temperature—it is best that patients with rosacea exercise indoors in air conditioning. If exercise takes place outside, it is best to exercise in the very early morning or after dusk to avoid heat and sun exposure. Exercise in a pool is a good choice, although chlorine might be a trigger, and the skin should be thoroughly rinsed after swimming.
- Hot beverages.
- Spicy foods.
- Emotional stress.
- Caffeinated beverages.
- Aged foods such as hard cheeses.

Not all these factors affect every patient with rosacea. Each individual is different, but heat and sun exposure seem to be factors in causing flushing in almost all rosacea patients. Scientists have determined that certain bacteria on the skin of patients with rosacea produce toxic proteins at higher skin temperatures. These toxic proteins may be responsible for the papules and pustules associated with rosacea.

## Skin-Care Triggers

Some skin-care products and ingredients have been associated with rosacea flares. In general, drying, alcohol-based products; products that evaporate quickly such as many toners and astringents; and any stimulating product containing stimulating essential oils, peppermint, menthol, or other ingredients that increase blood flow may cause a flare.

In general, many of same precautions should be taken for rosacea as for sensitive skin. Make sure any products used have been thoroughly irritancy-tested. Avoid toners, or use an alcohol-free toner that has been tested on sensitive skin. The avoidance of exfoliants, especially granular or rough scrubs, is a good rule. Anything that scrapes the skin can cause redness and a possible flare. Avoid rough sponges, drying and setting masks, or masks that release heat such as mineral masks or paraffin masks.

Any form of heat or extreme cold can trigger flushing. Teach your clients to use tepid water only when rinsing. Pat the face dry, rather than rubbing. Cotton or extremely soft cloths are best for cleansing.

Fragranced products have been known to cause flushing. Fragrance should be avoided when choosing skin-care products for clients with rosacea.

As with sensitive skin, any product that might damage barrier function, such as heavily foaming cleansers, or aggressive peeling and drying agents should be avoided.

## Subtypes of Rosacea

The National Rosacea Society is a nonprofit organization founded for research, education, and support of persons who have rosacea. The society estimates that as many as 14 million Americans have some form of rosacea. They conduct frequent surveys to determine factors that may trigger flares or flushing and assemble committees of dermatologists and other experts to conduct and interpret research about rosacea and its management. An expert committee of the society has divided rosacea into the following four subtypes:

**Erythematotelangiectatic** (ear-ith-theem-a-toe-tell-anj-ee-ec-tatic) **rosacea** (subtype 1) is characterized by diffuse facial redness, patchy redness in the nose and cheeks, and turns red extremely easily (Figure 14-4). Clients may or may not have distended capillaries (telangiectases). Persons with erythematotelangiectatic rosacea may have **transient erythema**, which means that the redness and symptoms can come and go. Facial swelling, skin roughness, dry-looking patches, tightness, and a grainy texture that feels much like fine sandpaper to the touch also may be seen. This grainy texture occurs primarily in the forehead and cheeks. The skin can sting and burn periodically.

**Papulopustular** (pap-u-lo-pus-chu-ler) **rosacea** (subtype 2) often resembles acne (Figure 14-5). The one difference is there are often no clogged pores or comedones present. These larger-than-normal pimples primarily occur on the nose and upper cheeks. There may be a lot of redness in the skin around the papules and pustules. There may be a dehydrated, crinkled appearance to the surface skin in these areas. Subjective symptoms of burning and stinging may also be present.

**Phymatous rosacea** (subtype 3) has a thickened appearance and results in an enlargement of the nose or other facial areas (Figure 14-6). An enlarged nose resulting from rosacea is known as **rhinophyma** (Figure 14-7 and Figure 14-8). The famous comedian W.C. Fields suffered from rhinophyma, with his well-known red, bulbous nose.

**Erythematotelangiectatic rosacea** is a subtype of rosacea that is characterized by diffuse, patchy redness, and a grainy texture.

**Transient erythema** is redness that comes and goes.

**Papulopustular rosacea** is a subtype of rosacea that often resembles acne vulgaris, with large red pustules and papules.

**Phymatous rosacea** is a subtype of rosacea in which the nose has a thickened appearance and the client sometimes has rhinophyma, which is a noticeable substantial enlargement of the nose.

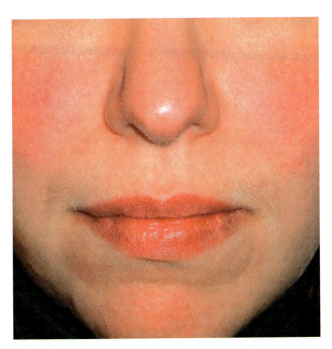

**Figure 14-4** Subtype 1: facial redness (erythematotelangiectatic rosacea). Flushing and persistent redness. Visible blood vessels may also appear (Courtesy National Rosacea Society)

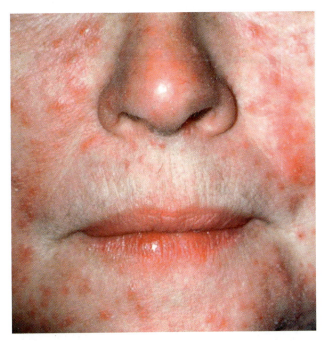

**Figure 14-5** Subtype 2: bumps and pimples (papulopustular rosacea). Persistent facial redness with bumps or pimples. Often seen following or with subtype 1 (Courtesy National Rosacea Society)

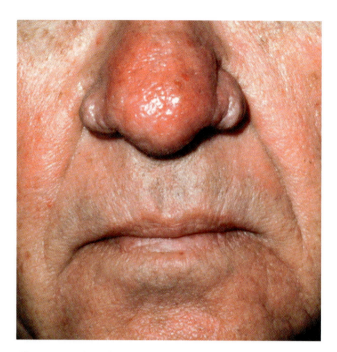

**Figure 14-6** Subtype 3: skin thickening (phyma-tous rosacea). Skin thickening and enlargement, usually around the nose
(Courtesy National Rosacea Society)

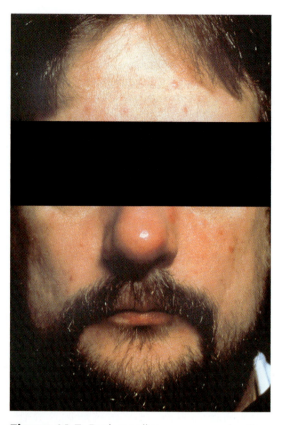

**Figure 14-7** Red, swollen noses can be the beginning of rhinophyma (Courtesy National Rosacea Society)

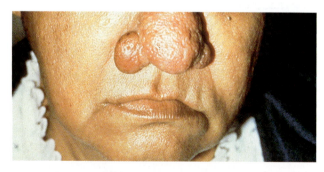

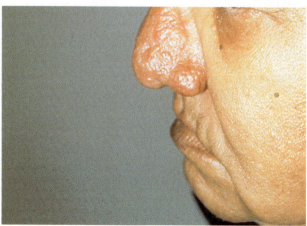

**Figure 14-8** Rhinophyma (Courtesy Rube J. Pardo, M.D., Ph.D.)

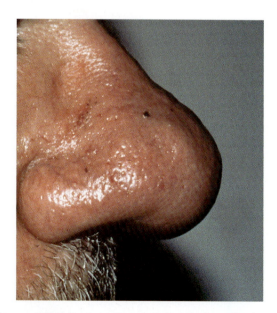

**Figure 14-9** Dark and red distended capillaries, enlarged pores, and enlargement of the nose are shown in this photo of rhinophyma. This nose will also have large amounts of sebaceous filaments and secretions (Courtesy National Rosacea Society)

Many people thought that his big, red nose was caused by alcoholism, but it was actually phymatous rosacea. Alcohol use can cause flares and flushing, but it does not directly cause the thickening of tissues associated with rhinophyma (Figure 14-9).

Phymatous rosacea can affect either women or men, but it is more prevalent in men. It is interesting to note that rosacea is more common in women, but phymatous rosacea is more common in men.

**Ocular rosacea** (subtype 4) occurs in the eye and eyelids, resulting in eye redness (bloodshot eyes), swollen eyelids, **chalazia** (small lumpy, cysts in the eyelids), **hordeolums** (better known as styes), eyelid skin telangiectases, stinging and burning, and other visual problems (Figure 14-10).

## Combinations of Subtypes

It is possible for a client to have more than one subtype of rosacea. Subtypes 1 and 2 are frequently seen together. Some patients with rosacea have all four subtypes.

There is another factor that may affect any subtype of rosacea, known as **granulomatous rosacea**. This is not a subtype; it is more of a factor that can affect the four basic subtypes. Granulomatous rosacea causes hard, nodular papules in the cheeks and around the mouth. They may be red, yellowish, or brown in color, and multiple papules will be identical in size and shape on an individual client.

## Rosacea—A Medical Condition

A physician, preferably a dermatologist, must make the diagnosis of rosacea. Because it is a medical condition, estheticians should not tell their clients they have rosacea, unless a doctor has officially diagnosed it.

That being said, estheticians see rosacea frequently in the salon. Clients may think they have acne blemishes or an allergy to a product. It is important that estheticians be familiar with the signs and symptoms of rosacea, so that they may refer the client to a dermatologist for diagnosis and medical treatment.

**Rhinophyma** is an enlarging of the nose often resulting from a severe form of acne rosacea.

**Ocular rosacea** is a subtype of rosacea that affects the eyes, resulting in eye redness, swollen eyelids and other eye lesions.

**Chalazia** are small, lumpy cysts in the eyelids.

**Hordeolums**, or styes, are infected tear ducts.

**Granulomatous rosacea** causes hard, nodular papules in any form of rosacea.

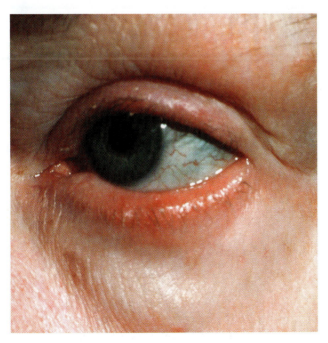

**Figure 14-10** Subtype 4: eye irritation (ocular rosacea). Watery and bloodshot appearance, irritation, burning, or stinging (Courtesy National Rosacea Society)

There are also many esthetic issues that accompany rosacea, and estheticians can certainly help with the appearance problems with rosacea and serve as educators to instruct their clients on proper skin care for rosacea, including products and activities that may trigger flares and should be avoided. Once the diagnosis has been made, and medical treatment has been prescribed, the esthetician can work with the rosacea patient to help determine the proper skin-care products and makeup to help reduce redness and avoid inflammatory products and treatments, and work with the dermatologist to help the client manage the rosacea flushing and, hopefully, avoid flares (Figure 14-11).

## Medical Treatment of Rosacea

The most common topical treatment drug in dermatological treatment of rosacea is **metronidazole**, commercially known as Metrogel®, Metrocream®, Metrolotion®, or Noritate®. **Sodium sulfacetamide** and **sulfur**, under the trade names of Klaron®, Sulfacet-R®, or Novacet®, are another type of topical medication for rosacea. The newest topical drug, as of this writing, is 15% **azelaic acid**, marketed as Finacea®.

**Metronidazole** is a medication used to control rosacea and decrease inflammation.

**Sodium sulfacetamide** is a topical drug agent used to treat rosacea.

**Sulfur** is a topical drug agent used to treat rosacea.

**Azelaic acid** is a topical drug agent used to treat rosacea.

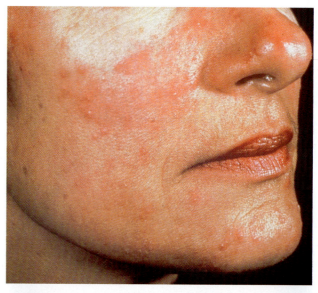

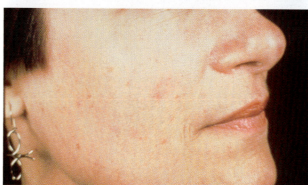

**Figure 14-11** Before and after rosacea treatment. Rosacea can be kept under control by using prescribed topical and/or oral medication, controlling flushing; avoiding heat, spicy foods, and other triggers; and using nonirritating skin care products. (Courtesy National Rosacea Society)

All of these prescription topicals have anti-inflammatory effects.

Oral antibiotics, such as **tetracycline**, **doxycycline**, and **minocycline**, are prescribed by dermatologists for patients with more severe rosacea. Occasionally, the use of laser treatment of telangectasias is used to help control flares and reduce redness and the appearance of these capillaries. In severe cases, a low dose of Accutane®, a drug normally used for grade 4 cystic acne, is also beneficial.

The goal in medical treatment of rosacea is to reduce inflammation; reduce or eliminate flares and flushing; and, in some cases, kill or reduce bacteria associated with papules and pustules.

Patients with rosacea also suffer occasionally from **seborrheic dermatitis**, a disorder caused by an inflammation of the sebaceous gland. The signs of seborrheic dermatitis include flaking and redness in oily areas of the face, especially the eyebrows, hairline, and the sides and the corners of the nose.

Surgical treatment of rosacea is sometimes necessary. Laser treatments may be used to obliterate telangiectasias. Laser resurfacing is sometimes used to remove extensive telangiectases. Removal of these telangiectases slows the progression or worsening of rosacea.

Laser and plastic surgery sometimes are used to reduce or remove excess tissues developed in patients with rhinophyma.

## THE ROLE OF THE ESTHETICIAN IN ROSACEA MANAGEMENT

As we have already discussed, rosacea is a medical condition, and a dermatologist or medical physician must make its diagnosis. Never tell a client he or she has rosacea, unless a medical diagnosis has been made.

However, you may often suspect that a client has rosacea. If you notice that a client has frequent flares of redness, has large papules and pustules without comedones, gets very red during treatment or has redness that is always present and never seems to fade, this client likely does have rosacea. Specific symptoms you may notice include the following:

1. Diffuse redness and distended capillaries, especially in the center of the face, such as the cheeks or nose.

2. Patches of redness in the cheek area, often accompanied by large pores or a grainy texture.

3. Enlarged appearance of the nose, bulbous structure, redness, with very prominent pore appearance of the nose, sometimes appearing rough and bumpy.

4. Turning red very easily or redness after drinking wine or alcohol or eating spicy foods.

5. Flushing that appears after exercise and does not go away quickly.

6. Flares of large, red, solid-looking, or "lumpy" papules and pustules on the cheeks, nose, and chin. Often, there are no comedones in these areas, as you might see in acne vulgaris.

7. Very dehydrated, sometimes flaking, red areas in the nose and cheeks. The skin may appear thick or swollen in these areas, and the client may complain of burning and stinging.

If you notice any of these signs during analysis, refer these clients to a dermatologist for diagnosis and treatment.

Estheticians can play a very important role in the management of rosacea. Educating clients about lifestyle triggers, helping them choose skin-care products that do not trigger flushing, and helping with makeup techniques to help camouflage redness are examples of how the esthetician can help.

**Tetracycline** is an oral antibiotic used to treat more severe rosacea and other acne-related conditions.

**Doxycycline** is an oral antibiotic used to treat more severe rosacea.

**Minocycline** is an oral antibiotic used to treat more severe rosacea and other acne-related conditions.

**Seborrheic dermatitis** is a skin disorder characterized by flaky, red, patchy skin primarily in the eyebrows, T-zone, and scalp. Seborrheic dermatitis is caused by inflammation of the sebaceous gland.

# CHOOSING SKIN-CARE PRODUCTS FOR CLIENTS WITH ROSACEA

In general, the same procedures should be followed as already discussed in the chapter on sensitive skin. The basic principle is to avoid exposure to any product that can cause redness or inflammation. This would include any product that has the potential to damage the barrier function or causes a stimulation of blood flow. Also, make sure that all products are noncomedogenic because exposure to fatty ingredients may worsen the condition, especially in clients with oily skin and rosacea.

Cleansers—Wash-off type cleansers are the best for rosacea skin. They are easy to rinse off and should rinse completely without leaving residues.

Keep in mind the skin type when choosing a cleanser. Oilier clients need cleansers that remove more sebum, but these should not be aggressive and stripping. Dry and dehydrated skin with rosacea needs less aggressive cleansers that foam less. Make sure the product is slightly acidic pH-balanced, particularly if no toner is used.

Toners—Toners can be a problem for patients with rosacea, and are the number one cosmetic trigger for flushing. Avoid any toner with alcohol or astringent ingredients. A nonalcoholic hydrating mist, with soothing ingredients may be tolerated better.

Moisturizers—Nonfragranced, lightweight hydrating moisturizers are the best tolerated. Again, follow the guidelines already discussed in the sensitive skin chapter. Addition of soothing agents like licorice extract, green tea, or silymarin may help reduce redness.

Sunscreens—Sunscreens are very important for patients with rosacea because sun exposure is a major flare trigger. Patients with rosacea, as all clients, should wear a sunscreen every day. Look for a fragrance-free sunscreen that contains a built-in hydrator and soothing ingredients, and check to make sure it has been irritancy-tested. Sunscreens that contain physical sunscreens like zinc oxide or titanium dioxide are the best choices for patients with rosacea.

Exfoliants—Exfoliants must be very carefully chosen, if used at all in patients with rosacea. Mechanical exfoliants, such as beaded scrubs or gommages, tend to aggravate flushing. Probably the best exfoliant is a gentle alphahydroxy (AHA) or betahydroxy (BHA) lotion, but even these can cause flushing in some patients with rosacea. NEVER apply an exfoliant during a rosacea flare.

In general, it is best to start the client on basic products first, and after a few weeks of successful use, add an AHA or BHA exfoliant lotion. Try lightly applying the lotion only every other day until you see how the client tolerates it.

## Soothing Products

There are products that are designed to help soothe sensitive skin, and some of these may be helpful in reducing redness and preventing flushing.

Many of these are antioxidants and are in serum form. Look for ingredients like green tea, white tea, grapeseed extract, and silymarin. These serums are usually used after cleansing and before application of a sunscreen or moisturizer.

## Medication Application

Do not forget that the client's topical medication will have to be applied at some point during the home care regimem. Usually these are applied after cleansing and are allowed to absorb for a few minutes before using a moisturizer or sunscreen. If in doubt, check with the client's dermatologist or pharmacist to know when this important step should take place.

# STEP-BY-STEP HOME CARE RECOMMENDATION FOR CLIENTS WITH ROSACEA

## Morning

1. Wet the face with tepid (body temperature) water. Apply a nonfragranced light foaming cleanser that is easily rinseable. Choose the cleanser carefully, based on the client's skin type and dehydration level. Nonfoaming or low-foaming cleanser may be used for drier skins. In clients with oilier skin, a slightly more aggressive foaming cleanser may help reduce oiliness. In clients experiencing flares, a nonfoaming cleanser is usually a better choice.

2. Apply a spray-type, nonalcoholic toner containing soothing agents and hydrators. Toners have been known to cause flushing, so make sure you choose a toner that has no stripping agents and no fragrance. Pat the skin with a clean, dry towel. It is important to emphasize to the client that the skin should be patted and not wiped with a rough towel that can abrade and cause flushing.

3. A soothing serum may be used to calm redness. These are often hydrating serums with soothing agents and antioxidants that are theorized to interfere with the inflammation cascade. Grapeseed extract and green tea are typical components.

4. Medication usually is typically applied at this step. Have the client check with her dermatologist to determine the exact application step for the medication.

5. A fragrance-free moisturizer, appropriate for the skin type and containing an SPF-15 or higher broad-spectrum sunscreen should be used. A product containing zinc oxide or titanium dioxide as a sunscreen agent is a good idea and is often less reactive than absorbing chemical sunscreens. The presence of soothing agents in the formula may also reduce redness tendencies.

## Evening

1. Makeup should be removed using a nonfoaming, fragrance-free cleansing milk. The client should apply this with the fingertips to slightly dampen skin. Use of cleansing sponges and other implements to apply cleanser may cause redness. After applying and lightly massaging the cleanser to dissolve makeup, wipe off the cleanser with cool, wet cotton pads. Splashes of tepid water will help remove any excess cleanser.

2. Apply toner as in the morning.

3. Apply soothing serum as in the morning.

4. Medication usually is applied at this step. Have the client check with her dermatologist to determine the exact application step for the medication.

5. A lightweight, fragrance-free hydrator with soothing agents should be applied lightly.

# SALON TREATMENT FOR PATIENTS WITH ROSACEA

Typically, the salon treatment used for sensitive skin discussed in the sensitive skin chapter is appropriate. The use of cool steam and nondrying products and the avoidance of stimulating, peeling, and stripping products are best. Keep every step mild and gentle. Extraction, although helpful for oilier rosacea skin, should be as gentle as possible and the duration should be short.

## LIGHT-EMITTING DIODE TREATMENT FOR REDNESS

**Light-emitting diode**, or **LED** treatment, is a fast-flashing light treatment that is often used to treat diffuse redness.

**Photomodulation** is the process of using light to treat conditions of the skin.

**Light-emitting diode (LED)** treatment is a procedure using fast-flashing lights to cause changes in the appearance of the skin. Also known as **photomodulation**, LED treatments use nonburning, low-wattage lights that flash at a rapid rate to energize activities of the skin. Unlike lasers and intense pulsed light, LED does not produce the intense heat that can cause damage to the dermis. LED is used to treat various sun damage symptoms.

LED light treatments have been used to treat diffuse redness in the skin. Although LED does not remove or ablate any skin or dilated capillaries, it can be used safely to minimize redness in clients with rosacea. LED is used by both esthetic clinics and dermatologists' offices. Usually, a series of treatments are administered over a period of weeks. Each machine varies as to treatment protocols.

## GET TO KNOW THE ROSACEA SKIN

Rosacea skins vary in sensitivity levels, oiliness or dryness, and what seems to cause flares. It is best to keep any treatment or home care very simple when first helping your client with rosacea. Pay attention to medications that have been prescribed by the dermatologist, and respect the doctor's instructions.

Have the client keep in close touch with you and monitor his or her progress carefully. You should always start slowly and gently, and can always try other treatments later, when you have established the sensitivity level of the client's skin.

## TOPICS FOR DISCUSSION

1. What might be some differences in procedures or products you would recommend for clients with oily versus dry rosacea? Why?
2. Why should you never tell a client he or she has rosacea?
3. Name several procedures or product types that should be avoided on clients with rosacea.
4. Discuss how medical and esthetics professionals can work together to best help a client with rosacea.

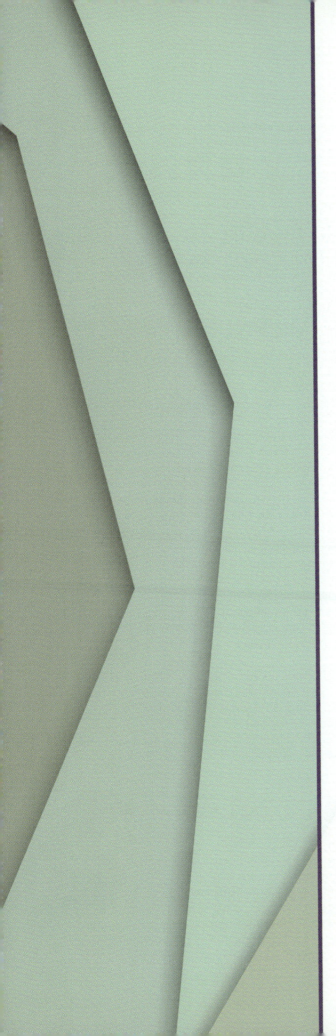

# CHAPTER 15

# Acne and the Esthetician

## OBJECTIVES. . .

In this chapter you will learn about factors that influence the development of different types of acne. You will learn to identify the different types of acne lesions and will learn about several acne-like medical conditions. You will learn how dermatologists treat acne and when you should refer a client to a dermatologist. A variety of treatments, ingredients, drugs, and products will also be studied.

**Acne** is a skin condition that results in inflammatory and noninflammatory lesions. Commonly associated with teenage and adolescent skin, it actually affects many age groups at different stages of life. There are many forms of acne and acne-related conditions that the esthetician sees every day. Although many forms of acne require the care of a dermatologist, many clients can benefit from esthetic treatments for problem skin.

**Acne** is a skin condition that results in inflammatory and noninflammatory lesions.

**Acne vulgaris** is the most common form of acne that is often associated with teenagers.

# COMMON ACNE

The most common form of acne is called **acne vulgaris**. This is the type of acne so often associated with teenagers. It usually begins at the inset of puberty, at which time teenagers begin producing larger amounts of sex hormones. (See the chapter on hormones.) These hormones cause stimulation of the sebaceous gland, which produces an overabundance of sebum.

# HEREDITARY FACTORS IN ACNE

**Hereditary** means a trait or condition is inherited from the parents; genetic.

We inherit certain genes from our parents that determine how our bodies, and our skin, function and behave. These are known as **hereditary** factors. If either of a child's parents had acne or excessively oily skin, there is a very good chance that the child also will have a strong tendency to develop acne.

**Retention hyperkeratosis** is the hereditary tendency of dead cells to stick to the sides of the follicle wall.

There are two major factors in acne development that are hereditary. As we learned earlier, the epidermal cells, particularly the corneum, are constantly shedding and being replaced by younger cells. **Retention hyperkeratosis** is a hereditary condition in which these cells are retained. The dead cells stick to the surface of the skin and begin lining the inside walls of the follicle. We will, for simplicity, refer to retention hyperkeratosis as "cell buildup." Much like wax tends to build up on the surface of furniture, the cells inside the follicle build up.

This process of buildup is complicated by the fact that the cells continue to push to the surface of the epidermis at a faster rate. *Hyper* means more than normal, so hyperkeratosis means the process of keratinization (turnover of cells) occurs at a rate much faster than normal.

Some researchers believe that retention hyperkeratosis is caused by an inability of the body to produce intercellular structures called lamellar granules. These granules are theorized to release an enzyme that causes dead cells to break away from the corneum in the normal manner. It has been determined that chronic acne patients do not have as many of these active structures present in their follicular cells.

**Oiliness** describes a larger than normal amount of sebum secreted onto the skin by the sebaceous glands.

The second major hereditary factor in the tendency to develop acne is **oiliness**. The amount of sebum produced by the skin is largely hereditary. People who have acne or excessively oily skin have inherited this tendency.

The excessive sebum "bathes" and "waxes over" the cell buildup. The sebum becomes sticky and solidifies, much like the fat in chicken broth hardens and solidifies when it is refrigerated.

**Microcomedo** is a small impaction formed by cells that have built up on the inside of the follicle wall.

When enough cells and waxy sebum build up in the bottom of the follicle, they form a small impaction called a **microcomedo**. Microcomedones (plural) are a mixture of dead cell buildup, bacteria, fatty acids from the sebum, and other cellular debris. They are the beginning phase of any acne lesion.

Microcomedones cannot be seen on the surface of the skin. They are deep in the follicles and can only be seen by microscopic examination of skin tissues (Figure 15-1).

# NONINFLAMMATORY AND INFLAMMATORY ACNE LESIONS

**Inflammatory** means swollen and red.

**Noninflammatory** means that the impaction is not red or inflamed.

As microcomedones continue to retain more and more dead cells and are coated by more and more sebum, they develop into larger, visible acne lesions. They may become either inflammatory or noninflammatory lesions. **Inflammatory** acne lesions are, like they sound, inflamed, meaning that they are red and swollen lesions. A typical acne pimple is an inflammatory lesion. **Noninflammatory** means that the impaction is not red or inflamed. Examples of noninflammatory acne lesions are **open comedones** (blackheads) and **closed comedones** (whiteheads) (Figure 15-2).

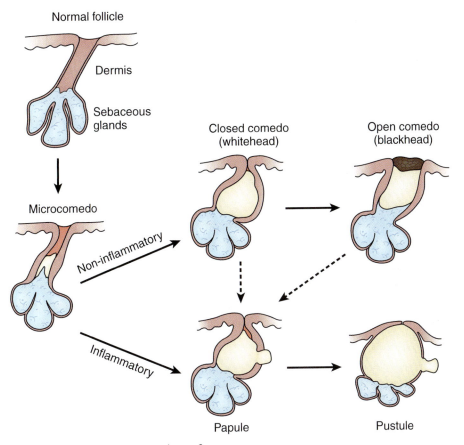

Normal follicle

Dermis

Sebaceous glands

Microcomedo

Non-inflammatory

Inflammatory

Closed comedo (whitehead)

Open comedo (blackhead)

Papule

Pustule

**Figure 15-1** The progression of acne

Open comedones occur when the follicle is large enough to hold all of the debris retained by the follicle. The **ostium**, or opening, in these follicles is dilated by the mass of the impaction, allowing the comedo to push toward the surface opening.

***Propionibacterium acnes (P. acnes)*** is the scientific name of the bacteria that causes acne vulgaris. These bacteria are **anaerobic**, which means they cannot survive in the presence of oxygen. These bacteria are constantly present in all follicles in small numbers. They are kept from reproducing to large numbers by the oxygen that is constantly aerating the open follicle. However, when the follicle gets blocked from oxygen circulation, these bacteria multiply in great numbers, feeding off the sebum produced by overactive sebaceous glands (Figure 15-3). Open comedones do not encourage development of this bacterial growth because the follicle opening is large enough to expose the follicle to oxygen. The oxygen is also what causes the "blackhead" to form at the exposed part of the impaction. This darkening is caused by the exposure of the top of the comedo to the oxygen in the air outside the follicle. The sebum turns a brown color, similar to the way mayonnaise will turn yellow if left out on a picnic table for a period of time. The darkness is also caused by clumps of **melanin** (skin pigment) present in the dead cells in the comedo. This theory is easily demonstrated by observing an extracted open comedo. It is a solid cylindrical plug, topped by a dark area that gets lighter as the deeper parts of the impaction are extracted.

Open comedones, therefore, rarely develop into inflammatory lesions. Unfortunately, the same cannot be said for closed comedones. Closed comedones have very small pore openings, which prevents oxygen from readily penetrating the follicle. The walls of the follicle stretch to hold the contents of the impaction, but the follicle

**Open comedones** are noninflammatory acne lesions usually called blackheads.

**Closed comedones** are noninflammatory acne lesions called whiteheads.

**Ostium** is the opening in follicles.

***Propionibacterium acnes (P. acnes)*** is the scientific name of the bacteria that cause acne vulgaris.

**Anaerobic** bacteria are bacteria that do not need oxygen to grow and survive.

**Melanin** is the pigment of the skin.

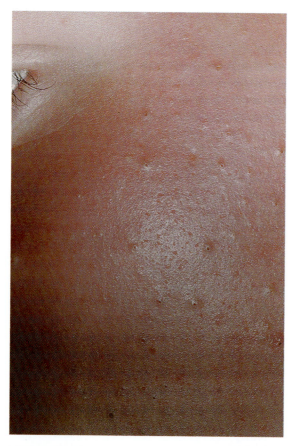

**Figure 15-2** Open and closed comedones (Courtesy Michael J. Bond, M.D.)

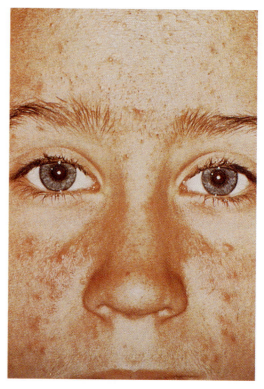

**Figure 15-3** The development of acne in a young girl (Courtesy Mark Lees Skin Care, Inc.)

opening does not. Because of this lack of oxygen, the lesions can easily become inflamed due to the increasing number of bacteria multiplying in the anaerobic environment.

Closed comedones are easily recognizable. They are frequently seen in adult women, often in the blush line of makeup users. They are small "underground" bumps and are not easily extracted. They are frequently associated with the use of comedogenic cosmetics. (See the chapter on comedogenicity.)

When enough bacteria form inside the closed comedo and the impaction becomes large enough, a small tear occurs in the follicle wall, which stimulates the immune system to investigate (See the chapter on the immune system), releasing white blood cells into the area. These white blood cells arrive via the blood vessels, causing the lesion to become red. This is an inflammatory lesion.

A **papule** is a red, sore bump without a "whitehead" (no pus) (Figure 15-4). This is the beginning of the "rescue" by the white blood cells. When enough white blood cells arrive, they may form a "clump" and rise to the surface, creating what is known as a **pustule** (Figure 15-5). *Pus* is the common name for this "clump" of white blood cells. For practical purposes, a papule is often described by the client as a large, red, sore bump that never "comes to a head." Papules seem sometimes to "magically disappear." This is because the immune system has "won the battle" and disposed of the impaction through enzymes and absorption, and the body has disposed of the remains through normal blood excretion. Papules affect the nerve endings more than pustules because they are deeper in the skin. This explains the soreness. Pustules have "migrated" the impaction toward the skin surface, dilating the follicle opening and relieving the pressure on the nerve endings, resulting in less pain.

**Papule** is a raised area on the skin that is generally smaller than 1 centimeter.

**Pustule** is a clump of white blood cells that have formed and risen to the surface of the skin.

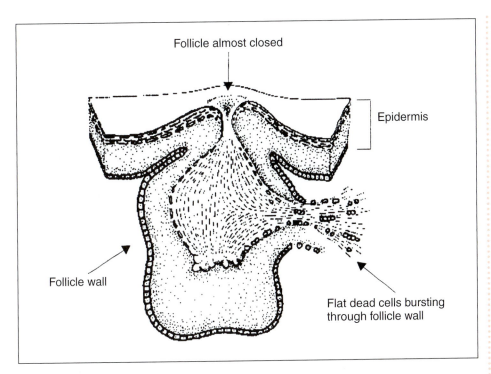

Follicle almost closed

Epidermis

Follicle wall

Flat dead cells bursting through follicle wall

**Figure 15-4** The papule

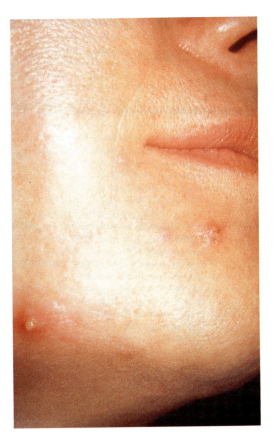

**Figure 15-5** The pustule (Courtesy Mark Lees Skin Care, Inc.)

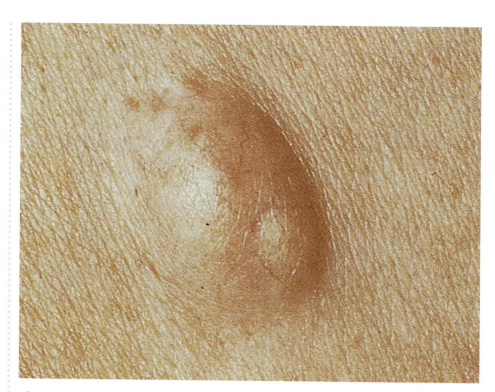

**Figure 15-6** The cyst (Courtesy Mark Lees Skin Care, Inc.)

**Nodule** is a raised lesion that is larger and deeper in the skin. A nodule looks like a lump, but the skin can be moved over the lesion.

**Cysts** are deep infections caused by the deep, massive invasion of white blood cells.

A **nodule** is similar to a papule, but it is deeper in the skin and feels very solid and sore. **Cysts** are deep infections caused by a deep, massive invasion of white blood cells. They are very pustular and very large (Figure 15-6).

## The Grades of Acne

Acne is "graded" by dermatologists on a four-point scale. (See Figure 15-7a–d.)

- ◆ **Grade 1 acne**—mostly open and closed comedones with an occasional pimple. Grade 1 acne is typical of a teenager just beginning puberty.
- ◆ **Grade 2 acne**—very large number of closed comedones, with occasional pustules or papules.
- ◆ **Grade 3 acne**—thought of by most people as "typical teenage acne." It involves large number of open and closed comedones and many papules and pustules as well. It is very inflamed and red.
- ◆ **Grade 4 acne**—commonly referred to as cystic acne, with many deep cysts and scar formation.

## Why Scars Form

Scars form when the skin, in a desperate attempt to heal itself, produces lots of collagen to try to compensate for the lack of normal skin functioning. This type of scar is usually raised. Acne "pit" scarring occurs from actual destruction of the tissue during the inflammatory process. Cystic acne is almost always associated with scarring (Figure 15-8).

## Hormones

**Androgens** are male hormones largely responsible for oily skin and acne.

Hormones, specifically male hormones, or **androgens**, are the mechanisms that cause stimulation of the sebaceous glands, which, in turn, produce more sebum. This sebum

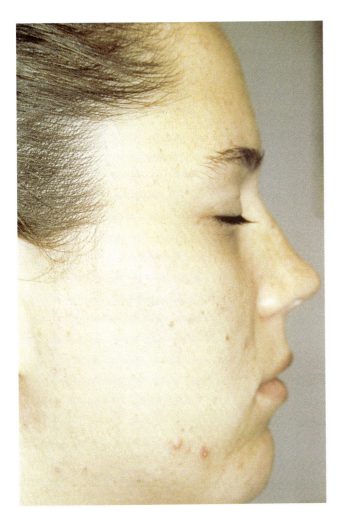

**Figure 15-7A** Grade 1 acne (Courtesy Mark Lees Skin Care, Inc.)

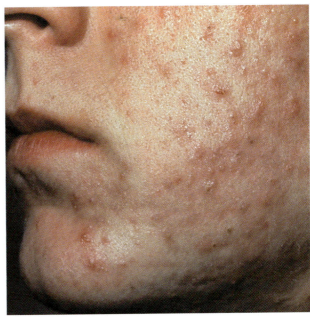

**Figure 15-7C** Grade 3 acne

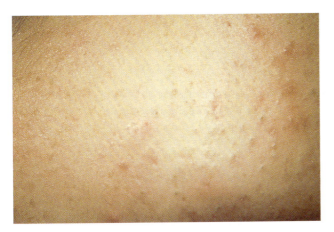

**Figure 15-7B** Grade 2 acne (Courtesy Mark Lees Skin Care, Inc.)

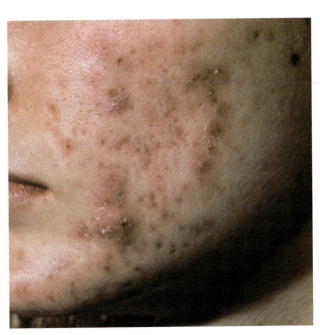

**Figure 15-7D** Grade 4 acne

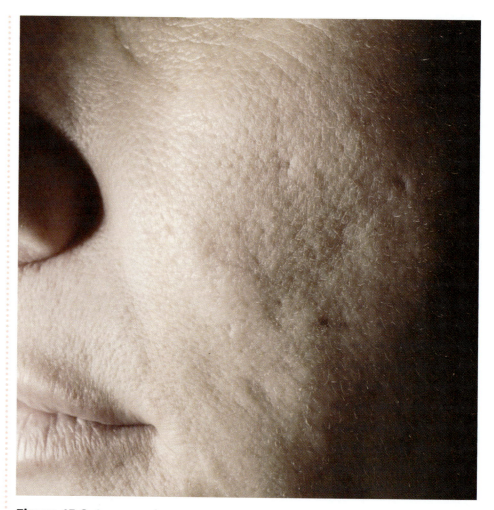

**Figure 15-8** Acne scarring

causes inflammation in the follicles, coating the cell buildup and providing a source of fatty acids, which is the food of *P. acnes* bacteria.

**Testosterone** is the male hormone responsible for the development of typical male characteristics.

**Dihydrotestosterone (DHT)** is a form of male hormone that stimulates the sebaceous glands to produce sebum.

**Testosterone**, an androgen, converts to **dihydrotestosterone (DHT)**, another form of male hormone, which "switches on" the oil gland. The oil gland is stimulated via receptor sites on the cells of the sebaceous glands, which are little "switches" that are "turned on" by hormonal stimulation.

As we discussed in the hormones chapter, males and females produce both male and female hormones, which are transported around the body via the circulatory system.

## Premenstrual, Hormonal, and Adult Acne

Premenstrual acne flares are often referred to as adult acne. Often, women who have never had problems with acne as a teenager suddenly develop a problem in their 20s or 30s. Although this can be related to comedogenic cosmetics, stress, and hereditary acne factors, hormones play a significant role in adult female acne.

Again, the male hormone, or androgen, flares in the bloodstream cause this type of flareup. Premenstrual flares are caused by a sudden predominance of androgen, which corresponds with the eventual loss of the egg during menses.

The elevation of testosterone in the bloodstream begins eight to ten days before a woman's period. This elevation is actually not an increase in androgen as much as a decrease in the female hormone estrogen. Nevertheless, there is suddenly a larger percentage of androgen in the bloodstream and therefore a sudden likely increase in stimulation of the sebaceous glands.

A sudden flow of sebum in the follicle causes **perifollicular inflammation**, inflammation around the inside of the follicle. This irritation causes swelling inside the follicle, decreasing the flow of oxygen to the lower part of the follicle and creating an "anaerobic pocket," an ideal environment for the *P. acnes* bacteria. The bacteria multiply, feeding off the sebum and causing a sudden flare of acne papules and pustules.

## Chin Acne

Many women suffer from premenstrual acne flares predominantly in the lower part of the face, the chin, and the jawline (Figure 15-9). Many researchers believe that this is the area most responsive to male hormone sebaceous stimulation. It is also believed that many women have very large sebaceous glands in these areas and relatively small follicles. When a sudden sebaceous stimulation occurs, these follicles fill very quickly, causing inflammation due to the large amount of sebum. Women who suffer from chronic chin acne should see a dermatologist. There are hormone treatments available to help this problem.

**Perifollicular inflammation** means inflammation around the inside of the follicle.

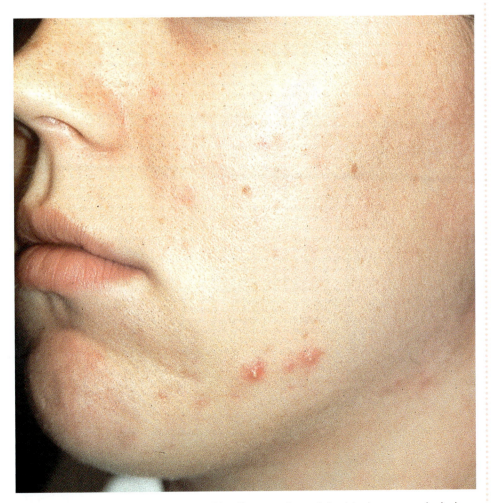

**Figure 15-9** Acne in the chin and jawline can be related to hormone imbalances (Courtesy Mark Lees Skin Care, Inc.)

## Stress

Stress is what causes "pimples on prom night." Many acne sufferers, as well as dermatologists and estheticians, have noticed acne flareups when a patient is under stress. A final exam at school, dating problems, financial problems, or difficulties at work seem to frequently accompany breakouts.

There is a fairly simple explanation for this relationship. Stress causes the brain to manufacture a hormone that, in turn, causes the adrenal gland to make more hormones, which causes an abundance of oil to be produced. The reaction is very similar to the premenstrual reaction.

## Birth Control Pills

Birth control pills can cause an androgenic flareup that can contribute to acne. When starting birth control pills the skin may get better or worse. The same may be true when discontinuing birth control pills. Women using birth control pills may find that their monthly premenstrual breakouts occur at different times in the cycle.

The reasoning here is simple. Birth control pills affect hormone levels and may affect different women in different ways. For more information, see the chapter on hormones. If your client seems to experience flares of acne when starting, stopping, or changing birth control pills, refer her to her doctor.

## Pregnancy

Pregnancy may also produce unpredictable flareups or clearing of acne. The usual course is that acne gets worse during the first three months of pregnancy, then gets dramatically better. The acne may flare up again after childbirth or after breastfeeding is discontinued. Theoretically, this is due to obvious hormone changes, but stress levels may be partially responsible.

## Menopause

During menopause, similar hormonal changes are very prominent and may cause flares. Because menopause is a time of more permanent hormonal change, some women will experience even more acne flares and other androgen-induced symptoms, such as facial hair growth.

## Treatment of Hormonal Acne

In many cases, hormonal acne flares can be handled using topical treatments to manage these flares. Regular deep cleansing facial treatments, as described later in this chapter, are helpful in decreasing the instances in many cases.

Many of these women also have very oily or oily combination skin. Proper use of a good rinseable foaming-type cleanser, gel-based 10 percent alphahydroxy acid used daily, and the elimination of comedogenic (clog-pore causing) products (see the chapter on comedogenicity) help to prevent comedones from forming and cut down on acne flares.

In chronic cases of hormonal acne, hormonal therapy using special kinds of birth control pills may be prescribed by a dermatologist, gynecologist, or family physician. Tricyclen® is a birth control pill approved by the Food and Drug Administration (FDA) as a management drug for hormonal acne. In extreme cases, chronic hormonal acne may also be a symptoms of more serious illnesses such as ovarian polycystic disease and adrenal growths. If you notice chronic hormonal breakouts that are not responsive to topical treatment, do not hesitate to suggest that the client consult her physician.

# Inflammatory versus Comedonal Acne

Many women also notice that premenstrual flares result in sore, inflamed papules. Hormonal acne is more inflammatory and less comedonal. In other words, it is the sudden irritation, rather than the traditional and slower buildup of cells in a comedo, that causes these papular lesions. The soreness is due to the swelling and relatively deep inflammation inside the follicle. This deep swelling is more likely to cause pressure on nerve endings, creating a painful lesion.

Inflammatory acne is not just caused by hormones. Acnegenic skin-care products that cause overnight flares of pimples are a good example of inflammatory acne. Overtreated skin that has had too many peeling agents, or peeling agents applied too often, will show signs of dry irritation and often flares of inflammatory acne. Be very observant of your clients' habits in these cases. Often they are overtreating their skin or may be using a new product that causes a flare.

Unfortunately, professional products are not immune from being acnegenic. "Natural" products also do not mean nonacnegenic. Check to make sure that the products you use and sell have been properly tested for irritancy to make sure they do not cause acnegenic or follicle irritancy reactions.

# The Beginning of Teenage Acne

The beginning of teenage acne is characterized by minor breakouts in the nose area. Small blackheads and clogged follicles, small papules, and small milia are found. The esthetician will only notice the beginning of visible pores in the nose and chin and sometimes the forehead. This is the beginning of adolescent pore structure, and usually, puberty and adolescence. Usually within six months more pimples will develop. Boys may notice small pimples in the lower cheeks. This may be caused by the beginning of beard hair growth. The hair is beginning to grow, but the follicle is not large enough to accommodate the hair.

This condition is known as **keratosis pilaris**, which essentially means there is a very small hair trying to force its way out of the follicle, resulting in irritation. This condition, which may affect girls or boys, is usually red or pink and has a "sandpaper" texture. It is often seen in the lower cheeks. If you look carefully at the area, you may notice very small whiteheads, responsible for the bumpy feel. Keratosis pilaris also frequently occurs on the upper arm and is more likely to affect adults in this area. Keratosis pilaris is best treated with alphahydroxy home care lotions and gels, and use of mild mechanical exfoliating cleansers helps bump off dead cells to allow the hair to come out. Salon treatment using softening and extraction techniques is also helpful (Figure 15-10).

Young teenagers should be treated every two to three months until breakouts become persistent. At that time regular treatments are recommended. Recommend a gentle, nonmedicated, foaming cleanser, a toner for oily/combination skin, and a mild gel of alphahydroxy or salicylic acid or 2½ percent benzoyl peroxide. Used regularly, these products will help prepubescent teens through this period. Teenagers usually do not need a moisturizer except in cold weather. Regular use of noncomedogenic, daily-use, broad-spectrum sunscreen is also advised.

# Lack of Care

Young teenagers may not be disciplined when it comes to a regular facial care routine. Gently explain to them the need for consistent care. They usually will take advice from you before they will from Mom at this age.

Teenagers are not the only age group that suffers from lack of skin hygiene. Even though acne is not caused by dirt, many adults neglect their skin. Sleeping in makeup is not only unhygienic, it also means that the night treatment is not applied. Explain

**Keratosis pilaris** is a condition in which the skin exhibits redness and irritation in patches, accompanied by a rough texture, and small pinpoint white papules that look like very small milia.

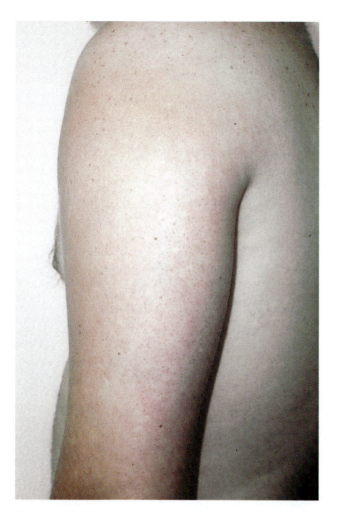
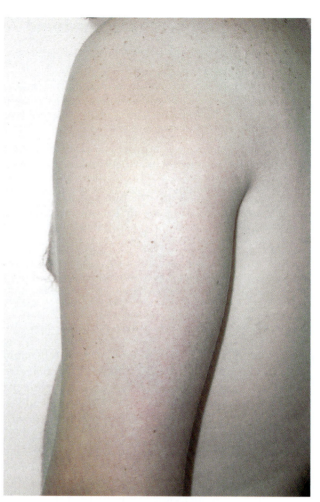

**Figure 15-10** Improvement in bumpy arms after using a glycolic hydrator (Courtesy Mark Lees Skin Care, Inc.)

to the client that she may come to have a treatment at the salon twice a month, but she is responsible for the other 60 times a month that the skin is cleansed and conditioned! Help her find simple routines that she enjoys doing. Teach her to clean her face as soon as she gets home for the evening. This is also a good time to floss her teeth, right after dinner. When she gets sleepy later in the evening, she can walk past the bathroom guilt-free!

## ENVIRONMENTAL FACTORS THAT INFLUENCE ACNE

### Heat and Humidity

There is no question that acne is more likely to flare up in the summer months when heat and humidity are high. Heat causes the skin to swell slightly, and humidity causes tremendous swelling of the outer epidermis. It is reasonable to assume that this could possibly exert enough pressure on the follicles to further complicate an already existing condition.

It has been observed over the years that people who live in tropical, warm climates with high humidity experience a fairly predictable seasonal pattern of flareups. Estheticians should bring this to the attention of their clients and encourage them to come to the salon more often for treatments during this type of weather if the client notices a consistent relationship.

## Sun Exposure

Although sun exposure may have an immediate drying effect on acne lesions, sun damages skin and is documented to cause more "cell buildup," which can add to or increase the chances of acne flareup.

Many patients with acne claim their acne improves with sun exposure. Tanning masks the redness, and as the buildup of tan cells occurs on the surface of the skin, acne may appear better. As soon as beach season is over, however, these same patients notice reoccurrence of their acne. What actually happens is that the tan fades and the cell buildup subsides, suddenly exposing a tremendous number of clogged follicles and closed comedones. The most unfortunate part of this situation is that these clients have a strong tendency to neglect treating their acne during beach season, making it more complicated when the tan fades. It is up to the esthetician to educate the client before sun season to avoid this problem.

## Greasy Workplaces

Patients with acne who work in environments where their skin is constantly exposed to large amounts of occlusive grease or airborne grease, such as that present in fast-food restaurants, may notice a strong flareup in their conditions. Occupations such as car mechanics and short-order cooks are good examples of such situations. It is best for these individuals to avoid working for prolonged periods of time under these conditions. Advise clients who must work in these types of jobs to cleanse their skin at regular intervals (about twice during an eight-hour period) with a mild cleanser that will remove the environmental oil without drying the skin too much.

## OVERCLEANING

Clients are constantly under the impression that acne is directly caused by lack of cleansing. Although keeping skin as clean as possible is certainly important, acne is not caused by dirt. In fact, acne can be aggravated by too much cleaning. Repeated exposure to detergents in facial cleansers, for example, can aggravate acne if the client is using the cleansers too often. Estheticians often find that their clients are cleaning the face numerous times daily (eight to ten times). This causes enough irritation to precipitate not only an acne aggravation, but other sensitivities as well. Instruct these clients to cleanse two or three times a day only.

## SELF-TRAUMA EXCORIATIONS

**Acne excoriée** is a condition in which the client constantly picks at the skin. An **excoriation** is a scrape or scratch on the skin, in this case caused by the client. Most of the time, these clients are scratching or picking at small closed comedones and papules. Often the raised portion of the acne lesion is literally scraped off the face, usually with the fingernails.

An esthetician will notice acne excoriée during skin analysis because the acne lesions are flat, red, and sometimes raw, where the client has scraped off the entire epidermis to the point of bleeding. They often look like a freshly scraped knee or a brush burn (Figure 15-11). Sometimes there are scabs, which these clients have trouble leaving alone. Sometimes the esthetician will notice round, dark, hyperpigmented lesions. This is hyperpigmentation, either caused by trauma, known as **post-inflammatory hyperpigmentation,** or from exposure to sun after the client has picked the lesions raw.

**Acne excoriée** is a condition in which a person picks at their acne lesions, causing scrapes and possible scars and hyperpigmentation.

**An excoriation** is a scrape or scratch on the skin.

**Post-inflammatory hyperpigmentation** describes dark melanin splotches caused by trauma to the skin; can result from acne pimples and papules.

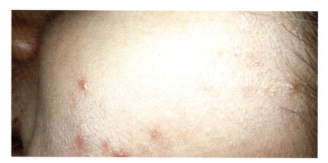

**Figure 15-11** Acne excoriée (Courtesy Mark Lees Skin Care, Inc.)

Clients who have obvious excoriated acne lesions should be told by the esthetician not to pick at the lesions. The lesions will never heal properly if the scabs are constantly being scratched off. Fingernails carry many germs that can cause other infections besides acne. Encourage "picker" clients to use a mask at home instead of picking, or tell them to call and move their treatment appointment to an earlier date. Suggest that they wear cotton gloves while reading or watching television. The touch of the glove material will signal them and make them aware when they are picking at their skin.

Clients sometimes absentmindedly pick at an occasional pimple. However, when clients constantly have several scraped areas on the face, this is a different situation. Some chronic pickers are often troubled mentally or suffer from a psychological disorder such as obsessive-compulsive disorder. Some may need referral to a psychologist or other mental health professional.

## NUTRITION AND DIET

There are numerous falsehoods regarding the effects of food on acne. Chocolate, nuts, seafood, greasy "teenage" foods such as burgers and french fries, pizza, and candy have all been falsely accused at one time of causing or worsening acne. Although some of these foods are not healthy in large quantities because they may be high in sugar, cholesterol, or triglycerides, they do not directly or indirectly cause acne. Many patients with acne and, unfortunately, some estheticians are still under the mistaken impression that these foods cause acne.

It is important to have a properly balanced diet to have good skin and good health. The food group that has consistently been implicated in aggravating acne conditions is iodides. Foods that are high in iodides include some types of shellfish, kelp, squid, asparagus, and iodized salt in salty foods. Iodine causes a follicular irritancy when ingested in large quantities. Consumed in reasonable quantities occasionally, these foods probably do not cause serious problems. It stands to reason, though, that excessive consumption of foods high in iodides can cause acne to flare up.

Milk and some milk products have been found to cause problems, primarily in females. The fat in milk does not appear to be associated with acne. It is theorized that the hormones present in milk (from the cow) are the probable culprits for causing acne flares. If your client experiences chronic acne and does not seem to clear through topical treatment, ask your client if she consumes a lot of milk or milk products. Milk is a very important part of the diet, especially for calcium needs of the body, and should not be discontinued unless the client associates a direct correlation between milk consumption and flares of acne.

Foods are NOT the major cause of acne. Unfortunately, many estheticians put too much emphasis on diet when treating problem skin, blaming foods when their treatments seem not to be working. Failure of the treatment plan is more likely to result from poor product choices or incomplete home care programs. If you are truly concerned about the client's diet, you should refer the client to her doctor or to a registered dietician.

Zinc supplements are furnished to some patients with acne by dermatologists. Prescribed in inflamed acne to reduce redness and inflammation, the usual dosage is 100 mg per day. It is best to check with a dermatologist before suggesting zinc supplements to your clients, because estheticians are not registered dieticians and therefore are not authorities on nutritional science. It is best to leave advice to the specialists in this area.

## ACNE AND COSMETICS

Probably the best service an esthetician can render to a patient with acne is helping the patient choose cosmetics and skin-care products that are noncomedogenic (see the chapter on comedogenicity).

So many factors cause or contribute to acne, but the esthetician has control over only a few. Heredity and hormones are not part of the practice of esthetics. Even though we may know a lot about these subjects, there is little the esthetician can do to control or affect these factors. Estheticians can temporarily reduce stress by administering soothing treatments, but the stress-reducing effects of these therapies are not long lasting when the client gets in an argument with the boss or forgets when a term paper is due.

The point here is that the only real factors over which estheticians have control are how the client cleanses the skin and what cosmetics and skin-care products the client uses routinely.

It is imperative that the esthetician fully understand comedogenicity for clients with acne or problem skin. It is the best service we can offer them. The client may come in for treatment only once a month, but she exposes herself to cosmetics and skin care up to 60 times a month.

The esthetician must eliminate all possible comedogenic factors from the home care and cosmetic regimen of the patient with acne. Cosmetics, skin care, and topical drugs are the only things that are in constant, direct contact with the skin.

## ACNE-RELATED CONDITIONS

**Seborrheic dermatitis** is a sometimes-chronic inflammation of the skin associated with oily skin and oily areas. Seborrheic dermatitis is characterized by dry-looking, flaky, crusty patches. Redness is often apparent under these flaky patches. Seborrheic dermatitis is most often seen in the T-zone of the face, eyebrows, hairline, inside the ears, along the sides of the nose, and the scalp (Figure 15-12). The exact cause of seborrheic dermatitis is unknown, but it is believed to be associated with a type of yeast called **pityrosporum ovale**.

Seborrheic dermatitis is often misdiagnosed by the client or an inexperienced esthetician as "dry skin"; it is actually an inflammation of the oil glands. Seborrheic dermatitis is best treated by a dermatologist, but the esthetician may be involved in choosing the correct skin-care program. Sometimes a flare may be triggered after a client first uses a cream or product that is too rich or fatty-based. It is, again, important to avoid fatty, comedogenic products. Suggest a gentle but thorough rinseable cleanser; toner; and a very light, noncomedogenic moisturizing fluid. Overmoisturizing can be a contributing factor to flares of seborrheic dermatitis. Sunscreen is important for all skin types. Fragranced products, essential oils, or stimulating products and products with drying alcohols may aggravate or cause seborrheic dermatitis to flare.

**Seborrheic dermatitis** is an inflammation of the sebaceous glands, resulting in patches of inflamed flakiness in oily areas of the skin.

**Pityrosporum ovale** is a type of yeast sometimes associated with seborrheic dermatitis.

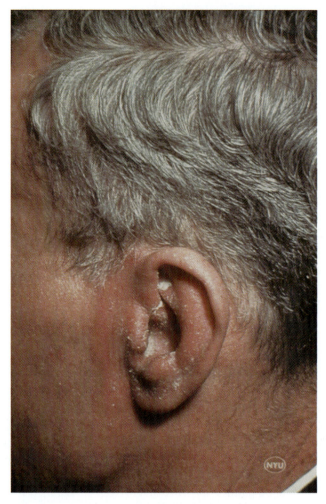

**Figure 15-12** Seborrheic dermatitis presents with red, flaky skin in oily areas of the face and most often affects the T-zone of the face, eyebrows, ears, scalp, and hairline (Reprinted with permission from the American Academy of Dermatology. All rights reserved)

Clients who suffer from seborrheic dermatitis are likely to experience flares as the seasons are changing. Lack of routine cleaning occasionally has been associated with the disorder. Dermatological treatment usually includes topical hydrocortisone, coal tar shampoos, salicylic acid, selenium sulfide, and zinc pyrithione. Antiyeast topicals and oral medications are used in severe cases.

In the salon, avoid excessive massage, stimulating treatments or products, and products with drying alcohol. Most peeling agents should be avoided when the seborrheic dermatitis is flared. Use soothing, nonirritating treatments, as if you were treating oily-sensitive skin. Gentle extraction of the areas affected is helpful.

## Perioral Dermatitis

**Perioral dermatitis** is dermatitis around the mouth.

**Perioral dermatitis**, which is dermatitis around the mouth, is also considered an acne-related disorder. Red papules and pustules in the mouth, nose, and chin area, usually small in size and in clusters of several lesions, are apparent. Almost always found in women, perioral dermatitis often occurs during the childbearing years, age 20 to 35 years (Figure 15-13).

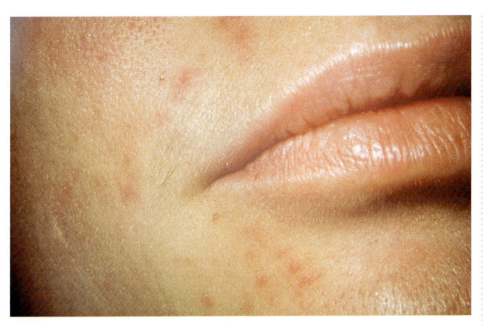

**Figure 15-13** Typical pattern of perioral dermatitis on the chin. Perioral dermatitis can also appear on the cheeks or anywhere around the mouth area
(Courtesy Mark Lees Skin Care, Inc.)

The condition is sometimes accompanied by scaliness and stinging dehydration. Moisturizers may complicate the condition. If a moisturizer is used, it should be water-based and noncomedogenic and used sparingly. Perioral dermatitis is, again, in the domain of the dermatologist. There is no known cause for perioral dermatitis. Because it is almost exclusively seen in females, it is thought to be somehow hormonally related.

Clients may report to you that their normal acne treatments are not working on this area of the face. This is not typical acne and needs medical referral. The usual course of treatment is oral antibiotics. Sometimes topical antibiotics or antibacterials are prescribed, but topicals are not usually effective. It is not unusual to have recurrences, and they must be treated again by the doctor.

Instruct the client not to touch or rub the area, because this can worsen the condition.

In the salon, avoid massage or overstimulation of the area. Esthetic treatments can help the client's other problems, but you must refer the client to a dermatologist for treatment of the perioral dermatitis. Home care for clients should emphasize lightweight, nonfatty, noncomedogenic, fragrance-free hydrating fluids or sunscreen/day creams. Stay away from any heavy-textured or oily product. Mild foaming cleansers and toners designed for oily to combination skin are appropriate.

# CONCEPTS OF ACNE TREATMENT

There are several basic concepts in esthetic treatment of acne, acne-prone, and clog-prone skin.

## Follicular Exfoliation

Many estheticians make the mistake of giving deep-cleansing facials, carefully and skillfully removing sebaceous filaments (clogged pores) and open and closed comedones, but they never make an effort to have the client treat the areas on a daily basis at home to prevent new lesion development. They treat only the visible lesions, forgetting about

**Follicular exfoliants** are chemical ingredients that slough the inside of the follicle, shedding and preventing cell buildup that can cause comedones and acne lesions.

the hundreds of microcomedones that lie under the surface of any acneic skin. We must always remember that the microcomedo is the primary lesion of acne. If we do not control the development of the microcomedo, we cannot control the problem skin.

The key to controlling the microcomedo is the daily use of **follicular exfoliants**. These are chemicals that cause the inside of the follicle to exfoliate, breaking loose cell buildup and solidified sebum, loosening clogged pores, and drying visible acne lesions. The client must use some type of these exfoliant products at home every day. The real value in using these chemicals is that they break up the microcomedones that already exist and keep the hyperkeratosis from accumulating to form new microcomedones.

We cannot forget that there is not a *cure* for acne. We are battling hereditary factors. Just because we clear a face does not mean it will stay clear unless daily care is taken by the client at home to keep the cell buildup broken up and to prevent new microcomedones from developing, therefore preventing new *visible* acne lesions. The client must treat the skin *every day*, even if the skin seems perfectly clear.

These exfoliants are *not* scrub cleansers. They are keratolytics that cause dead skin to shed by loosening them from each other. Over-the-counter (OTC) drug forms of these exfoliants include benzoyl peroxide, **sulfur**, **resorcinol**, and **salicylic acid**. Exfoliant performance ingredients include **glycolic acid**, **lactic acid**, other alpha- and betahydroxy acids, and enzymes. Prescription keratolytics include tretinoin (Retin-A®), adapalene (Differin®), tazarotene (Tazorac®), and azelaic acid (Azelex®).

Clients should not use more than one type of exfoliant agent at a time, especially if using the prescription exfoliant because they are much more aggressive. Double exfoliation is NOT a good idea. It will strip the barrier function and make the skin very red and suddenly incredibly sensitive. Also, do not use any salon exfoliation treatments, such as microdermabrasion or alphahydroxy acid (AHA) peels, in combination with these prescription drugs, unless approved by the physician treating the patient.

**Sulfur** is an exfoliant and an antibacterial.

**Resorcinol** is a peeling agent, usually coupled with sulfur, used in acne treatments and drying lotions.

**Salicylic acid** is a betahydroxy acid ingredient used for exfoliating and for its antibacterial properties.

**Glycolic acid** is an alphahydroxy acid used in acne treatment as a follicular exfoliant.

**Lactic acid** is an alphahydroxy acid used as an exfoliant.

**Enzymes** are naturally occurring chemical substances that help to dissolve cell buildup.

**Tazarotene** is a topical prescription retinoid (vitamin A derivative) used to treat acne. It is commercially known as Tazorac®.

## Oil Control

Controlling and dispersing the large volume of sebum involved with acne is helpful in preventing lesion development. Daily home use of foaming, detergent-type cleansers helps disperse this excess oil. Carefully choose a cleanser for your client that has the right amount of detergent for her skin type and sensitivity.

Oil control can also be achieved with the use of oil control cosmetics, which may be lotions, gels, or actual color cosmetics that contain ingredients that help to absorb excess oil. They remedy shine problems more than they have a therapeutic effect. These should be used in conjunction with, not instead of, a good, foaming, rinseable cleanser.

## Avoidance of Oils and Comedogenic Products

As discussed in the comedogenicity chapter, there are many cosmetic and topical agents that are fatty materials that can contribute to the worsening of acne or clogged pores when used on acne-prone and clog-prone skin types. All of these fatty agents must be strictly avoided when treating any skin that is already overproducing sebum.

## Antimicrobials and Antibiotics

**Erythromycin** is an antibiotic used topically for medical acne treatment.

These drug chemicals kill acne bacteria. OTC antimicrobials include benzoyl peroxide, sulfur, and salicylic acid. Prescription topical antibiotics include clindamycin (Cleocin-T®) and **erythromycin**. Prescription oral antibiotics are taken by mouth and are prescribed in more severe cases of acne. Common oral antibiotics used for acne include tetracycline, minocycline, and erythromycin.

# TREATMENT PRODUCTS AND INGREDIENTS FOR ACNE

## Benzoyl Peroxide

**Benzoyl peroxide** works well on most forms of acne vulgaris and occasional pimples. Benzoyl peroxide works by peeling off excess cell buildup, temporarily dilating the follicles, and breaking up follicle impactions and debris. Benzoyl peroxide also releases oxygen in the follicle, helping to kill bacteria. Benzoyl peroxide is available in a variety of bases, from drying clay bases to masks, creams, gels, and lotions. The lotions and gels are most frequently used by estheticians.

Benzoyl peroxide normally is made in three strengths:

◆ 2½ percent for mild acne and thin, sensitive skin

◆ 5 percent for moderate acne

◆ 10 percent for more severe acne

Additional strengths are available by physician's prescription. Scrubs and foaming washes containing benzoyl peroxide are also widely used. Unfortunately, many people are or become allergic to benzoyl peroxide. Benzoyl peroxide is also a bleach and may bleach fabric and hair if contact is made. Benzoyl peroxide may also be used in the treatment room as a treatment after extraction.

### Recommended Usage of Benzoyl Peroxide

1. First and most important, check to see if the client has ever experienced an allergy to benzoyl peroxide. Many clients will overuse a benzoyl peroxide product, resulting in peeling and irritation, which the client may assume is an allergy. When in doubt, don't use it.

2. Benzoyl peroxide may be used as a keratolytic to loosen impactions (open and closed comedones), or as a treatment for papules and pustules. Therefore, benzoyl peroxide can be used on present pimples or used as a preventative for development of future lesions.

3. Benzoyl peroxide can be a very aggressive drying agent. Visible peeling of skin will often occur. Some clients, especially older women, will confuse this peeling with "aging." Tightness of the peeling skin may accentuate lines and wrinkles for a short period of time. As the dead skin buildup is removed, the visible peeling lessens or subsides with continual use of benzoyl peroxide. Unfortunately, these clients will often stop using the benzoyl peroxide just as it is beginning to work. It is best to explain this peeling procedure to the client at the first consultation before it actually begins. Explain that the peeling will be temporary and is not the same type of drying that occurs with aging. Many older clients find that, with continued use of a peeling agent, their aging skin looks better and their acne is controlled. With many clients, especially older ones, it is good to recommend a light, noncomedogenic moisturizer that they can use to combat the visible flaking and peeling from drying agents, which will make the skin more comfortable as well as make the drying areas look smoother.

4. Occasionally, a client will call complaining of severe itching, burning, urticaria (hives), and rash. This is most likely an allergic reaction. Tell the client to discontinue treatment immediately. Severe allergic reactions should be seen by a dermatologist. Overuse of benzoyl peroxide products, as previously discussed, can cause an irritation reaction similar in appearance. The client should wait until the irritation completely subsides before trying benzoyl peroxide again. The client should then try applying the benzoyl peroxide to a small area for the

**Benzoyl peroxide** is a frequently used acne medication; both an exfoliant and antiseptic.

first day or two of application. If the irritation returns to the small test area, she should completely discontinue use.

5. Benzoyl peroxide should be used with extreme caution on clients with very dark or black skin. It is recommended not to exceed 5 percent benzoyl peroxide in these clients. The area around the mouth should be treated very lightly, because occasionally African-American clients will experience darkening (hyperpigmentation) of this area.

## Sulfur and Resorcinol

Sulfur and resorcinol are often combined in an acne-drying product. These products are usually available in gels, creams, masks, and clay-based "spot" treatment products. They are ideal for use when a client is allergic to benzoyl peroxide products. These products are also irritants and can cause irritations or allergic reactions. They can be used in the same way as benzoyl peroxide products. They help peel away excessive cell accumulations and loosen follicle impactions. They do not, however, release oxygen as benzoyl peroxide does. As a general rule, they are not quite as aggressive as benzoyl peroxide, but they are also less irritating. Although benzoyl peroxide is usually the more effective treatment, sulfur–resorcinol products are very helpful in drying acne lesions. If an allergy occurs, follow the same procedures as recommended for benzoyl peroxide.

## Salicylic Acid

Probably the mildest of the drying agents, this chemical is ideal for use on older, drier skin types. It usually comes in lotion form and can be incorporated in a moisturizing base. It is available in various strengths. Many companies automatically include salicylic acid in their moisturizers for problem skin. In thin or sensitive skin, it is often used as a day treatment, whereas benzoyl peroxide or sulfur-resorcinol is used as a night treatment.

Some people are very allergic to salicylates, the family of salicylic acid-type products. Salicylic acid, in its oral form, is aspirin. If your client is allergic to aspirin, avoid using salicylic acid.

## Glycolic and Alphahydroxy Acids

Alphahydroxy acid at 8 to 10 percent in a gel base is very effective at helping remove impactions. Alphahydroxy acids help acne by removing dead cell buildup and loosening impactions in the skin. Coupled with salicylic acid, and in more serious acne, benzoyl peroxide or sulfur and resorcinol, this treatment can really help clogged skin and problem acne. After the acne has cleared, regular use can help keep follicles clearer of hyperkeratosis, helping to prevent comedones and other acne lesions.

## PRODUCTS FOR HOME CARE FOR CLIENTS WITH ACNE

Scrubs and washes are very popular treatment cleansers for the acne patient. There are several types of these rinseable cleansers available.

The base of most of these washes is water and a mild-to-aggressive detergent. These detergents are surfactants that help remove excess oil from the skin's surface, which helps keep the oil from further clogging follicles. Examples of detergents are ammonium lauryl sulfate and disodium lauryl sulfosuccinate (a milder detergent used for more sensitive skin and less drying).

Acne medications such as benzoyl peroxide, sulfur–resorcinol, glycolic acid, and salicylic acid are sometimes added to these detergent bases. These are referred to as **medicated cleansers**. They can be considerably more active than regular cosmetic detergent cleansers. For extremely oily, problem skin, these medicated cleansers sometimes contain small, bead-like granules made of polyethylene or ground nuts, seeds, or hulls. These **exfoliating cleansers** help to mechanically remove surface cell buildup, helping the detergents or medication penetrate the surface better. However, they can be very abrasive on red, sensitive, thin skin, and are not recommended for patients using Retin-A or Accutane or patients using any other prescription peeling agent. They should only be used on the thickest, oiliest skin types.

Cleansing milks for acne are generally only recommended for makeup removal. Their use should be followed by a mild-to-moderate detergent cleanser to remove any traces of the cleansing milk. These cleansing milks are generally used at night only and should be made of noncomedogenic ingredients.

## Astringents and Toners

Astringents and toners are usually recommended for clients with acne to use after cleansing. These toners are helpful in controlling surface oils and in lowering the pH after cleansing. They are always water-based, with astringent chemicals such as witch hazel, isopropyl or SD alcohol, lemon extract, or citric acid. Some toners are made with antiseptics such as salicylic acid, which also exfoliates the skin.

Toners containing more aggressive drying agents such as alcohol and salicylic acid should be avoided on sensitive skin or the skin of someone using Retin-A or other prescription peeling agents.

## Day Treatment for Acne-Prone Skin

Acne and oily skin are not immune from sun damage. In fact, sun protection is often neglected in the patient with acne. The use of peeling agents increases this need for suncreen protection.

Advise your client to use an SPF-15 or higher, lightweight, broad-spectrum screen that has been tested for comedogenicity and follicle irritancy. This should be applied every morning after an application of 8 to 10 percent alphahydroxy gel.

## Night Treatments

Medicated gels have already been briefly discussed. These gels or creams contain peeling agents to help remove cell buildup and are extremely beneficial to clients with acne. They contain benzoyl peroxide, salicylic acid, sulfur, resorcinol, or glycolic acid. The exfoliant gel should be applied very lightly all over the face, even in areas where there is no current acne flares. Remember, we must prevent the development of microcomedones to prevent the recurrence of acne.

Hydrating fluids are sometimes needed by clients with acne to combat flaking caused by the medicated gels. Adult patients with acne frequently require the use of these hydrating fluids. A good hydrating fluid for problem skin is extremely light in texture and made without comedogenic ingredients. They are often alternated with peeling treatments and used on skin with acne tendencies and during colder seasons.

## Masks for Acne

Masks for clients with acne are almost always in a clay-type drying base. The clay most frequently used is **bentonite**, which has excellent oil-absorbing qualities.

**Medicated cleansers** are acne cleansers, in which medications such as benzoyl peroxide, sulfur-resorcinol, and salicylic acid have been added.

**Exfoliating cleansers** are acne cleansers in which small, bead-like granules made of polyethylene or ground nuts, seeds, or hulls have been added.

**Cleansing milk** is an emollient, non-foaming cleanser, generally used for makeup removal.

**Bentonite** is an oil-absorbing clay frequently used in clay cleansing masks.

Masks for acne are frequently also medicated, containing benzoyl peroxide, sulfur, or sulfurated lime. They are available in a variety of strengths. Camphor is a popular ingredient for more sensitive and adult skins, because it is less drying than the keratolytic agents. Some clay masks also contain a mechanical granule such as pumice or polyethylene to help exfoliate during application and rinsing.

Masks should be applied for 15 to 20 minutes after night cleansing. After drying, they should be removed by wetting the mask, then gently wiping off with a very soft cloth or sponge. Toner and night treatment should then be applied.

Masks are used two or three times a week, depending on the client's condition and oiliness. Weather and climate may also influence use frequency.

## Home Care Treatment for Beginning Teenage Acne

1. Wash the face thoroughly with rinseable foaming cleanser. Use a sponge or soft cloth to help exfoliate surface cells. Rinse thoroughly.
2. Apply mild antiseptic toner with a damp cotton ball or gauze to the entire face.
3. Apply an 8 to 10 percent alphahydroxy gel to the entire face, avoiding the eye area. Please explain to the teenager that it is normal for this to sting slightly when first applied.
4. After the alphahydroxy has absorbed, apply a noncomedogenic, lightweight broad-spectrum SPF-15 sunscreen. Most sun damage occurs before age 18; therefore, sunscreen must be used daily!

### Night Treatment

1. Remove any makeup thoroughly with noncomedogenic cleansing milk.
2. Wash face thoroughly with rinseable cleanser. Apply toner.
3. Apply alphahydroxy gel as in the morning treatment.
4. Apply a small amount of $2\frac{1}{2}$ or 5 percent benzoyl peroxide gel to clogged areas. Gently massage until the gel penetrates. Apply additional dabs of gel to individual raised lesions (papules and pustules). The only medication seen should be on the lesions. Excessive peeling may result, particularly in young, sensitive skin, if too much medication gel is used.

## Salon Treatment

Salon treatment should be administered whenever clogs and comedones are present. Sometimes treatment is necessary only every month or two during the very beginning stages of the teenage years. Treatment should be more frequent when apparent blemishes are more frequent. Parents should be consulted and advised when treating very young skin, so that they may advise children at home. It is often best to consult with the young client without the parent present and then discreetly talk to the parent afterwards. Teenagers will often perform home care better if they do not feel "supervised." It is important to advise parents to bring the young client in as soon as pimples start to develop. Unfortunately, many parents neglect a child's acne, thinking they will "outgrow it," until the teenager has a more serious condition. "An ounce of prevention is worth a pound of cure!"

## Home Care Treatment for Grade 1 Acne

### Morning

1. Wash the face with granular (nongranular if sensitive or thin skin) medicated cleanser, with wet fingertips, then with a wet sponge or very soft cloth. Rinse thoroughly with room temperature water.
2. Apply moderate strength toner to the entire face (except eyes). Allow to dry briefly.

3. Apply an 8 to 10 percent alphahydroxy gel to the entire face, avoiding the eye area.

4. After the alphahydroxy has absorbed, apply a noncomedogenic, lightweight, broad-spectrum SPF-15 sunscreen.

**Afternoon.** It is sometimes advisable in very oily skins to repeat the morning procedure in the mid-afternoon, or after school for teenagers. Cleansing should be repeated in the afternoon if working in a greasy environment or after exercising.

**Evening**

1. Remove makeup thoroughly with noncomedogenic cleansing milk.

2. Wash the face again with medicated cleanser. Nonmedicated foaming cleanser can be substituted if the skin is irritated, sensitive, or peeling.

3. Apply toner as in the morning.

4. Apply alphahydroxy gel as in the morning.

5. Apply 5 percent benzoyl peroxide, sulfur–resorcinol, or salicylic gel or lotion to all clogged and oily areas lightly. This treatment should penetrate almost immediately. Apply additional dabs to pimples and raised lesions. It is important that the client understand that they are not only to treat raised lesions. Treating unaffected but oily areas routinely with light applications will help break up "cell buildup" and help prevent future lesions (Figures 15-14A, 15-14B).

**Frequency of Salon Treatments.** Weekly or biweekly treatments are advised until the acne clears substantially. This normally takes between three and six months. After clearing, the client should be treated every three to four weeks in the salon and should use masks two to three times a week at home. The client should be reminded that acne is a controllable, not curable, condition and that upkeep is very important.

## Home Care for Grade 2 Acne

The home care routine is the same as for grade 1 acne; however, avoid very strong toners. Remember, there are usually many closed comedones in grade 2 acne. These lesions have smaller pore openings, and astringents may prevent these follicle openings from loosening with home care therapy.

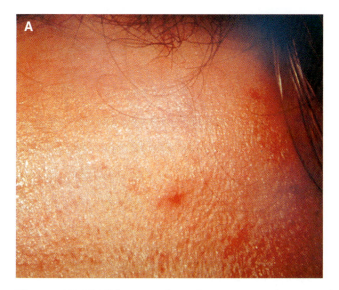 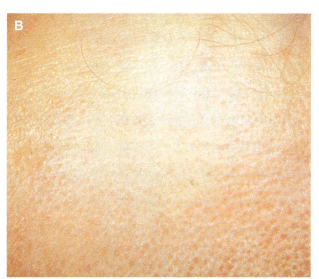

**Figure 15-14** This case of grade I acne was improved significantly in only six weeks of home care by eliminating comedogenic products, using daily follicular exfoliants to loosen and prevent hyperkeratosis, and using an effective foaming cleanser to control sebum (Courtesy Mark Lees Skin Care, Inc.)

Grade 2 acne is one of the hardest types to clear. It requires diligent attention from both client and esthetician. Treatments in the salon should be weekly or bi-weekly. Extensive extraction is necessary. After the first consultation, allow the client to use products two weeks before the second salon treatment. The closed comedones usually will be much easier to extract after two weeks of proper home care. It is especially important that these clients avoid comedogenic products. The esthetician should check every product carefully for comedogenic ingredients (Figures 15-15A–D, Figures 15-16A–D).

## Home Care for Grade 3 Acne

Most grade 3 acne cases should be seen by both the dermatologist and the esthetician. The esthetician must pay careful attention to the dermatologist's instructions and prescriptions. Benzoyl peroxide granular washes, stronger astringents, and 10 percent benzoyl peroxide gel may be used, if they are not contraindicated by the dermatologist. Oral medication is often required for these clients. They will also need help choosing noncomedogenic products and makeup.

Treatment is advised weekly, unless otherwise directed by the dermatologist. Once clear, the client should be seen for salon treatment every three to four weeks.

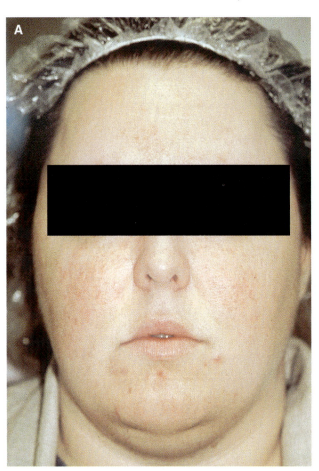
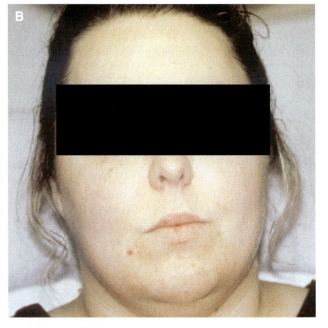

**Figure 15-15** This client had problem skin for 15 years and was using comedogenic product before starting treatment. All comedogenic products, including makeup, were eliminated and replaced with non-comedogenic products. Home care included sunscreen, hydrator, a 10 percent alpha/betahydroxy gel, a drying lotion for blemishes, a sulfur-based mask, and effective surfactant cleansers. No salon treatment was performed. Results photographed after six weeks of home care. Note improvements in redness, comedones, texture, and coloration (Courtesy Mark Lees Skin Care, Inc.)

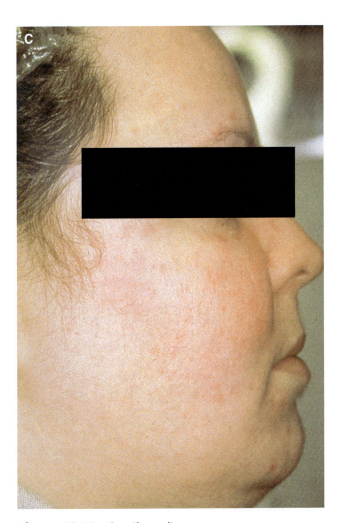

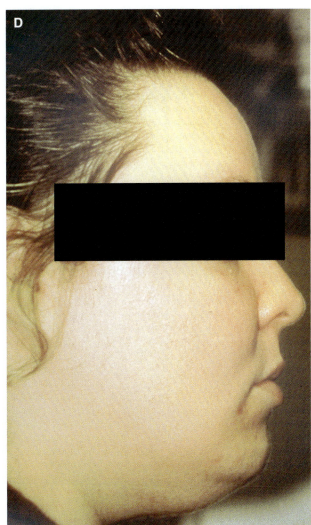

**Figure 15-15** *(Continued)*

## Home Care for Grade 4 (Cystic) Acne

Grade 4 acne always requires a dermatologist. This is the oiliest and worst acne condition. Home care should be the same as for grade 3 acne, again following any specific instructions from the dermatologist. Salon treatment should be frequent to help prevent lesions by removing clogs and open and closed comedones. Be very careful if cysts or nodules are present during treatment. Refer the client to the dermatologist immediately for treatment of any cysts, nodules, or deep papules. Again, avoidance of comedogenic ingredients is a must for these clients.

## DRUGS OFTEN PRESCRIBED BY THE DERMATOLOGIST FOR ACNE TREATMENT

### Retin-A, Retinoids, and Other Prescription Keratolytics

**Tretinoin**, better known as Retin-A, is a vitamin A acid that was developed in the late 1960s at the University of Pennsylvania by a team of researchers headed by Dr. Albert

**Tretinoin** is a form of vitamin A acid, also known as Retin-A, a prescription drug for treating acne.

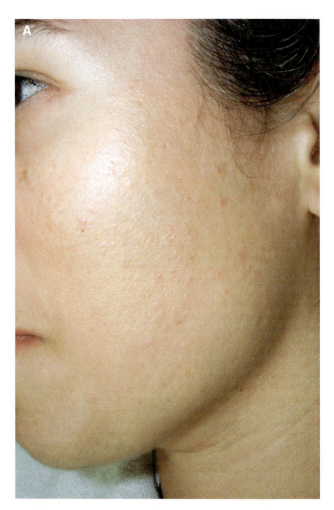
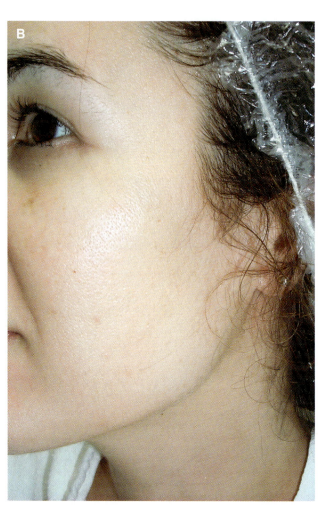

**Figure 15-16** Grade 2 acne. This client improved significantly after several months of esthetic treatment
(Courtesy Mark Lees Skin Care, Inc.)

**Clindamycin** is a topical prescription antibiotic used for acne treatment.

Kligman. Retin-A works by helping "flush out" follicular debris, helping to clear the follicles of comedones. It also is an excellent drying agent for oily skin and pimples. It is used extensively as a prescription in all grades of acne and is often used for other skin problems (see the chapter on the new science of aging skin treatment). Tretinoin requires a physician's prescription, because it is a potent topical acid. It is available in cream, gel, and liquid forms.

Because it is a powerful keratolytic, it is usually not used with other keratolytics such as benzoyl peroxide, sulfur–resorcinol, alphahydroxy, or salicylic acid, except by dermatologist recommendation. Occasional cases do well with benzoyl peroxide and Retin-A. This is a dermatological decision. Do not add keratolytics to a Retin-A user's regimen without consulting the dermatologist.

Tretinoin, also known as retinoic acid, does not have a substantial direct effect on bacteria within the follicle, however. It is often used with a topical antibiotic called **clindamycin** (trade name Cleocin-T™), which is a powerful antibiotic. It is in an alcohol base and by itself can be quite drying. The theory here is to use a powerful "follicle flusher" along with an antibiotic to kill bacteria and remove comedones and impactions. Because Retin-A is such a powerful keratolytic, it is also an irritant. It is not unusual for clients beginning Retin-A to experience flaking, dry skin, redness, irritation, and slight discomfort. The prescribed dosage varies with the client

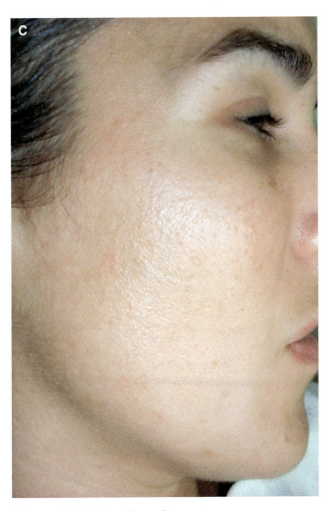

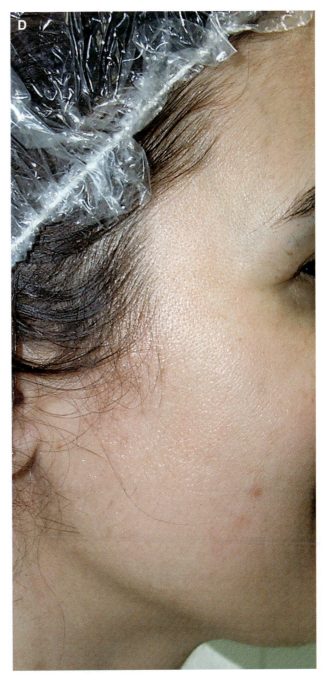

**Figure 15-16** *(Continued)*

and the dermatologist, but many dermatologists start patients on Retin-A every third night, slowly increasing the frequency to nightly applications.

Because of the irritating side effects of this drug, clients often find that their present skin-care program and cosmetics may be irritating or overdrying. It is up to the esthetician to work with the client or dermatologist to find products that work with retinoic acid therapy.

**Adapalene**, commercially known as Differin®, is a chemical cousin of retinoic acid. Adapalene produces similar effects and side effects as tretinoin, but it is reputed to be less irritating in some patients. Tazarotene, commercially known as Tazorac®, is yet another retinoid approved by the FDA for acne treatment. Again, it is an aggressive peeling agent, and the same precautions should be followed.

**Adapalene** is a form of vitamin A, also known as Differin®, that is a topical prescription drug used for acne treatment.

**Azelaic acid** is a form of acid, also known as Azelex®, a topical prescription drug used for acne treatment.

**Azelaic acid**, commercially known as Azelex®, is a different type of acidic agent that helps flush follicular debris. Azelaic acid also has a melanin suppressive effect on hyperpigmented skin but is not, at the time of this writing, officially approved as a melanin suppressor for prescription drug use. It is approved for acne treatment.

## Products for Users of Retinoic Acid and Other Prescription Exfoliators

1. First, eliminate any other keratolytics from the client's home-care program. As discussed previously, avoid benzoyl peroxide, sulfur, resorcinol, salicylic, and glycolic acid. Use these products with clients using Retin-A only with the approval of the dermatologist.
2. Eliminate high alcohol products, particularly those containing isopropyl alcohol.
3. Avoid fragranced products.
4. Avoid spicy, stimulating products.
5. Avoid large amounts of citric acid.
6. Eliminate essential oils from the regimen. Large amounts of many plant extracts may cause further irritation.
7. Sometimes it is necessary to totally eliminate the use of astringents or fresheners, particularly during the first six to eight weeks of Retin-A therapy.
8. Encourage the use of sunscreens, because Retin-A also makes the skin photosensitive.
9. Eliminate the use of granular scrub cleansers or tight drying masks, particularly during the first part of the Retin-A therapy. Later in the therapy (six to eight weeks), a gentle granular exfoliant, diluted with cleansing milk, may be beneficial in helping to remove dry, dead cells.
10. Highly stripping cleansers, soaps, and abrasives must be discontinued.

## Basic Home Care for Clients Using Tretinoin and Other Prescription Peeling Agents for Acne

### Morning

1. Cleanse the face with a gentle foaming cleanser for oily or combination skin.
2. Apply a gentle, nonalcoholic toner if not too irritated from beginning treatment.
3. Apply a noncomedogenic SPF-15 sunscreen. If using clindamycin, apply sunscreen after clindamycin application or follow the dermatologist's specific instructions.

### Evening

1. Remove makeup with a gentle cleansing milk. Extremely oily skin may need to be washed gently with a foaming cleanser. Apply toner if not too sensitive.
2. Wait 20 minutes.
3. Apply the topical drug as directed by a physician.

If the skin is very dehydrated, a light, nonfragranced, noncomedogenic, hydrating fluid may be applied 20 minutes later. Check to make sure that this is approved by the physician. If Retin-A is used on alternate nights, the client may choose to use the same noncomedogenic hydrating fluid on alternate nights to combat dehydration.

## Salon Treatment Changes for Clients Using Prescription Peeling Agents

1. Do not use wax on these patients. Waxing is extremely irritating to retinized skin. Electrolysis is usually acceptable to continue.

2. Avoid enzyme treatment, particularly when starting the prescription. After eight weeks or so, these may be acceptable.

3. Do not use mechanical abrasion; or microdermabrasion, brushing, or "rub off" type masks.

4. Avoid all keratolytics previously discussed during treatment.

5. Camphor masks can usually be tolerated if the skin is not red and irritated.

6. Avoid excessive massage.

7. Electrical therapy should be shortened in duration and performed at a lower intensity.

8. Avoid heavy, thick creams, as with all clients with acne.

## Accutane

Accutane is a cousin of retinoic acid. It is an oral medication prescribed for patients with severe, chronic, grades 3 and 4 acne with multiple cysts. It is very useful when treating this type of patient.

Accutane has numerous side effects, including severe drying of the skin and mucous membranes, nosebleeds, and severely dry, cracked lips. More severe side effects include birth defects in children of women who take Accutane during their childbearing years. Many doctors insist on a pregnancy test for women planning to undergo Accutane therapy. Other side effects include muscle aches. Periodic blood, kidney, and liver function tests are administered during Accutane therapy. Accutane has been associated with depression and occasionally suicide. These incidences, although rare, have caused some controversy and more investigation about the drug.

Clients considering Accutane therapy should thoroughly discuss the possible side effects with the dermatologist before starting the drug. Although Accutane seems to have alot of side effects, for grade 4 cystic and severe acne sufferers, it can be the only drug that makes a difference.

**Skin Care for the Accutane Patient.** Follow the same precautions as recommended for patients taking Retin-A. No waxing *on any part of the body* should be done during or for several months after Accutane is discontinued. You may need to administer soothing hydrating treatments to the Accutane patient, using light, noncomedogenic, hydrating fluids and gentle gel or cream masks.

Again, avoid all keratolytics, excessive massage, and any stimulating treatments. Extractions on patients taking Accutane should be extremely gentle, because the skin becomes extremely thin and fragile and reddens and bruises easily.

Help the client taking Accutane with light hydrating fluids and gentle cleanser. This may be the first time this client has ever used a moisturizer. Take some time to reinstruct the client in the uses of the new products.

After Accutane therapy, the skin usually returns to being somewhat oily; rarely is it as oily as it was before treatment. Within two or three months after Accutane is discontinued, reevaluate the skin and recommend the correct home-care regimen.

## DERMATOLOGICAL TREATMENT OF CYSTS

The dermatologist treats cysts by a number of different methods. Extraction is used, using a small incision to drain the cyst. This technique is known as acne surgery.

Sometimes the dermatologist injects the cyst with a steroid. The steroid usually clears the lesion in between one and three days of injection. It is an extremely effective treatment for cysts. The doctor usually also prescribes an oral antibiotic for these patients. Avoid pressure or extraction around a freshly treated cyst. Sometimes the dermatologist will suggest avoiding facial treatment until the cyst is completely healed.

## LIGHT THERAPY FOR ACNE

**Photodynamic therapy** is a medical treatment using intense types of light. Similar to laser, an extremely focused blue light in a very specific spectrum is used. The blue light reacts with chemicals called **porphyrins**, naturally given off by acne bacteria. The reaction of the blue light with the porphyrins kills acne bacteria. In some cases, a special drug gel, **5-aminolevulinic acid**, also known as **Levulan**® or **Kerastick**®, is applied to the skin. The blue light reacts with the aminolevulinic acid to release intense forms of oxygen, creating free radicals that kill the acne bacteria.

Photodynamic therapy is particularly effective for back or chest acne, but it also can be used on the face. It is a good choice of treatment for stubborn acne that does not respond well to other therapies. It is still not a cure for acne, but it may be able to keep acne under control, particularly in resistant cases. It is a relatively expensive treatment choice, especially compared with traditional therapies.

## ANALYSIS TECHNIQUE FOR ACNE OR PROBLEM SKIN

Before treating problem skin, the esthetician should take a thorough health history of the client. This is best accomplished by having the client fill out a health form. On your form you should include the following:

1. Client name, address, and phone numbers.

2. The client's occupation. This tells you if the client is in a high-stress job or if the client is employed in a situation where there is constant exposure to "greasy air," such as a fast-food restaurant.

3. Is the client already seeing a dermatologist? If so, was medication prescribed? Is the client using the medication as instructed by the dermatologist? (Often a client is not using the medication correctly or has discontinued it because of excessive drying or irritation. Do not interfere with a doctor's prescription or attempt to instruct about medication! Refer your client back to the dermatologist for further instruction. Never instruct a client to discontinue prescribed medication!) If questions arise, call and consult with the dermatologist.

4. How long has the client experienced problem skin? (This may tell you if it is a long-term hereditary problem or if it is caused by short-term factors such as comedogenic cosmetics, hormones, drugs, stress, etc.)

5. When does the client have flareups? Shortly before her period? During stressful times?

6. Is the client under a lot of stress?

7. What cosmetics and skin-care products does the client use presently? Request that the client bring in products presently used. This will allow you to check for comedogenic products and to see what steps the client is taking to help.

8. Is the client using birth control pills, and what type?

9. Has the client had any history of hormone problems? Is she experiencing menopause? Is she taking prescribed hormones?

10. Is she pregnant?

**Photodynamic therapy (PDT)** is a medical treatment using intense types of light.

**Porphyrins** are chemicals produced by acne bacteria during normal metabolic processes. These chemicals can react with blue light and become toxic to the bacteria.

**5-aminolevulinic acid**, also known as **Levulan**® or **Kerastick**®, is a drug chemical that is used when administering photodynamic therapy.

11. Does the client have allergies to any cosmetics, foods, or drugs?
12. Does the client have any other health problems or use any other form of medication?
13. Does the client eat a balanced diet?
14. Does the client take vitamin supplements?
15. Does the client have a history of acne in the family?
16. How often does the client clean the skin and with what product?
17. Does the client pick at acne lesions?
18. The client's age. Sometimes this will indicate the nature of the problem.

These standard questions should also be asked on the preliminary form completed on the first visit. It is generally recommended that any client who has not visited in six months fill out a new health evaluation form. Make sure you check for any other health problems or contraindications for home care or salon treatments (such as electrical therapy, heart problems, etc.) just as you would on any client.

## Hands-On Analysis

Remove the client's makeup and cleanse the skin's surface thoroughly. Analyze the client's skin through a magnifying lamp. It is a good idea at some point in the beginning of analysis to look at the skin with the client in a magnifying mirror. The best way to accomplish this is to use one of the two-way mirror devices available through equipment manufacturers. This interaction will allow the client to see what you are describing. Explain each type of problem to the client as thoroughly and simply as possible. Remember, the client is a consumer, not a professional. The bottom line of interest for the client is how you can help with beauty problems and problem skin.

Ask the client lots of questions about any skin problems:

◆ How often are you having breakouts?
◆ Where do they occur?
◆ Do they seem to come at certain times of the month?
◆ What do the blemishes look like when they occur?
◆ Do you normally have more or less breakout than this?
◆ Explain what you are doing now at home.

Even though the client may have written some of these answers down on the health form, it's a good idea to discuss them. Clients sometimes forget to write something down, or the esthetician may discover that the client is doing something incorrectly. This is also a good opportunity to review any experiences that the client has had with previous esthetic or dermatological treatment.

While observing the skin under the magnifying lamp, make detailed, written notes of any problems and any discussion you have with the client. You should particularly note the following:

1. Number of lesions.
2. What type of lesions? Open comedones? Closed comedones? Papules? Pustules? Nodules? Cysts?
3. Chin breakouts, particularly if isolated to that area.
4. Breakout around the mouth, isolated to that area. (This could possibly be perioral dermatitis.)
5. Flaking in the hairline, sides of nose, eyebrows, and ear areas. (Possibly seborrheic dermatitis.)
6. What is the thickness of the skin? Is it sensitive? Does it turn red easily?

7. Are the unaffected follicles clogged and enlarged? (This is indication of generally oily skin.)

8. Large red pustules and surrounding redness in the nose area. (Possibly rosacea.)

9. Flat red lesions that look like scraped skin, sometimes with scabs. (Client is probably scraping with the fingernails.)

10. Scarring—make special notes of any existing scarring, icepick scars, raised (hypertrophic) scars, and any scars from cyst removal.

11. Macules, which are lesions that have healed but are still red or tan in color. They are flat and are most often found in the fleshy areas of the face, such as the cheeks.

12. Is there any surface flaking or dehydration? Is the skin tight or pliable?

13. What grade of acne exists?

The esthetician must check to see if any client with rosacea, seborrheic dermatitis, perioral dermatitis, or cysts is seeing a dermatologist. These conditions are dermatologic, not esthetic. It is not the esthetician's place to diagnose or suggest these conditions to the client. Simply suggest that the client see a dermatologist. After the client sees the doctor, call the doctor and discuss esthetic concerns or arrange for the client to obtain a letter from the doctor.

## Salon Treatments

Before discussing salon treatments, a few important procedures and precautions should be discussed:

1. Do not use any product or ingredient to which the client is allergic.

2. Extraction should never last more than 10 or 15 minutes in one session. If you are uncomfortable with extraction procedures, omit this step completely. Extraction is probably the most important part of esthetic salon treatment, but it can also be the most harmful if done improperly. Never extract a lesion you are not sure about. Open and closed comedones and pustules are the only lesions that the esthetician should extract. Leave papules, nodules, and cysts alone!

3. The esthetician should wear disposable latex gloves during the entire acne treatment.

4. If lancets are used they must be sterile and disposable.

5. Active acne should never be massaged. After the acne is completely cleared, then consider a light massage.

6. Clients should be told not to wear makeup for at least two hours after treatment.

7. Skin that has been exposed to Retin-A or other prescription peeling agents should not be exfoliated. Eliminate the use of all keratolytics, including benzoyl peroxide, salicylic acid, sulfur, resorcinol, or glycolic acid, for clients using Retin-A.

8. Be careful how much you extract on the first visit. As the client begins home care, the impactions will be much softer and easier to extract and a lot more comfortable for the client. Explain this so the client will understand that you will do more extraction on the second visit, when the client has been using the correct products for a week or two.

## Basic Salon Acne Treatment

1. Thoroughly cleanse and analyze.

2. Re-cleanse with a foaming cleanser.

3. Apply a desincrusting pre-mask. Begin the steam treatment during the pre-mask. Allow to sit for eight minutes.

4. Remove the pre-mask. Proceed with galvanic desincrustation as normal, about five minutes in duration.

5. Begin extraction in the chin area first, moving up the face, and finishing at the forehead. This will avoid contact with my blood or fluids. As previously mentioned, the esthetician should wear latex disposable gloves during extraction and throughout the remainder of treatment.

6. After extraction, apply a generous amount of antibacterial toner to the entire area extracted.

7. Unfold a 12-ply piece of gauze and place across the client's entire face. Avoiding the eye area, apply high-frequency current to the client's face (through the gauze) for about one to two minutes. Remove the gauze.

8. Apply a small amount of 5 percent benzoyl peroxide to the extracted areas.

9. Apply a drying mask with camphor. (For more severe conditions, you may use a sulfur drying mask or benzoyl peroxide mask.) Avoid the eye areas.

10. Allow the mask to sit for about 15 minutes. Wet the mask well with a cold spray solution of toner to loosen before removal. Remove with wet sponges or a soft cloth. Spray the face again with toner mixture to remove any excess mask.

11. Apply a small amount of sunscreen to finish the treatment.

## Alternative Treatment #1 for Acne

This treatment is effective for thicker skin types with grades 2 and 3 acne.

1. Thoroughly cleanse and analyze.

2. Re-cleanse with an alkaline pre-mask or an alkaline rinseable cleanser.

3. Apply a soft-setting enzyme treatment to help dissolve surface cell buildup and dilate follicles. Begin the steam treatment during the enzyme treatment. Allow to sit for eight minutes.

4. Remove the enzyme treatment. Proceed with galvanic desincrustation as normal, about five minutes in duration.

5. If you are using a lancet, begin dilating the follicle openings of the closed comedones in the chin area, moving up the face to the cheeks and finishing on the forehead. Proceed with extraction. Gently dilate the top of any follicles with pustules with separate lancets. Extract pustules.

6. After extraction, apply a generous amount of antibacterial toner to the entire area extracted.

7. Unfold a 12-ply piece of gauze and place across the client's entire face. Avoiding the eye area, apply high-frequency current to the client's face (through the gauze) for about one to two minutes. Remove the gauze.

8. Apply a small amount of 5 percent benzoyl peroxide to extracted areas.

9. Apply a drying sulfur or benzoyl peroxide mask, avoiding the eye area. For more sensitive skins, apply a drying mask with camphor.

10. Allow the mask to sit for about 15 minutes. Wet the mask well with a cold spray solution of toner to loosen before removal. Remove with wet sponges or a soft cloth. Spray the face again with toner mixture to remove any excess mask.

11. Apply a small amount of sunscreen to finish the treatment.

## USING GLYCOLIC AND OTHER PEELS FOR ACNE

Use of exfoliant peels such as glycolic or salicylic or mixed acid 30 percent AHA peels can be beneficial in drying, exfoliating, and speeding up results in chronic acne and very oily, clogged skin. The client should be using a 10 percent AHA at home for at least two weeks before starting the use of these light peels.

AHA peels can be used between extraction facial visits, and if the skin is not too sensitive, peels can be performed at the beginning of a regular facial treatment.

Microdermabrasion may be used in cases of clogged, oily skin, but it is not recommended for papular, pustular, or inflammatory acne. Microdermabrasion should not be used in addition to any other form of exfoliation or peel.

No form of peels should be performed on clients using prescription keratolytic drugs, unless approved by their dermatologist.

## Treatment for Clients Who Have Recently Begun Using Retin-A or Other Prescription Peeling Agents

1. Thoroughly cleanse and analyze, paying particular attention to any red or sensitive areas.

2. If the skin is red or sensitive, apply a light, noncomedogenic hydrating fluid. Proceed with steam for five to eight minutes. Be very careful not to get the skin hot from the steam. Cool steam, is a good choice here. For skin that appears noninflamed, apply a desincrustant pre-mask instead of the dehydrating fluid.

3. Remove the pre-mask or hydrating fluid. Galvanic is best avoided on clients just beginning Retin-A treatment.

4. Begin extraction gently in the same chin to forehead pattern.

5. Apply a generous amount of antibacterial nonalcoholic toner on a cool, wet, cotton pad or soft cloth. Apply to all extracted areas. If you prefer, you may use a diluted cold spray toner solution.

6. Apply a noncomedogenic hydrating fluid. Cover with gauze and proceed with high frequency (mushroom attachment) for one to two minutes.

7. Apply a cool, soothing treatment with aloe, azulene, bisabolol, or chamomile. Gel masks are very beneficial and gentle, as long as they are free of alcohol and fragrance. For thicker skins, you may try a light application of light-setting, clay-based camphor mask.

8. Do not allow to sit for more than five to seven minutes. Remove the mask by thoroughly wetting it with cold spray, then gently wiping with cool, wet cotton or soft cloths.

9. Apply a light, noncomedogenic moisturizer with sunscreen.

## TOPICS FOR DISCUSSION

1. What is acne?

2. Trace the development of the comedo.

3. Explain how hormones affect acne.

4. Name some environmental factors influencing acne development.

5. Explain various cleansers, toners, and treatment creams and lotions available for acne and their action on the skin.

6. Discuss some acne-related conditions that should be referred to the dermatologist.

7. What are some questions that should be asked of the client during the first consultation?

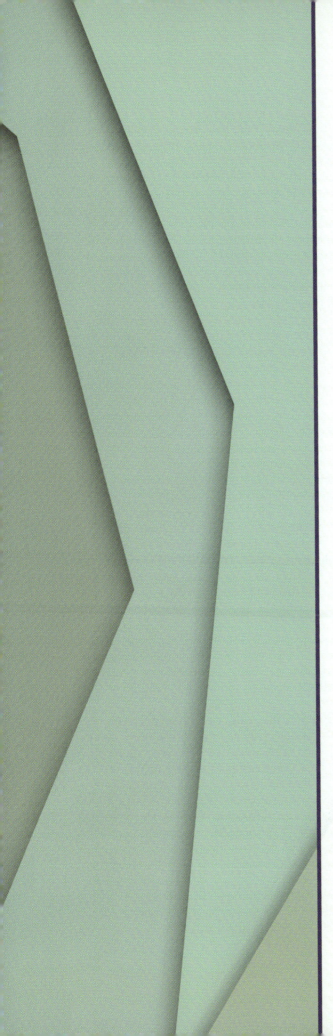

CHAPTER **16**

# Comedogenicity

## OBJECTIVES. . .

Many ingredients used in cosmetics can make acne worse and can contribute to the development of comedones of all types.

**Comedogenicity** is the tendency of topical substances to cause the development of comedones, possibly leading to or worsening acne eruptions. Multiple comedones, both open and closed, can lead to the formation of inflammatory acne lesions. Dermatologists began scientific documentation in 1941 of topically induced acneiform eruptions in chlorinated hydrocarbons in occupational acne in workers handling certain chemicals.

Comedogenicity is a particularly important subject for the esthetician to understand, because the esthetics profession specializes in keeping skin healthy and clean and advising clients about cosmetic treatment preparations. It is a vital part of the esthetician's job to prevent potential reactions on their clients' skin and to educate clients about preventative treatment techniques, including avoiding treatments or products that may not be right for their skin.

In this chapter you will learn about these ingredients and how they affect the skin. You will learn how to check ingredient lists for possible comedogenic ingredients. You will also learn about the many products that are helpful for clog-prone, oily, and acne-prone skin.

**Comedogenicity** is the tendency of topical substances to cause the development of comedones, possibly leading to or worsening acne eruptions.

# BACKGROUND

For many years, dermatologists often told women who had acne or problem skin to avoid using makeup. Many doctors said this as a blanket statement and encouraged women with acne to avoid all cosmetics.

These doctors noticed that women often did not respond to traditional acne therapy. They also noticed that many of the women continued to use makeup and cosmetics on a regular basis.

These dermatologists did not know at the time specifically why the cosmetics caused acne to become worse or not to improve during treatment. Many thought that the cosmetics sat on the skin and occluded aeration of the follicles, not allowing oxygen to penetrate the follicles. Others were aware that many of the cosmetics had a high fat or oil content. It seemed to make sense that oily skin that developed acne lesions easily did not need additional oil from outside.

These theories made sense, and some studies touched on the subject of cosmetics and hair products aggravating acne, but it wasn't until the early 1970s that doctors published studies that showed increased retention hyperkeratosis or a buildup of cells within the follicle in patients using some types of cosmetics.

It was discovered that the use of certain ingredients within cosmetics was more likely to cause a pronounced buildup of cells within the follicle. This buildup lined the follicle walls, and when enough was accumulated, it began forming a microcomedo. The microcomedo eventually evolved into an open or closed comedone and then possibly into an inflammatory acne lesion, such as a papule or pustule.

The acne-prone women who used the cosmetics in question already had a predisposition to clog development. In other words, they already had a tendency to develop clogged pores from hereditary retention hyperkeratosis and oiliness.

**Acne cosmetica** is acne caused or worsened by the use of comedogenic or inflammatory cosmetics or skin care products.

**Comedogenic** means the tendency of a topical ingredient or product to increase the buildup of dead cells within the follicle, eventually causing comedone formation.

**Noncomedogenic** means that the ingredient or product does not cause excessive follicular hyperkeratosis and therefore is unlikely to cause comedone development.

The doctors coined a term for this condition, **acne cosmetica**, meaning "cosmetic acne." They were able to correlate excessive buildup of dead cells within the follicles of patients using certain cosmetics. These cosmetics were said to be **comedogenic**. Comedogenic means the tendency of a topical ingredient or product to increase the buildup of dead cells within the follicle, eventually causing comedone formation. **Noncomedogenic** means that the ingredient or product does not cause excessive follicular hyperkeratosis and therefore is unlikely to cause comedone development.

There are two basic types of reactions that are cosmetic-induced acne aggravators. First is true comedogenesis, which can take up to several months to occur, resulting in comedo formation. Comedogenic products essentially cause increased follicular hyperkeratosis, combining with sebaceous secretions and resulting in solidified plugs or comedones.

The second is a perifollicular irritation that can cause an acute eruption of papules or pustules in a very short period of time. Clients, from time to time, will experience an overnight flare of pimples when using a new cream or even after a salon facial treatment. It is this irritant type of reaction that can cause overnight flares. The irritation from the chemical or product will cause follicular inflammation or swelling, creating a narrowing of the follicle thus creating an anaerobic pocket, which is ideal for acne bacteria to flourish. This is known as an **acnegenic** reaction. The product or ingredient causing the inflammation is known as an acnegenic ingredient or product. The term acnegenic is probably a more appropriate term than comedogenic, because the term acnegenic can actually encompass both comedogenic and follicular irritant reactions.

**Acnegenic** refers to the tendency of a topical substance, usually a cosmetic or skin care product, to cause inflammation or aggravate acne.

Irritant reactions and true comedogenic reactions can be evaluated by microscopic examination of follicles exposed to the ingredients or of the finished product and checking for inflammation or thickening of the follicle wall.

The development of comedones through comedogenic product exposure can take months to occur. Acnegenic reactions due to perifollicular irritation can occur very quickly.

## Analysis of Acne Cosmetica

Acne cosmetica is most often characterized by multiple open and closed comedones. These may be all over the face, or in isolated areas where a certain product is being used, or where the skin is oily and susceptible to comedo development.

Acne cosmetica often looks like bumpiness just under the surface of the skin. This can be particularly apparent in the chin or cheeks. You may also notice that the client wears a lot of makeup, uses very oily products, or tends to try many different skin-care and cosmetic products.

Ask the client the following questions:

1. Do you notice worsening of the acne after using certain products?
2. Do you notice excessive oiliness when using certain products?
3. Is one area more clogged than others?
4. Are there many clogged pores and comedones, or just papules without comedones?
5. Do pimples seem to flare during certain times of the month?
6. How long have you had this problem?

Following are some scenarios that may be helpful in determining causes of flares or comedones.

Clients reporting a recent worsening may be able to pinpoint a new or fairly new product as the culprit. Comedones can take up to 6 months to form, so you must help the client remember any product changes in the last 6 months. Sudden flares of papules are more likely to indicate acnegenicity or a follicle-irritating product. Follicle irritation can cause an overnight flare. This can be connected to a very recent product addition.

Flares of acne without comedones are **inflammatory acne** and can result from hormonal flares or acnegenic products causing follicle irritation. Some medications may contribute to flares also.

Worsening of acne after using certain products also indicates that the products may be acnegenic. Excessive oiliness when using a particular product can indicate that an oily emollient is present in the products. This oiliness tends to worsen when the product has been worn for an hour or two and body temperature has caused the product to feel more oily.

If one area is more clogged than another, this may indicate an isolated comedogenic product or an area of the skin that is more prone to comedo development. **Blushline acne**, characterized by multiple closed comedones, is a good example of acne in an isolated area.

When the rest of the face is clear, the clogged T-zone indicates a tendency of the skin to clog in this area. Careful monitoring of products applied to this area is needed.

Bumpiness in the skin of the forehead and around the hairline is known as **pomade acne**. This occurs when comedogenic or irritating hair products, usually styling gels, conditioners, scalp oils, or sprays, coat the surface of the skin around the hairline. Pomade acne is often seen in teenagers who use many hair gels and on African-American clients, who often use scalp oils.

If the client reports worsening during certain times of the month, hormonal factors are likely playing a role in acne-prone skin. Sudden stimulation of the sebaceous

**Inflammatory acne** are flares of acne without comedones, and can result from hormonal flares or acnegenic products causing follicle irritation.

**Blushline acne** is a type of acne cosmetica, with multiple closed comedones in the blushline; caused by comedogenic pressing agents and/or dyes in the blush.

**Pomade acne** is bumpiness in the skin of the forehead and around the hairline.

glands from flares of male hormones produces sebum, irritating the follicle walls. Even though the client's acne flare may be hormonal, it is still important to make sure the client avoids comedogenic products.

## TESTING FOR COMEDOGENICITY

Researchers have developed a test for comedogenicity using the inside of a rabbit's ear. Cosmetic or drug topical products were applied to the inside of the ear, because the follicles inside the rabbit ear develop comedones much faster than human skin. Within three weeks most cosmetics can be tested using the rabbit ear method.

The procedure for rabbit ear assays, as they are called by the scientific community, is really quite simple. A product is applied to the inside of one ear of a male albino rabbit at least 12 weeks old. The reason for the specific sex and age of the rabbit is due to the size of these particular animals' follicles, which are better for evaluation of comedo development.

The other ear of the rabbit is left alone, as a control. A *control* is an experimental factor that remains the same throughout the experiment. Scientists can compare the two ears at the end of the three-week period to determine the difference seen in the follicles of the skin of the two different ears of the rabbit model.

The product is applied to the test area daily for three weeks. Each day the ear is observed for obvious changes to the skin and checked carefully for comedo formation.

If after three weeks there are no comedones, the product testing is finished. However, to be absolutely sure there is no excessive follicular hyperkeratosis, small tissue samples are taken surgically from the skin of the ear and examined under a microscope. Any hyperkeratosis will be obvious as it lines the follicle walls. At the same time the follicle is examined for irritation that might cause immediate acne reactions due to follicle irritation. The test is not fully complete if this microscopic test is not run. This test is called a **histopathological** study (Figure 16-1).

**Histopathological** refers to microscopic examination of tissue to determine causes of disease or abnormality.

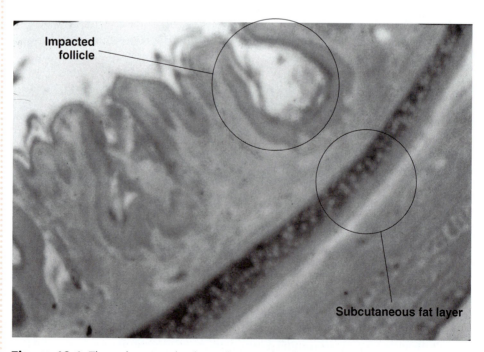

**Figure 16-1** The microscopic view of retention hyperkeratosis shows excessive cell buildup and swelling. This slide represents a positive test for comedogenicity

If comedo formation is detected, it is rated on a scale of 0 to 3. A score of 0 means that no comedones formed. A score of 3 means that the product or ingredient is comedogenic. Only products with overall scores of 0 on all rabbits tested are claimed to be noncomedogenic.

The hyperkeratosis and inflammation within the follicle found during the histopathological examination are rated on the same scale. Although most follicles will develop a small amount of irritation and keratosis while being tested, large amounts of keratosis may indicate a delayed comedogenic reaction. In other words, a high test score in the histopathology report may indicate that longer exposure time to the product or ingredient may cause comedo development or that the test material causes sufficient irritation within the follicle to possibly promote sudden acne flares.

Materials that are found to be both noncomedogenic and show no significant irritancy or retention hyperkeratosis within the histopathological examination are said to be nonacnegenic.

A few scientists and physicians use a five-point scale. Both tests are run using scores of 0 to 5, rather than 0 to 3. If you look at various studies, you will notice that both scales are used, but the three-point scale is more often used and is the standard widely accepted by the cosmetic industry. If you look at comedogenicity studies or charts, you will notice that one rating number is followed by a slash mark and then a 3 or a 5. As an example you may see a rating of 2/3. This means that out of 3 possible points, the product or ingredient tested had a rating of 2, making it significantly comedogenic. Scores of 3/3, 4/5, or 5/5 indicate highly comedogenic materials or products.

A score of 1/3, 1/5, or 2/5 means that the product or material showed comedogenic results in the rabbit ear but not as strong as a material with a higher score.

Remember, clients who are subject to easy development of clogged pores, comedones, and other acne lesions must first hereditarily develop retention hyperkeratosis. A client who does not develop clogged pores easily and has fairly oil-dry skin may show no reaction when treated with a product that has a low score of comedogenicity of approximately 1/3 or 2/5. Clients who easily develop acne flareups may be much more sensitive to even a mildly comedogenic material.

## OTHER TESTS

Tests for comedogenicity can also be run on humans, most often human backs. The product or ingredient to be tested is applied and occluded with a patch or bandage. This is repeated on a daily basis for a specified amount of time. The skin is observed for comedo development by scientists or dermatologists. The skin can also be **biopsied**, which means a tissue sample is removed, using a **cyanoacrylate** biopsy. Cyanoacrylate, the main ingredient in powerful household glues, is applied to the skin. When peeled off, the content of the follicle is attached to the chemical. The tissue sample can then be examined under a microscope for follicular debris and hyperkeratosis.

Many scientists believe that the rabbit ear assay is a much more accurate test for determining comedogenicity. There are several reasons for this opinion. First, the rabbit ear forms comedones much faster than human skin, making the testing procedure much faster and therefore more economical. Second, rabbit ear skin is very sensitive to comedo development. Human skin develops clogged pores much more slowly. The skin on the back of a human may not necessarily develop retention hyperkeratosis hereditarily. Third, and probably most important, a rabbit can be easily controlled, and there are very few variables involved with testing. The rabbit is in a controlled environment, with a controlled diet and climate. Humans, however, are not confined, and you must consider literally hundreds of variables when you interpret test results. As examples, human models may have different diets, different environments, and different activities.

**Biopsied** refers to removal of a small sample of tissue for microscopic or other examination.

**Cyanoacrylate** is a synthetic polymer, commonly known as "super glue."

Because of these variables, many scientists believe that human studies are not as reliable or as accurate as rabbit ear studies.

The American Academy of Dermatology issued extensive guidelines for the scientific evaluation of products for comedogenicity and follicle irritancy. These tests involve applying finished products to skin and observing any comedo development, carefully examining histological follicle biopsies for hyperkeratosis and perifollicular inflammation. The best confirmation of noncomedogenicity and nonirritancy is to have documentation by an independent test laboratory. Ask manufacturers how they determine if their products are noncomedogenic and nonirritating to follicles. Are the products tested by an independent laboratory, and what type of tests are run? Unfortunately, some companies make a noncomedogenic claim and have no tests to document their claim!

The bottom line of these guidelines is that for a true assessment of comedogenicity, the final skin-care or cosmetic product should be scientifically evaluated using this accepted protocol.

## TYPES OF INGREDIENTS THAT ARE OFTEN COMEDOGENIC

The frequent culprit in the most comedogenic products is the spreading agent or vehicle. A good example of this would be a foundation or moisturizer with a comedogenic vehicle. These ingredients are used to apply the skin-care or cosmetic product to smooth, serve as an emollient or sebum replacement in alipidic (oil-dry) skin types, or add an elegant feel to the product. Oily skin areas are, of course, not alipidic. Because some of these emollients are designed to mimic human sebum, it is no wonder that some of these ingredients add to the problem of cell buildup and comedo development. Unfortunately, the vehicle often makes up the greatest part of the product, so when comedogenic ingredients are present in the vehicle, they can be present in fairly substantial quantities.

A second culprit is the emollient ingredient. Certain emollient fats, oils, waxes, fatty alcohols, fatty acids, and esters are the most common comedogenic ingredients, and many of these can be either vehicle or emollient ingredients. These ingredients often have waxy or sebum-like textures, and because of their oily and heavy texture they are generally not appropriate for a skin that is already producing too much sebum.

Think of the dead corneum cells constantly shedding from the walls of the follicles as flakes of oatmeal lining a drinking glass. Because of the hereditary tendency to retain cells and because of this type of skin's oiliness, the flakes of dead cells naturally stick to the follicle walls.

Now imagine pouring oil down the sides of this glass filled with oatmeal. Imagine how oil would make the oatmeal sticky and clump together.

This may be a very rough metaphor, but it does illustrate the point. Many of the fats, oils, esters, and emollient ingredients used in cosmetics do penetrate the follicles of already clog-prone individuals, adding fatty substances to the follicles of the skin that is already burdened with too much sebum and cell buildup.

These ingredients are considered comedogenic. Their purpose in cosmetics is to lubricate or serve as a spreading agent. Although this may be helpful to truly dry skins that do not produce enough oil, it is bad for clog-prone skin. Unfortunately, not all comedogenic ingredients feel greasy or oily. In fact, some actually feel lightweight, confusing clients and estheticians alike. This is why it is so important that estheticians understand comedogenic and acnegenic principles, to prevent client use of the wrong products and to have available for purchase noncomedogenic and nonirritating formulations. Again, the bottom line is to make sure your products have been properly tested by an independent laboratory to ensure that they are truly noncomedogenic and nonacnegenic.

# Emollients and Oils

Emollients that often clog pores are derived from fats or waxes of animal or vegetable origin. We will divide these substances into several categories.

**Oils.** Many vegetable and animal oils are comedogenic. Coconut oil, cocoa butter, peach kernel oil, linseed oil, grape seed oil, olive oil, and sesame oil are comedogenic oils. Less comedogenic or noncomedogenic oils include avocado oil, safflower oil, castor oil, jojoba oil, and sunflower oil. Mineral oil is also noncomedogenic.

**Other Waxes and Fats.** Beeswax is noncomedogenic, particularly in small quantities of concentration, as it is often used. Emulsifying wax, carnauba wax, and candelilla wax, often used in lipstick, are noncomedogenic. Petrolatum is also noncomedogenic. However, because petrolatum is relatively greasy, it is not used often in cosmetics for oily and clog-prone skin, especially in large concentrations.

**Fatty Acids.** Probably the most comedogenic group of cosmetic chemicals is the fatty acids. Fatty acids, which are used to give cosmetics a creamy consistency, are often comedogenic. These substances are derived from animal and plant oils and include oleic acid, lauric acid, isostearic acid, palmitic acid, and myristic acid. Capric acid, caprylic acid, and behenic acid are less comedogenic but still should not be used in large concentrations for oily, problem skin.

**Esters.** The fatty esters obtained from combining alcohols with fatty acids are also often comedogenic. These esters are often used in cosmetics because they feel less oily than raw fatty acids. However, their chemical alteration to an ester often renders them comedogenic. The esters that are comedogenic include isopropyl myristate, very well known as a highly comedogenic ingredient. Other comedogenic esters are isopropyl palmitate, octyl palmitate, isopropyl isostearate, decyl oleate, sorbitan oleate, isopropyl lanolate, iosopropyl linoleate, butyl stearate, and myristyl myristate.

**Fatty Alcohols.** Fatty alcohols are used in cosmetics as emollients. They are generally less comedogenic than their parent acids or esters. The comedogenic fatty alcohols include oleyl alcohol, isostearyl alcohol, and octyldodecanol.

**Lanolin.** Lanolin is derived from sheep sebum. It is an excellent emollient, and in its purest form, in a small quantity, does not cause many problems for clog-prone skin. However, chemically altered lanolins, such as lanolic acid, isopropyl lanolate, and acetylated lanolin alcohol, are comedogenic.

**Performance Agents.** It is interesting that most extracts, pigments, humectants, and other performance agents are noncomedogenic ingredients. Emollients and fatty-type ingredients create the most problems. The other ingredients that create problems are inorganic pigments, specifically the red dyes.

Some ingredients, including some natural ingredients, may be irritating and still are not comedogenic, creating the possibility of an overnight type of acnegenic reaction.

**The Red Dyes.** Almost every red dye is comedogenic. This explains why you may often notice closed comedones on women's cheekbones. Red dyes are frequently used in blushes.

These dyes are derivatives of coal tar. Coal tar is extremely comedogenic. Red dyes are used in blush, lipsticks, powders, foundations, and skin-care products. They are not permitted to be used in eyeshadows. Coal tar is known to be a major eye irritant and is not safe for use in the eye area.

Unfortunately, many of the beautiful shades of blush or lipstick cannot be made without D & C red dyes. There is a red color in an organic pigment called carmine and in certain colors of iron oxide that are noncomedogenic. Carmine is more expensive to use than D & C red dyes and does not produce as vivid red colors.

Because of these facts, you may correctly assume that, in general, the more red a product is, the more likely it is to contain D & C red dyes and the more likely it is to be comedogenic. Again, these dyes do not produce problems for many clients who are not acne prone. However, they should be avoided in oily and acne-prone clients. Some cosmetics companies do manufacture blushes that are free of coal tar dyes.

## CHEMISTRY BEHIND COMEDOGENICITY

The chemical reasons why certain cosmetic ingredients are comedogenic are not fully understood. It is certainly logical that the fats that simulate human sebum could potentially cause problems for oily, problem skin. It is believed that the size of the molecule has a great deal to do with comedogenic potential. The larger the molecule, the less likely it is to be comedogenic. This explains why some fatty acids become more or less comedogenic when they are altered chemically. When a large molecular structure is added to a fatty acid, it tends to become less comedogenic. When a fat is broken down to a smaller molecule, it is more comedogenic. This is theorized to be linked to the size of the molecule and its ability to penetrate the follicle. It makes sense that smaller fatty molecules penetrate more easily into the follicle and therefore may cause more problems.

## Concentration of Comedogenic Ingredients

The amount of comedogenic ingredients used within a particular cosmetic formulation may also have an effect on the overall comedogenicity of the product. Moisturizers with large amounts of known comedogenic ingredients are more likely to be comedogenic than products with less concentration of comedogenic ingredients.

Controversy continues over the amount of comedogenic ingredients that should be used in cosmetics. Some scientists believe that as long as comedogenic ingredients make up less than 5 percent of the product, there will be no effect on the comedogenicity. The flaw in this idea is that neither the consumer nor the esthetician knows exactly how much comedogenic chemical is used in any particular product, because no cosmetic company publishes its percentages on the label. This makes this theory impossible to use practically.

The other argument against this theory is that known comedogenic ingredients should simply not be used in products that are designed for clog-prone, oily, or acne-prone skin. Again, the bottom line is to have the finished product tested. There are now many good noncomedogenic emollients and vehicle ingredients available.

## Pressing Agents

Besides the problem with D & C red dyes, the other problem with blushes, as well as pressed powders, is the pressing agent. Emollients are added to talc and other products to create cake-type blush and powder. Pressed powder is an example. By mixing the powder with a sticky emollient, a pressed cake forms, which is usually marketed as a compact or powder blush.

If a comedogenic emollient is used to press the powder or blush, the product may indeed cause or increase comedone development. If a blush with D & C red dyes is pressed with a comedogenic agent, you get a "double-whammy" as far as comedogenicity is concerned!

Zinc stearate, octyldodecyl stearoyl stearate, and mineral oil are safe ingredients to use in pressing powders. They do not cause clogging and make good pressing agents.

The other problem with pressing agents is that they involve mixing a fat, which is liquid or semiliquid, with a nonsoluble powder. This means that, unlike moisturizers, which are usually water-based and always liquid, there are no liquid ingredients to "water down" the comedogenic effects of the emollient pressing agent.

Because of this, comedogenic powders tend to be very comedogenic because the skin is more directly exposed to the concentrated emollient.

## Loose Powders

Loose powders are not immune from comedogenicity just because they are not in a cake form. Emollients are also added to loose powders to give them a silky texture and to help them adhere to the skin. Check powders carefully to make sure they are free of both comedogenic emollients and coal tar-derived D & C red dyes.

## Skin-Care Products

Skin-care products are often comedogenic, particularly many types of moisturizers, lotions, fluids, and creams. They may be made with comedogenic emollients or other fatty ingredients. If you are treating a clog-prone client, check ingredients carefully (Figure 16-2).

## The Controversy Over Ingredient Lists

Some scientists have objected to comedogenic ingredient lists (like the one included here). Their objection is based on the theory that mixtures of ingredients may not be as harmful as the individual ingredient's test score indicates.

Although it is true that the bottom line is to have the final product tested, many companies do not test their products or publish the results of testing.

Testing for comedogenicity can be expensive and time-consuming. This is an additional expense for the company. Theoretically, claims testing should always be performed by an independent testing firm. By having testing performed outside the cosmetic company, the test results will be more likely to be accurate, reliable, and nonbiased. The reason lists like this one exist is so that estheticians and consumers can check the labels of their skin-care products and cosmetics for comedogenic ingredients. Even though this may not always be the most scientific or accurate method of determining potential comedogenicity, it is certainly the most practical for helping clients choose the right products.

## COMEDOGENIC PRODUCT ANALYSIS

When you consult with a client who has acne or develops clogged pores easily, ask the client to bring in the products being used currently, so that you may check them for comedogenic ingredients.

Consumers today have heard the word *noncomedogenic*, but they generally are not aware of the variety of cosmetic ingredients that are comedogenic. One of the most important duties of the esthetician is to educate consumers about cosmetic chemistry. Although your clients do not need to know everything in this chapter, they will appreciate your knowledge about comedogenic ingredients and products, as well as the advice you can give about eliminating comedogenic products from home skin-care and cosmetic routines.

Although you cannot run a comedogenicity test on every product that your client might bring in, you can check the products for comedogenic ingredients content. Check each ingredient against charts like the one here. Companies that produce noncomedogenic cosmetics often have charts available that list ingredients and their comedogenic levels. On request, many of these same companies will be glad to share their comedogenic studies on their own products with you.

---

### Common Comedogenic Ingredients

**Highly Comedogenic
(4-5/5 or 5/3)**

Linseed Oil
Olive Oil
Cocoa Butter
Oleic Acid
Coal Tar
Isopropyl Isostearate
Squalene
Isopropyl Myristate
Myristyl Myristate
Acetylated Lanolin
Isopropyl Palmitate
Isopropyl Linoleate
Oleyl Alcohol
Octyl Palmitate
Isostearic Acid
Myreth 3 Myristate
Butyl Stearate
Lanolic Acid

**Moderately Comedogenic
(3-4/5 or 2/3)**

Decyl Oleate
Sorbitan Oleate
Myristyl Lactate
Coconut Oil
Grape Seed Oil
Sesame Oil
Hexylene Glycol
Tocopherol
Isostearyl Neopentanoate
Most D & C Red Pigments
Octyldodecanol
Peanut Oil
Lauric Acid
Mink Oil

**Mildly Comedogenic
(2-3/5 or 1/3)**

Corn Oil
Safflower Oil
Lauryl Alcohol
Lanolin Alcohol
Glyceral Stearate
Lanolin
Sunflower Oil
Avocado Oil
Mineral Oil
(Please note that mildly comedogenic
ingredients are generally not a problem when
used in diluted concentrations. Check to see
their ranking of concentration on the ingredient
label.)

**Noncomedogenic**

Glycerin
Squalane
Sorbitol
Sodium PCA
Zinc Stearate
Octyldodecyl Stearate
SD Alcohol
Propylene Glycol
Allantoin
Panthenol
Water
Iron Oxides
Dimethicone
Cyclomethicone
Polysorbates
Cetyl Palmitate
Propylene Glycol Dicaprate/Dicaprylate
Jojoba Oil
Isopropyl Alcohol
Sodium Hyaluronate
Octylmethoxycinnimate
Oxybenzone
Petrolatum
Butylene Glycol
Tridecyl Stearate
Tridecyl Trimellitate
Octyldodecyl Stearoyl Stearate
Phenyl Trimethicone

**Figure 16-2** Chart of common comedogenic ingredients

Returning to your product analysis, check with your clients to see what products they are routinely using. Clients will often bring in products that they are not actually using. It is important that your client is honest with you regarding daily habits.

Begin by checking your client's moisturizers and treatment preparations. The most important products to observe are products that remain on clog-prone areas of the face for prolonged periods of time. These include day creams, night treatment creams, moisturizers, hydrators, sunscreens, foundations, powders, blushes, and any other specialty products that the client uses that stay on the face for long periods of time.

Cleansers and toners should also be noncomedogenic, but these products do not stay on the face for eight hours at a time. Cleansers should be very easily rinseable and should not leave residues on the face. Superfatted soaps, for example, tend to leave a film on the face. Often the fat added to these soaps is comedogenic. Toner can also be made with fats, particularly if they are designed for extra dry, alipidic skin.

A good noncomedogenic cleanser should be made with noncomedogenic emulsifiers. Many contain a detergent. They may vary in strength, but many will be on the stronger side, because most skin types that develop clogs easily are also predominantly oily, making thorough cleansing a necessity. These detergent cleansers will do a good job of cleansing surface oil and debris. The cleansers may be too strong for very dry skin, but most alipidic skins do not clog easily.

A foaming cleanser is often used. These cleansers are extremely rinseable and leave the skin feeling very clean, a feeling clients often describe as "squeaky." There is nothing wrong with this feeling, as long as the cleanser does not have a high pH, stripping off too much oil and creating impaired barrier function. Most oily clients like to feel superclean. They enjoy and will use a foaming-type cleanser, particularly if they use soap on a regular basis. In short, foaming cleansers give the client the feeling of using soap without the undesirable effects of some soaps. Foaming cleansers are also convenient and can be used in the shower or bath easily.

Toners should be, as previously discussed, free of fats. They should have moderately strong astringent action, helping to remove excess oils and cell buildup. Some may contain an antibacterial, and some of the stronger ones for oily skin may contain a mild peeling agent like salicylic acid. Cleansing milk can be used for makeup removal but should be easily removed and should not leave a residue on the skin. For oilier skin, clients may want to use a foaming cleanser after removal of makeup with a cleansing milk. Cold cream type of cleansers should not be used for clog-prone skin because they leave too much of a residue and do not remove enough oil from the surface.

## Sunscreens and Day Creams

When most people think of sunscreens, they imagine greasy, coconut-fragranced oils and creams worn at the beach. Obviously, many of these oily products are comedogenic, and many clients may associate them with a previous acnegenic experience.

Sunscreens are now made for daily use and are much more lightweight than the beach products many of us remember. Still, it is important to check to make sure that the sunscreens you are using and selling to acne-prone clients are truly noncomedogenic and are also lightweight in texture for those clients with oily and combination skin.

Sunscreens for oily skin are usually in a light lotion, blended with hydrators and/or silicones such as dimethicone to help prevent dehydration. Like all sunscreens, they should be broad spectrum, screening both UVA (ultraviolet A) and UVB light. It cannot be stressed enough that day sunscreens be very comfortable for the user. They cannot be sticky, and they must perform well under makeup.

## Night Treatments

There are two basic types of night treatments for clogged and problem skin: hydrators and exfoliating products.

Hydrating creams or fluids are made for skin that is clogged or acne prone but still dehydrated—in other words, skin that really needs hydration but also breaks out easily. These fluids are water-based, very light in texture, noncomedogenic, free of the offending ingredients we have discussed and they contain hydrating agents that will not clog, such as sodium PCA, glycerin, sorbitol, or hyaluronic acid. These agents hydrate without causing clog development and may be used in products without high levels of fatty emollients. Exfoliating treatment products and fluids are designed to help exfoliate excess dead cell buildup to break loose impactions. These products contain peeling agents such as benzoyl peroxide, salicylic acid, glycolic acid, resorcinol, sulfur, or a combination of these. They should be used in a lightweight vehicle base that is noncomedogenic. For more information on how to use these acne treatments, please see Chapter 15.

## Foundations for Clog-Prone Skin

Foundation makeup for clogged and acne-prone skin must be noncomedogenic, preferably in a "fat-free," water-based liquid. As a general rule, liquid foundations are the only appropriate type of foundation for clogged and acne-prone skin. The foundation should be completely free of comedogenic ingredients and should be very lightweight. Coverage can still be attained if you look for foundations that contain a lot of talc and pigment. Many of these foundations contain some sort of evaporating agent, like witch hazel, to help control surface oiliness. These foundations often dry to a matte finish, a good characteristic for oily skin. Some of the newer foundations contain silicones such as cyclomethicone as a spreading agent. These foundations are good for older clients with acne problems, because they do not dry as matte.

Recently, loose powder makeup foundation, also known as **mineral makeup**, has been developed. Called mineral makeup because it largely comprises earth-based ingredients, this product contains coverage pigments like zinc oxide and titanium dioxide, both also physical sunscreens.

The powder is often blended with some sort of binder, usually a fatty substance, to help it adhere to the skin. Mineral makeup provides good coverage, but it should be checked for comedogenic binders that may serve as spreading agents to help the powder adhere to the skin.

## Other Products That May Be Comedogenic

Hair products and many kinds of face creams may contain comedogenic agents. The purposes of these creams, or claims, may vary greatly. They may not fall into the categories just mentioned. Check all products that come in contact with clog-prone areas.

Some items such as lipstick, eyeshadows, and other products need not be noncomedogenic because they are not being used in clog- or acne-prone areas. The only reason you may want to check these is if the client has an isolated clogged area, such as the lipline (you should check her lipstick or lip conditioner), or if the client is using the product in an area for which it was not intended (i.e., using a hair conditioner on the face). Hair conditioners and styling products often contain fats, oils, and other comedogenic ingredients. They are not designed to be used on the face.

Eye creams or concealers can be a factor in cosmetic acne. Because of gravity, these products may "drift" on to the upper cheeks while being worn. If comedogenic, they could cause problems for acne-prone areas.

Comedogenic ingredients are also sometimes used in ointments and prescription topical drugs. Although you should never tell a client to discontinue the use of a prescribed drug, you should be aware that some topical medications can be comedogenic.

## DEHYDRATED, CLOGGED SKIN

Many women, particularly mature women, suffer from dehydrated skin that is also clogged. This is caused by the client mistaking dehydrated skin for dry skin. In other words, the client actually has dehydrated (water-dry) skin but mistakenly uses products designed for dry (oil-dry) skin. These products designed for mature alipidic skin are often full of fatty acids, esters, waxes, oils, and fats. In the attempt to treat their dehydrated skin or wrinkles, they expose oily areas to the excessive fats and oils present in these emollient products.

Unfortunately, these clients have often been misdiagnosed by a cosmetic salesperson, or more unfortunately, a poorly educated esthetician. Many women have a fear of "dry skin," because they fear aging and associate "dry skin" with aging. They do not understand that aging is not caused by "dryness" but by hereditary factors and sun damage. They attempt to treat aging with oils.

**Mineral makeup**, another term for loose powder makeup foundation, largely comprises earth-based ingredients. This product contains coverage pigments like zinc oxide and titanium dioxide, both of which are also physical sunscreens.

It is very important to educate this client about dehydration versus oil dryness. Explain to clients that dehydration makes the skin look dry and flaky, but this does not mean that they need oil; they need water!

Hydration can be achieved in one of two ways. Hydrating active agents can be used to increase the water level of the surface cells, easing dehydration and flaking and making the skin look smoother and softer and feel better.

Adding oily products to this type of skin keeps the skin from further dehydration, but it does not necessarily add significant water to the surface cells. Fatty, oily products often contain comedogenic ingredients. While these clients attempt to "moisturize," they actually cause clogged pores to form, possibly developing into acne, and are not best treating their dehydrated skin.

Almost all hydrating active agents are noncomedogenic. Many emollient-active agents for oil-dry skin are comedogenic. Retrain clients to use noncomedogenic products with noncomedogenic emollient ingredients, and use good noncomedogenic hydrating agents such as sorbitol, sodium PCA, glycerin, or hyaluronic acid. Make sure you check the vehicle ingredients for comedogenic ingredients. Most often the spreading agents are comedogenic.

Avoid using overdrying peeling agents on these clients. Psychologically they will feel that their skin is even more dry, particularly in the first few days of treatment. It is important to make sure that the client is comfortable to ensure compliance with the new program.

## Heavy Creams

Many heavy creams can make acne-prone or oily clog-prone skin worse. Some of these creams are not actually comedogenic, but they contain large amounts of oils or petrolatum. They are simply too heavy for these oily-skinned clients. Although neither petrolatum or mineral oil is particularly comedogenic, they are not appropriate in large concentrations for oily, clogged, or acne-prone skin.

## Oil-Free and Water-Based

The "oil-free" and "water-based" claims are often made for products supposedly designed for oily skin. Neither of these two terms mean the same thing as *noncomedogenic*. *Oil-free* means, technically, that there are no oils in the product. That doesn't mean that there are no fatty esters, fatty acids, or other comedogenic ingredients.

*Water-based* simply means that the main ingredient is water, which might be mixed with comedogenic ingredients. The bottom line is, check the product carefully for comedogenic ingredients.

## CLINICAL COMEDOGENICS

Some clients will have a sudden acne flareup when introduced to certain new products. Although there can be many reasons for this reaction, occasionally even a non-comedogenic product can cause an acne flareup due to irritation of the follicles. If your client reports such a flareup, advise your client to try the cream again after a short time. If the reaction continues, the client should discontinue use of the product.

## Checklist of Products

The following products should be checked during a comedogenic analysis:

- ◆ Cleansers, washes, and soaps
- ◆ Toners, fresheners, and astringents
- ◆ Day creams, moisturizers, and sunscreens

- Night fluids, creams, specialty products, and ampoules
- Foundation makeup
- Blush
- Any other product that is being used over a clog-prone area of the face for a prolonged period of time

## Checklist of Analysis Procedures

1. Analyze the skin and the areas that have comedones, clogged pores, sebaceous filaments, or other acne lesions.
2. Check the client's current products for comedogenic ingredients.
3. Are the products the client is using really correct for the skin type, or is the client using products for oil-dry skin when the skin is actually dehydrated?
4. Is the client using fluids and lotions or creams?
5. Are the products the client is using simply too heavy for the skin?
6. Is the client skipping steps that should be done?
7. If the products the client uses contain comedogenic ingredients, are they high or low on the ingredient list? If the client has a minimal number of clogged pores, it may not be caused by the products. Remember, in order to have a comedogenic reaction, you must have comedogenic products and a skin type that tends to clog due to hereditary oiliness and hyperkeratosis.

## CLIENT PRODUCT ANALYSIS

As we have previously discussed, you should ask a client who is clog prone to bring in all products for analysis on the first visit. First, check the products with the checklist for analysis.

After checking the products for correct skin type, and so forth, begin checking the products for comedogenic ingredients. Let's look at a typical label. You have already established that the client is definitely clog prone. Here are the products the client is using:

**Product:** Cleansing Cream. Ingredients: Mineral oil, purified water, beeswax, sodium borate, isopropyl palmitate, petrolatum, stearyl alcohol, lanolin alcohol, ceteareth-20, magnesium aluminum silicate, sodium dehydroacetate, methyl paraben, propyl paraben, D & C red # 6.

**Analysis:** More than comedogenic, this cleansing cream is simply much too greasy and heavy for oily, clog-prone skin. It contains isopropyl palmitate, a known comedogenic ingredient. However, the ingredient is fairly low on the ingredient list. It also contains D & C red # 6, which is not very comedogenic compared to other D & C red dyes and is present in a fairly small quantity. The biggest problem with this cleanser is that it is oil based, very heavy, and is probably not being rinsed off well, which can be a real problem for oily, clog-prone skin. This cleanser is a good cleanser for drier skin types or for those who wear heavy or theatrical makeup and need a thorough oil-based cleanser. It should be replaced for your client with a rinseable foaming cleanser and/or a nongreasy cleansing milk.

**Product:** Day Protectant. Ingredients: Water, isopropyl palmitate, isopropyl myristate, mineral oil, propylene glycol, proplyene glycol stearate, stearic acid, magnesium aluminum silicate, oleic acid, cellulose gum, methyl paraben, propyl paraben, fragrance.

**Analysis:** This day cream is loaded with potentially comedogenic ingredients. Isopropyl myristate, isopropyl palmitate, and oleic acid are all comedogenic chemicals. Isopropyl myristate and isopropyl palmitate are extremely high on the ingredient list, indicating a fairly large concentration of these problem agents. This cream is left on the face all day, creating a true exposure time. This day cream should only be used on skin types that are not clog prone. Your client should discontinue this product.

**Product:** Liquid makeup. Ingredients: Water, propylene glycol, SD alcohol 40, titanium dioxide, talc, witch hazel extract, zinc oxide, magnesium aluminum silicate, methyl paraben, propyl paraben; may contain iron oxides, ultramarine blue.

**Analysis:** This is an excellent example of a noncomedogenic product. It contains no comedogenic ingredients and no real emollient fats. It contains witch hazel and SD alcohol as mild drying agents—a plus for oily skins. This makeup is safe enough to be used on acne. Your client made a good choice here and should continue to use this product.

**Product:** Loose powder. Ingredients: talc, myristyl myristate, zinc stearate, fragrance, methyl paraben, propyl paraben, iron oxides, fragrance.

**Analysis:** This product would be acceptable if it did not have myristyl myristate as a pressing agent. It should not be used on oily, acne, or clogged skin.

These are only a few examples of how to do a comedogenic analysis. Use your head and the facts you have been taught. The bottom line of all of this testing and analysis is: Is your client's skin developing clogged pores? If it is, something is not working correctly!

You should of course have available to your clients an entire range of noncomedogenic products. When purchasing products for your salon, remember to check carefully for the ingredients and testing procedures we have discussed throughout this chapter.

## TOPICS FOR DISCUSSION

1. Discuss testing for comedogenicity.
2. Discuss the difference between noncomedogenic and nonacnegenic products.
3. Discuss the concentration of possible comedogenic ingredients in a product and how this may affect comedogenicity.
4. Why are comedogenic ingredient lists controversial?
5. Discuss the various types of products for clog-prone skin. What should you look for in a day cream? Night treatment? Foundation?
6. Discuss treatment of adult, mature, clogged, and dehydrated skin.
7. Why is it important to test the final product for comedogenicity and irritancy?

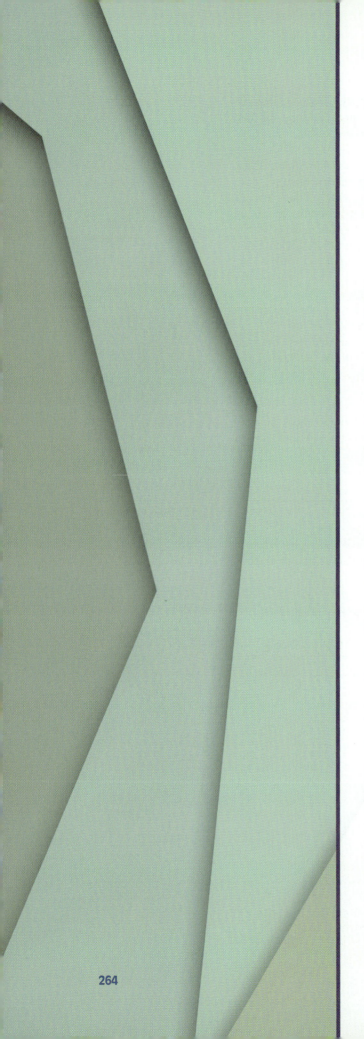

# CHAPTER 17

# Extraction

## OBJECTIVES. . .

Extraction is an extremely important part of the esthetician's skills, and it is a difficult process to master.

With proper hands-on supervision, this chapter will help the esthetician learn about extraction procedures for many different types of follicle impactions. Different methods of extraction will be discussed as well as specific unusual problems that may be encountered during extraction.

**Extraction** refers to the removal of dead cells, sebum, bacteria, and other debris from the skin's follicles. This expulsion technique is probably the most important function of a facial treatment. The solid mass of sebum, dead cells, and other matter stuck in the follicles are both an esthetic and a physiological problem. Besides being unsightly, failure to treat these lesions may lead to more serious acne and health problems, not to mention permanent scarring.

Extraction techniques cannot be learned by simply studying a book. You must have hands-on training in all areas of extraction, taught by a well-qualified instructor. Do not attempt any of the procedures outlined in this chapter without the supervision and hands-on demonstration of a qualified, licensed instructor.

Extraction is a very important part of the esthetics profession and is possibly the most important service that estheticians perform. It can also be an uncomfortable and unsafe procedure if performed incorrectly.

Some states do not allow the use of lancets for extraction. Check with your esthetics instructor or school for laws governing the use of lancets by estheticians in your state.

## ANALYSIS OF THE NEED FOR EXTRACTION

Almost every skin that you will see under the magnifying lamp will need at least some extraction. Even dry, older skin will be likely to have some clogged follicles in the nose area. Observe your client's skin closely under a magnifying lamp. Check all areas of the face well, including behind and in front of the ears, the neck, and the jawline.

### Understanding Clogged Pores

All clogged pores (follicles) and comedones have several developmental factors.

**Retention hyperkeratosis**, a hereditary factor, refers to the tendency of dead skin cells (corneocytes) not to shed in a regular and uniform manner. These dead cells accumulate inside the follicle, lining the walls.

Sebum production levels are also hereditary, and in clog-prone individuals, overactive glands secrete excess sebum, coating the buildup of cells. As sebum becomes exposed to air (oxygen), the sebum oxidizes and forms a semisolid mass; any sebum exposed to the oxygen turns dark, creating the black part of the "blackhead."

Sebum is basically a complex of fatty materials and can solidify similarly to the way chicken fat turns solid when refrigerated. It is this solidification that helps form the impaction in the follicle.

**Sebaceous filaments** are the small clogged pores many clients have on their noses. These are not classic comedones; they mostly just oxidized sebum and very little cell buildup. This explains their frequent occurrence and presence on many clients' skin.

**Open comedones** are classic "blackheads," with a distinctly dilated follicle opening. They contain a mix of keratinized cells and solidified sebum.

**Closed comedones** appear as small bumps just underneath the skin. They are frequently found in the cheekbone area, especially in the blushline. They are often associated with comedogenic skin-care and makeup products, hence their frequent appearance in the blushline from blushes pressed with comedogenic fats or use of coal tar–derived red dyes. They are frequently found just under the corners of the mouth. The difference between closed and open comedones is that in the closed comedo, the follicle is not uniformly dilated. The follicle opening, or **ostium**, is barely visible, even when examining the skin with a magnifying lamp.

### Analysis

After thoroughly removing all makeup using a light, nonfragranced cleansing milk, examine the skin carefully using a magnifying lamp. Do not tone the skin before analysis, because this will make the pores look smaller and will also constrict them for proper extraction. Spread the skin taut between your fingers and observe all areas, moving down the face and continuing the spreading movement and observation. Look for clogged pores (follicles), small white bumps just under the skin (closed comedones), large dilated open comedones, papules, and pustules. Carefully note the size of the pores and the location. This pattern will determine the type of skin (oily, combination, etc.). Clogged pores are rarely found on a truly dry or **alipidic** (does not produce enough sebum) skin. Because oil-dry skin does not produce much sebum and therefore has very small pores, it is very unlikely to suffer from comedones or clogged pores.

On combination skin you will likely see small clogged pores through the T-zone area and scattered larger clogged pores or blackheads. In any area you may see small

---

**Extraction** refers to the removal of dead cells, sebum, bacteria, and other debris from the skin's follicles.

**Retention hyperkeratosis** refers to an overabundance of sebum that often begins at the time teenagers begin producing larger amounts of sex hormones.

**Sebaceous filaments** are small impacted follicles on the nose and other facial areas caused by oxidized, solidified sebum.

**Open comedones** are noninflammatory acne lesions usually called blackheads.

**Closed comedones** are noninflammatory acne lesions called whiteheads.

**Ostium** is the opening in follicles.

**Alipidic** means "lack of lipids." These skin types do not produce enough lipids.

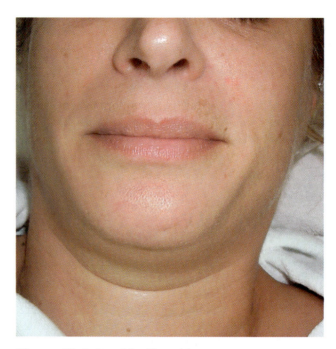

**Figure 17-1** Combination skin (Courtesy Mark Lees Skin Care, Inc.)

white bumps or closed comedones, milia (whiteheads), pustules, and papules associated with acne. The width of the T-zone will determine the oiliness of the area and therefore the number of clogged pores. Clogged pores are always a sign of an oily area (Figure 17-1).

The perimeter of the face is an ideal place for clogged pores and acne lesions to form. These are areas your clients often miss while cleansing. You can think of these areas as "cobwebs" in the corner of a room! (See Figure 17-2.)

Think about your client doing at-home cleaning. The client is not a skin-care specialist and probably does not take the time or care cleaning as you would cleaning

---

**Examination Procedures for Extraction**

1. Cleanse the skin well.
2. Using a magnifying lamp, examine the skin, observing areas with enlarged pores and noting areas with smaller and larger pores.
3. Combination skin—Note enlarged pores through the T-zone, indicating oilier skin, or smaller pores around the edges of the face, indicating less oil production. The width of the oily T-zone determines whether the skin is oily-combination or dry-combination. The wider the visible enlarged pore structure, the oilier the skin is.
4. Clogged pores, comedones, closed comedones, papules, and pustules are more likely to be seen in the oilier areas.
5. The small clogged pores in the nose are usually sebaceous filaments, not open comedones; they are simply follicles filled with oxidized sebum.
6. IN THE OILY AREAS . . . Pull the skin taut with the thumb and forefinger and observe any small white bumps under the skin. These are closed comedones.
7. Check the perimeter of the face well, including the chin, jawline, the neck, and in front of and behind the ears.

**Figure 17-2** Examination procedures

your own face. The client applies the cleanser and massages it but does not notice the remnants of cleanser or makeup left in front of the ears, in the hairline, and under the jawline. The client may also omit toner as a follow-up in these areas.

Failure to remove makeup and cleanser in these areas means that dead cells build up here as well as emollients and ingredients left from the cleanser. Clogs will inevitably form.

The first thing you should do when you encounter "perimeter acne" is to gently make the client aware of it and why it is probably there. Instruct your client to pay extra attention to cleaning these areas and to use toner after cleansing. You may also suggest that a foaming cleanser be used as a second cleanser after makeup removal. This not only helps remove any emollients left from a cleansing milk, but the foam itself is very obvious when it is still on the face or in one of those hidden corners! Your client will see the foam and rinse off the area.

## Continuing the Analysis . . .

Gently spread the skin with your thumb and forefinger. Move the fingers across the face, constantly spreading the skin gently. Observe if there are any small white bumps that are only visible when the skin is pulled taut. These are often closed comedones and can be seen on any area of the face, but they especially can be hidden in the chin area, just under the lower lip, and under the chin and jawline.

Check the skin for sebaceous filaments, which are not really open comedones. They are what most clients refer to as "clogged pores." These are follicles that have filled with sebum, sometimes over a very short period of time. They are most noticeable on the nose but can appear in any area. On very oily skin, they can literally seem to be in every single area (Figures 17-3A, 17-3B).

Sebaceous filaments indicate an oily area. They are not nearly as large or dilated as an open comedo, but they are basically the same type of lesion. The only real difference is that a sebaceous filament is mostly sebum, whereas a real open comedo is dilated, is much larger, and is filled with many dead cells. An open comedo may take weeks to form, but sebaceous filaments may form in just a few days. The debris extracted from a sebaceous filament will be much smaller than that of an open comedo, and you will also notice that the plug is not as deep or as solid (Figure 17-4).

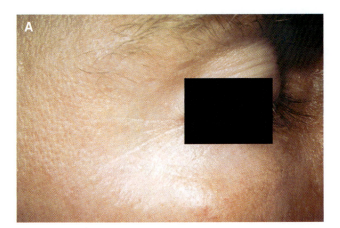 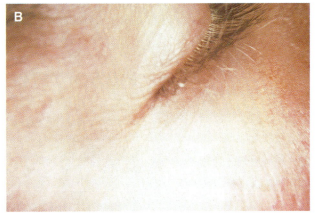

**Figure 17-3** Treatment for clogged, dehydrated skin includes noncomedogenic hydration fluid and sunscreen with low levels of emollient, along with an alphahydroxy acid gel. This home care was used for six weeks in this case study. Note the differences in texture, tone, clarity, and even coloration (Courtesy Mark Lees Skin Care, Inc.)

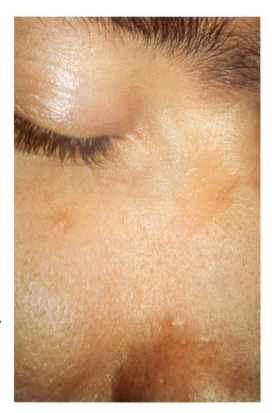

**Figure 17-4** Sebaceous filaments, often called clogged pores, are follicles filled with solidified sebum. The black tip is oxidized sebum in the top of the follicle (Courtesy Mark Lees Skin Care, Inc.)

## OPEN COMEDONES

Open comedones may appear anywhere on the face. They are most noticeable in acne conditions and in clients who have neglected their skin for a long time. They are also frequently observed in young adolescents who have a budding adolescent acne problem but may not be cleaning well and have not taken a true interest in their personal appearance yet.

Open comedones can certainly appear in any skin type, but they are more prevalent in the previously mentioned situations. Clients who are very conscientious will be aware of these lesions and will either have them extracted or attempt to do so themselves. Open comedones are often about the size of a pinhead. They have a large black top, hence the term *blackhead*. Open comedones are the easiest lesions to extract.

## PRESOFTENING BEFORE EXTRACTION

The procedure you follow before extraction will significantly help loosen follicle impactions, making extractions less difficult for the esthetician and less uncomfortable for the client. The skin must be pretreated before extraction. This pretreatment will help soften the accumulations in the follicles as well as the surface of the skin, making the skin more soft and flexible during the extraction procedure.

### Desincrustation

**Desincrustation** refers to the process of softening the skin and sebaceous impaction by applying a chemical that helps liquify the sebum, reducing hard, solid plugs to a softer consistency. This technique softens clogs significantly. The chemical used for this procedure is usually an anionic surfactant. Thus, desincrustation solutions usually have a higher, or more alkaline, pH.

**Desincrustation** refers to the process of softening the skin and sebaceous impaction by applying a chemical that helps liquify the sebum, reducing hard, solid plugs to a softer consistency.

Desincrustation solutions are usually either liquids or a soft gel-cream consistency, often referred to as a pre-mask.

The liquid is applied to the affected areas of the face after preliminary cleansing or is sometimes poured onto cotton compresses and then applied to the face.

The "pre-masks" can be applied to the face either with a brush or your hands. Pre-masks have a thicker consistency than liquid solutions. They can be seen on the skin, whereas liquids cannot. Being careful to follow manufacturer's instructions, allow the solution or pre-mask to sit on the face for 5 to 10 minutes. Steam treatment is frequently used at the same time. Steaming does not "open the pores"; however, it does hydrate the surface, helping to make the skin considerably more flexible for extraction. Galvanic desincrustation may be applied over the pre-mask or liquid, depending on the manufacturer's instructions. Galvanic treatment with a desincrustant chemical provides for better penetration of the product and better reduction of the plug due to chemical reactions produced by the electricity within the follicle. (See *Milady's Standard Fundamentals for Estheticians* or *Milady's Comprehensive Training for Estheticians* for further explanation and instructions for use of galvanic current.)

The oilier and more impacted the skin, the better it is to use galvanic treatment. Some clients who have a minimal number of clogged follicles and more dehydrated skin may find galvanic treatment to be too drying. It is a good idea to use galvanic treatment routinely on acne conditions, provided there are no medical contraindications for use.

After the "soak" period with desincrustation solution or pre-mask or galvanic treatment is completed, remove the desincrustant product well and proceed with extraction.

Desincrustant chemicals are often slippery and must be removed thoroughly before extraction. Otherwise the skin will be too slippery for extraction procedures.

## OTHER PRE-EXTRACTION PROCEDURES

The use of a brushing machine may help loosen dead cells, particularly on skin that is both dehydrated and clogged.

The electric rotating brush should be gently applied after steaming. The brush should be used over a layer of emulsion-type cleanser to prevent too much scratching of the face during the brushing procedure. Do not use the brush on acne, couperose, or sensitive skin. (For further instruction on brushing, see *Milady's Standard Fundamentals for Estheticians* or *Milady's Comprehensive Training for Estheticians*.)

Suction, or vacuuming, may be performed with a skin suction machine after desincrustation or steaming. Suction may help to further loosen impactions that have already been loosened with desincrustation. Suction removes very little debris from the follicle, but the procedure feels good to the client and has a nice psychological effect. Again, suction should not be used on sensitive or couperose skin or acne. See *Milady's Standard Fundamentals for Estheticians* or *Milady's Comprehensive Training for Estheticians* for instruction on suction machines.

### Enzyme Peels and Alphahydroxy Exfoliation to Ease Extraction

Using light peeling treatments performed with enzymes or alphahydroxy acids (AHAs) can help remove dead surface cell buildup, loosening clogged pores and other impactions. Clients who use AHAs at home, such as a 10 percent AHA gel, on a daily basis significantly loosen comedones and sebaceous filaments. Two weeks of home care using AHA gels, or in more severe cases, AHA gels and benzoyl peroxide gels, can make a huge difference in the ease of extraction.

Clients who have had two weeks of AHA at home are safe to have a 30 percent AHA performed at the beginning of their extraction treatment. Treatments of 30 percent AHA exfoliation help to loosen and slightly dilate follicle openings.

Enzyme treatments using pancreatin or papain also can help remove dead cell buildup from the skin surface blocking follicle openings. Clients who are both dehydrated and clogged may particularly benefit from an enzyme treatment prior to extraction. Enzymes are normally applied during the steam treatment for an eight to twelve minute period. For further information on how to use enzymes, see the chapter on chemical peeling and exfoliation procedures.

Peeling the surface of the skin helps remove dead cells and helps to dilate follicle openings, but it does not significantly affect the hardened sebum in the follicles. Desincrustation products are designed to work on the fatty plugs, as opposed to enzymes and AHAs, which work more on dead cell buildup. After exfoliation, it may still be necessary to use a desincrustant to soften the sebaceous impactions.

## HYGIENE AND EXTRACTION

It is very important to always wear gloves during extraction. It is generally good practice to wear gloves throughout the treatment, especially if there are any acne lesions present. Please review the chapter on hygiene and sterilization techniques before beginning extraction.

## EXTRACTION OF OPEN COMEDONES

After presoftening the accumulations, remove all products from the skin, leaving the face moist but not wet. Wet skin or skin that still has product on it is impossible to extract. Take two cotton swabs. Hold them as you would hold two pencils. It is best to use the type of swab that has a soft, flexible plastic stick. These plastic cotton swabs are much easier to work with and will snap if too much pressure is applied, a built-in safety feature (Figure 17-5).

Place a swab on each side of the open comedo. Gently press down on the swabs and then gently move the swabs closer together, with the tips touching the skin. This will have a lifting effect on the solid plug. Keep applying gentle pressure until you see the plug come out of the follicle. If the plug does not come out easily, move the swabs to another angle around the sides of the comedo and repeat the procedure. Once the plug is out, continue to press gently on the sides of the follicle to make sure all of the debris has been removed. When working around the sides of the nose, place one cotton swab under the cartilage of the nostril, and the other swab on the side of the nose. Using the two swabs, gently arch the cartilage of the nostril and slowly but firmly slide the lower swab upward toward the other swab. This is a great technique for extracting sebaceous filaments in the nose area. The technique may need to be repeated.

### Finger Technique

Wrap your gloved forefingers in damp cotton. Using the same gentle downward and inward pressure technique, attempt to extract the comedo. Work your fingers all around the comedo with the same pressure technique.

Cotton swabs are easier for many people because they are smaller than fingers. It is the consensus of clients that the cotton swab technique is more comfortable and more efficient.

### Extractor Technique

Comedo extractors are best to use on nonfleshy parts of the face, such as the forehead or cheekbones, or on clients whose skin does not have a fleshy thickness that can be

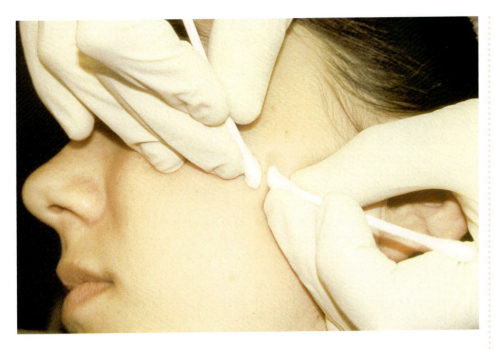

**Figure 17-5** Cotton swabs are used to gently extract comedones and sebaceous filaments by gently lifting and slightly twisting the skin. Careful preparation of the skin with desincrustation is essential for ease in extraction (Courtesy Mark Lees Skin Care, Inc.)

physically manipulated. Comedo extractors should never be used on thin, fragile, sensitive, or couperose skin.

Place the extractor over the open comedo, with the hole in the extractor directly over the comedo. It is very important that the lesion be smaller than the hole in the metal extractor. If the lesion is wider than the hole in the extractor, do not use the extractor. Either try a large extractor or try the cotton swab method.

Assuming that the comedo can easily fit into the hole in the extractor, gently press straight down on the extractor, using the leverage of the handle end to exert pressure. The plug should come out of the follicle and be noticeable inside the hole of the extractor. It is a good idea to follow this extraction procedure with another gentle expression of the follicle with the cotton swabs to check for any further debris that might be trapped in the follicle.

Remember when using a metal extractor that the extractor is metal and is not flexible. The use of a comedo extractor can be very painful for the client, particularly if used over the entire face. They should be reserved for use on bony areas or non-fleshy skin. In general, comedone extractors are more uncomfortable than using finger or cotton swab extraction techniques.

Comedo extractors are available in a variety of sizes. Some are made with a slight bend for better leverage. Some are made with a round hole, and some have an oval or rectangular hole. You should have some of each type available, and you will, over time, develop a feel for which is appropriate to use. Comedo extractors must be sterilized after each client. Plastic disposable extractors are breakable and are generally not advised. See the chapter on hygiene and sterilization techniques for sterile and aseptic procedure.

## CLOSED COMEDONES

Closed comedones appear as small bumps just underneath the surface of the skin. They can be found on any area of the face, but are frequently found on the cheeks, jawline, and chin. Often you will see a large number of closed comedones on the cheekbones of female clients. These are often caused by a comedogenic reaction to a blush. The closed comedo is just beneath the skin and normally has a very small follicle opening.

If you look carefully through a magnifying lamp, you may detect a very small opening in the top of the closed comedo. Often, these follicles must be dilated with a lancet before extraction.

## EXTRACTION OF CLOSED COMEDONES

Closed comedones are the most difficult of any lesion to extract, because they are just beneath the surface of the skin, have a very small pore opening, and may vary greatly in size. If you can see the opening of the follicle well and the white area surrounding the opening does not appear to be very large, you may attempt to extract the area by using the cotton swab technique. Make sure you have softened the area well with a desincrustant. Place the tip of the cotton swabs on either side of the closed comedo, being careful to make sure you are clear about the border of the lesion. In other words, make sure you have the entire comedo within the placement of your swabs. Failure to do so may result in extracting only part of the comedo. Gently press down on the swabs and then gently turn them inward while pulling the skin taut with the outside fingers. A solid white stream of sebaceous material will emerge from the comedo. Continue to gently press the area until no more material emerges.

In many closed comedones, follicle dilation is necessary. This procedure is performed for three reasons. Dilation of the follicle allows more room for the sebaceous material to emerge. Secondly, dilation of the closed comedo relieves pressure on the follicle walls, helping to avoid follicle wall rupture during extraction. Finally, relieving the pressure on the lesion by lancet dilation makes the extraction procedure much more comfortable for the client.

To dilate the follicle, find the small opening in the top of the closed comedo. Using a sterile, disposable lancet, gently dilate this follicle opening by gently pressing the tip of the lancet through the follicle opening. DO NOT attempt to force the lancet into the follicle (Figure 17-6).

After the follicle is dilated, extract the comedo using the cotton swab technique. Waiting a few seconds after lancet dilation sometimes helps to expel the debris. Relief of the pressure accomplished by dilation will often cause some "self-expelling" action.

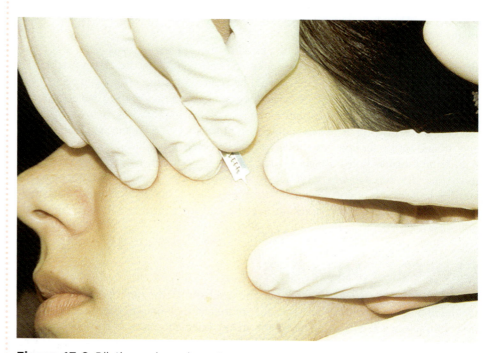

**Figure 17-6** Dilation using a lancet (Courtesy Mark Lees Skin Care, Inc.)

This will help make the extraction process easier. It is not advisable to use comedo extractors on closed comedones. Closed comedones are often found in fleshy areas of the face, making use of an extractor cumbersome and difficult. Second, closed comedones often have a larger diameter than that of the opening in a comedo extractor, making the use of the extractor unsafe and inappropriate.

## EXTRACTION OF PUSTULES

Pustules are raised, inflammatory acne lesions. They have a "head" that is filled with pus. Most of the pustule and its contents are above the surface of the skin.

To extract a pustule, gently place the tip of a sterile disposable lancet against the side of the pustule. Bracing the outside of your hand against the face, gently "lift" the very top of the pustule away with the lancet. This procedure is similar to removing a splinter from your finger, except that the lesion is above the skin. Because you are strictly removing dead cells from the top of the pustule, this procedure should not be very uncomfortable to the client.

When the top of this dead cell layer has been removed, the pus will begin to emerge from the follicle opening. Placing two cotton swabs on the sides of the lesion, gently press downward and inward on the swabs, being careful to hold the area taut with the outside fingers. The rest of the impaction should emerge from the follicle. Following the pus will be the emergence of the actual comedo, often referred to as the "core." This part of the extracted material will look much like the debris extracted from an open or closed comedo, except that these impactions will be slightly harder and more dense.

It is not unusual for a small amount of bleeding to occur while extracting pustules. Remember, the follicle wall has ruptured in a pustule, allowing blood to come into the follicle. A slight amount of red blood appearing after extracting a pustule indicates that there is no more debris or sebum present in the follicle.

Papules, nodules, and cysts are deep inflammatory lesions and are the domain of the dermatologist. Do not attempt to extract these lesions. Although papules will often develop into pustules or dissipate without treatment, cysts and nodules should be referred to the dermatologist for treatment.

## FACIAL TREATMENT BEFORE AND AFTER EXTRACTION

We have discussed the actual extraction procedures used in removing debris from the follicles. Treatment before and after extraction is very important to help ease the extraction process by softening the follicle accumulations, to treat the area after extraction to prevent infection, and to help further dry the lesions. The following is a suggested treatment in which extraction takes place. This treatment is known in the esthetics industry as "deep-pore cleansing."

1. Completely remove all the makeup from the face with a liquid cleanser.
2. Analyze the skin under the magnifying lamp. Check all areas of the face for clogged pores (sebaceous filaments), open and closed comedones, milia, and pustules. At the same time, of course, check for other disorders of the skin.
3. Apply steam treatment to the face with a vapor machine in the usual manner. Apply a desincrustant pre-mask, desincrustation lotion compresses, or enzyme treatment to the skin.
4. Remove the desincrustant or enzyme treatment after allowing the treatment to sit on the face for about eight to ten minutes, or the time prescribed by the product manufacturer.

5. Galvanic desincrustation treatment may be used to further loosen the debris in the follicle, especially in cases of multiple impactions or acne.

6. Suction may be used, providing that there are no contraindications, as previously discussed.

7. Begin extraction in the chin and jawline area first, working upward on the face. This order of extraction helps the esthetician avoid contaminating the hands or other areas of the face from debris extracted from the lower part of the face. It is the most hygienic and aseptic pattern of treatment.

8. After extraction is completed, apply an antiseptic toner to the face with damp sponges or cotton pads. This will help kill any bacteria on the surface of the skin. It will also lower the pH from the use of the alkaline desincrustant treatment.

9. Apply the appropriate treatment for the particular skin type. An ampoule or antiseptic lotion may be appropriate. Benzoyl peroxide or salicylic acid can be used on oilier and acne-prone skin.

10. Apply high frequency over the face. This also further helps kill surface bacteria. Using a piece of gauze over the face while extracting helps intensify the frequency treatment and helps the electrode move easily across the skin.

11. Apply a drying clay-based mask to the area that was extracted. A mask containing sulfur, salicylic acid, or benzoyl peroxide may be used for acne. A bentonite-based mask with camphor may be more appropriate for oily or more sensitive clogged areas. The mask should be allowed to dry completely, usually for about 15 to 20 minutes.

12. Remove the mask with damp, soft cloths, sponges, or cotton pads. Apply more toner after mask removal.

13. Apply a noncomedogenic hydrating sunscreen.

It is strongly advised that clients not wear makeup for about two hours after extraction. Extraction can be slightly irritating, and application of makeup to freshly extracted areas may be more irritating.

## EXTRACTION OF MILIA

**Milia** are small deposits of sebum between the follicle and the corneum.

**Milia** are small deposits of sebum between the follicle and the corneum (Figure 17-7). A milium is not the same as a comedo. The sebaceous material is trapped above the skin's surface, covered with a layer of dead cells. Milia may occur for several reasons. Milia is frequently seen on older, mature skin (Figure 17-8). This may be associated with the use of heavy creams loaded with emollients for treating dry, dehydrated skin. Injuries to the skin sometimes also cause milia to develop. Dermabrasion by a plastic surgeon is often followed by a large number of milia forming. This will be discussed more in detail in the chapter on treating the cosmetic surgery patient.

To extract a milium, make sure that it is large enough to be extracted. Milia are almost always perfectly round in shape and are found on any area of the face, but especially the cheeks and the forehead. A milium must be large enough to easily lift off the top with a lancet. This is about the size of the heads of two pins. Make sure that you are absolutely positive that the lesion is a milium. Other types of skin lesions look like milia, including some types of skin growths. Check the shape carefully. The milium should not have any capillaries running through it. If the lesion has a capillary associated with it, leave it alone. Also, if the milium seems to give you any resistance while using the lancet, leave it alone. The dead cell layer on the top of a milium is very thin. Milia are easily treated with a lancet and should not give any resistance to pressure from the lancet.

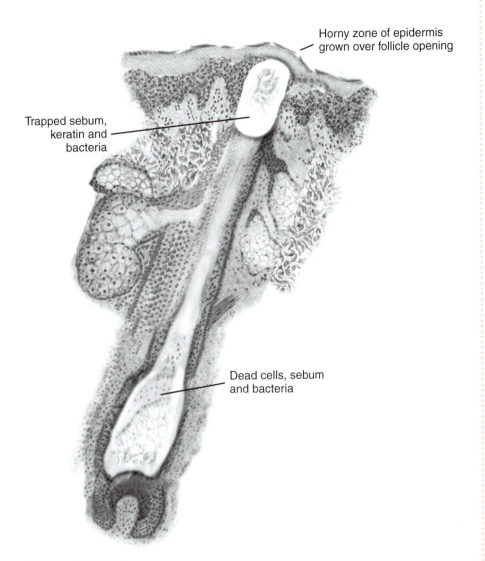

Horny zone of epidermis
grown over follicle opening

Trapped sebum,
keratin and
bacteria

Dead cells, sebum
and bacteria

**Figure 17-7** Milia

Gently spread the skin taut around the milium with your fingertips. Using a sterile disposable lancet, gently lift off the top cell layers from the milium. Gently place the lancet against the side of the top of the milium. The lancet should slide easily into the top. These are all dead cells in the elevated part of the milium, so the client should barely feel the lancet at all.

You should barely see the opening you have created in the top of the milium. Sometimes a very small amount of sebaceous material will emerge from the side of the milium where you have lifted the dead skin. After the lancet procedure is complete, place a cotton swab on both sides of the milium and gently press and lift on the milium. You may find it helpful to put slightly more pressure on the "unopened" side of the milium. This pressure will help the sebaceous material exit the follicle easier.

If the milium does not extract easily, you may try lifting more dead cells with the lancet. Sometimes when the milium is small enough, it is easier to use a comedo extractor, particularly on nonfleshy areas of the face such as the forehead. Place the

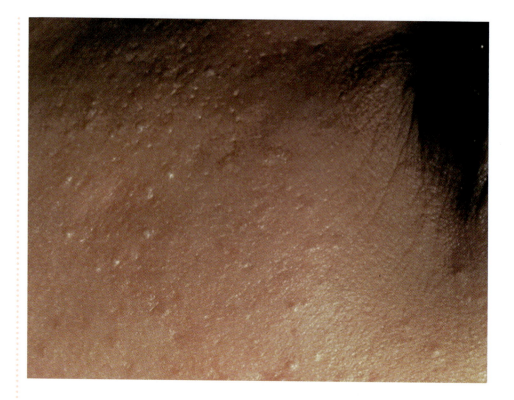

**Figure 17-8** Milia are often seen around the eye area, forehead, and cheeks, as seen in this photo (Courtesy Mark Lees Skin Care, Inc.)

## Some General Rules for Extraction

1. Always wear disposable latex or vinyl gloves during extraction and throughout the remainder of the treatment.

2. Do not extract for more than ten minutes in any single treatment. More than ten minutes of extraction is too stimulating for most skin types and can be very uncomfortable.

3. Reduce discomfort of the client by keeping the skin pulled taut during extraction and only extracting very small areas at a time.

4. Never attempt extraction if you have not had hands-on experience with a qualified instructor.

5. The biggest mistake made in extraction is failure to properly presoften impactions. Make sure you are using the correct products for this important phase of the treatment.

6. Always use an antiseptic, low pH toner, or special after-extraction product after completing your extraction procedures. This is important to reduce the chance of infection, soothe the skin, reduce redness, and reestablish the proper pH.

7. Do not use any alphahydroxy acid or betahydroxy acid products immediately after treatment, especially salon concentrations. Clients may use a low percentage AHA that evening, if recommended.

comedo extractor over the milium. Gently press down on the unopened side of the milium, moving the extractor very slowly toward the open side of the milium. You should see the emerging sebaceous material.

If the milium does not respond to treatment, do not continue attempting to extract it! You must have lots of experience to extract milia. Do not extract milia until you have been given hands-on instruction by a qualified licensed instructor.

# LESIONS AROUND THE EYES

Many clients will complain of small milia-like lesions around the eye area. Some of these lesions are milia. Some are other types of skin growth or lesions called xanthalasmas. **Xanthalasmas** are much larger and flatter than milia, have a yellowish appearance, are below the skin's surface, and may have irregular shape. They are rarely round like a milium. These lesions should be referred to a dermatologist—they are not in the domain of the esthetician. Xanthalasmas can sometimes be indicative of other diseases or disorders, such as high cholesterol. Refer the client to a dermatologist for treatment and follow-up (Figure 17-9).

**Syringomas** are small pinpoint lesions that occur under the eyes. These are actually small cysts on the sudoriferous glands. They may look like very small milia and are usually in multiple numbers. They are thought to be hereditary or possibly caused by sun damage. They are generally not extractable and should be referred to a dermatologist or an ophthalmologist for treatment.

Other small milia in the eye area are often associated with the use of heavy eye creams, concealers, and other eye cosmetics that are thick, heavy, and loaded with fatty emollients. This can cause a buildup of dead cells in the area. Advise the client to switch to a lighter eye cream or a gel-type treatment. These have fewer or lesser concentrations of emollients.

Improper cleansing has also been associated with milia development around the eyes. Clients who do not remove their eye makeup well on a nightly basis have a tendency to develop milia. These clients leave traces of makeup or do not remove the eye makeup at all. Instruct the client about the correct procedure to remove eye makeup and make sure she is using a proper eye makeup remover.

Clients who are very rough in removing their eye makeup may also suffer from milia development around the eyes. Injuries and excessive manipulation of the eyelid tissue have been associated with milia development.

Do not attempt to remove milia found on the eyelids. This tissue is extremely difficult to handle properly and is extremely fragile. Refer this client to an opthalmologist or dermatologist and give proper home care advice. Sometimes milia will disappear after the adjustment of proper home care.

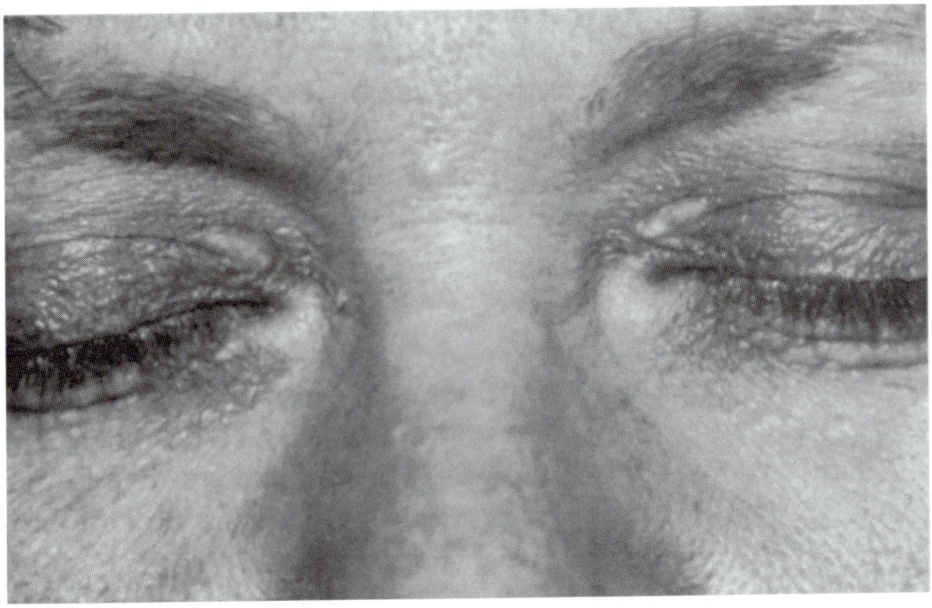

**Xanthalasmas** are much flatter than milia, have a yellowish appearance, are below the skin's surface, and may have irregular shape.

**Syringomas** are small pinpoint lesions that occur under the eyes.

**Figure 17-9** Xanthalasma (Courtesy Timothy G. Berger, M.D.)

## TREATING CLOGGED AND DEHYDRATED SKIN

Skin that is both clogged and dehydrated is extremely difficult to treat. The client's skin will feel dry but is actually oily and dehydrated. The follicle will become "crimped shut" from the tightness of the surface dehydration, making extraction difficult, if not impossible.

You should avoid heavily drying products. Products that are made with high levels of humectants and low levels of emollients are appropriate for this skin problem. The hydrating agents will help hydrate the skin's surface, making it less dry feeling and more pliable so that extraction is more easily accomplished.

To treat this type of skin, apply a hydrating fluid during salon steam treatment. Allow to steam with the humectant-based hydrating fluid for eight to ten minutes. This water from the steam and the humectant will help soften the skin, hydrate the surface, and reduce the "crimped" effect on the follicles.

After this procedure, proceed with extraction. Follow extraction with a toner and then apply hydrating fluid to the skin before applying a gentle, clay-based drying mask. Applying a drying clay-based mask without applying a hydration fluid can be overdrying to this type of skin problem. Clients should be instructed to use the hydrating treatment with the mask at home too. Twice-a-week application will help clear the clogged pores.

The client with both dehydrated skin and clogged pores often is middle aged, trying desperately to "fight aging" through the use of heavy moisturizing and believing that he or she is "drying up" with age. These heavier, and often comedogenic, cosmetics clog the skin while the client attempts to treat the wrinkles and lines associated with aging, dehydrating, and sun damage.

This client needs lots of education about the aging process, sun damage, and comedogenic cosmetics. It is up to the esthetician to provide this education and help the client find a product program that helps dehydration but will not be clogging to this clog-prone skin condition.

## SOLAR BLACKHEADS

In older clients, often men, you will find a concentration of large open comedones around the eye area. Although the development of these huge blackheads is similar to acne-related blackheads, these lesions are caused by excessive long-term sun exposure. This condition is called Favre-Racouchot syndrome. More on this condition will be discussed in the chapter on sun and sun damage (Figure 17-10).

Extraction of solar comedones must be done very gently. This type of skin often has extremely fragile capillaries, also associated with excessive sun exposure and damage. This sun-damaged skin bruises easily, and it is easy to cause redness that lasts for days after treatment. You must be extremely gentle while treating this fragile skin.

Begin by cleansing or steaming the skin. Applying a fluid hydrating agent while steaming will help loosen the impactions and make the skin more pliable. Very gently extract the lesions with the cotton swab technique. Do not attempt to remove every single clog in one session. Advise the client to have weekly treatments in the salon until the problem is clear and then regular monthly treatments to prevent or control their return. Favre-Racouchot is a chronic problem, and this client will often have other sun-related skin problems. There are medical treatments for Favre-Racouchot syndrome and other sun-damage conditions.

## DURATION OF EXTRACTION

Extraction should not be performed for more than 10 to 15 minutes on any client during one treatment visit. Extraction that is longer than this can be painful and traumatic

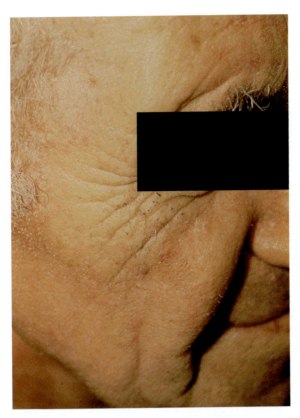

**Figure 17-10** Favre Racouchot (senile solar comedones) in a typical pattern on an individual with sun damage (Courtesy Rube J. Pardo, M.D., Ph.D.)

to both the client and the skin. You will, of course, have to assess the needs and the duration for each client as an individual.

Clogged skin should never be massaged, at least not for prolonged periods of time. Avoid massage on excessively clogged skin, until such time that the skin is almost completely clear of clogged pores and any other type of acne lesion. As a general rule, if you take 10 minutes or more for extraction on a client, that client should not be massaged. Massaging of the clogged skin will simply stimulate more oil production and apply pressure to clogs, forcing them to become more impacted in the skin.

## TOPICS FOR DISCUSSION

1. Discuss extraction—can any skin type need extractions?
2. Why is it important to presoften the skin before extraction? What are some techniques used to presoften the skin for extraction?
3. Describe the extraction process for closed comedones. When is follicle dilation necessary? Describe the extraction procedure for pustules.
4. Describe the order of facial treatment procedures involved in a deep-cleansing treatment.
5. Discuss problem impactions around the eyes. Which should be referred to the dermatologist?
6. What are some special procedures used for treating clogged skin that is also dehydrated?

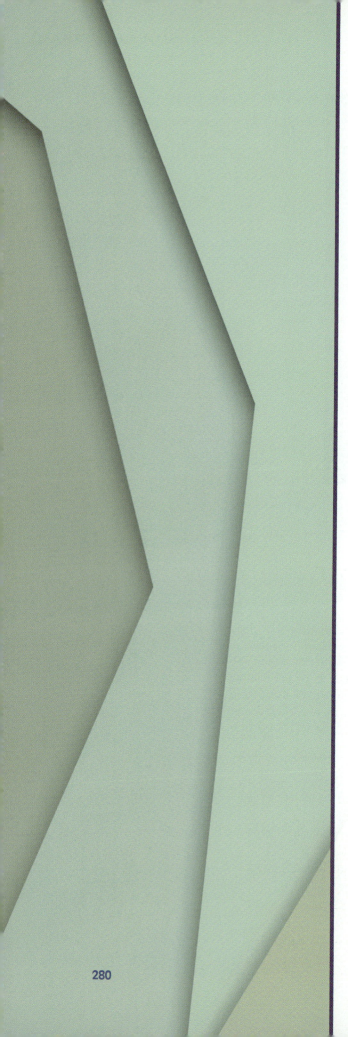

# 18

# The Intrinsic Aging Process

## OBJECTIVES. . .

Aging is a process that almost every person fears. Some changes in the skin inevitably happen as years pass. In this chapter we will discuss the way the skin changes as it becomes older and some of the ways we can manipulate these changes to make the skin look better.

It is the natural order of life that matter changes as it ages. Skin is not immune to this natural law.

We must take a minute to differentiate between two major types of factors that contribute to aging skin. **Extrinsic** aging factors are the effect of outside influences on the skin's health. The very best example here is sun exposure, known to be the major factor in premature skin aging, as well as skin cancer development. Many medical and cosmetic scientists now believe that 85 percent of the aging process is due to extrinsic factors.

**Intrinsic** aging is the part of the aging process that is due to the actual passing of the years, wearing out of the body, and hereditary factors. Expression lines are an example of intrinsic facial aging. Regardless of our sun protection habits, we still "fold" our faces in expression, and this eventually leads to wrinkles in the skin due to repetitive movement of the skin in the same way.

It is important to separate between the two types of aging factors when analyzing and treating aging skin, so we may determine which symptoms are caused by intrinsic or extrinsic factors. There is also, inevitably, some overlap of the two. This chapter will mostly deal with intrinsic aging factors but will mention some symptoms, normally associated by the consumer with passing of the years, that are actually extrinsic and preventable.

A human baby has beautiful, supple, smooth skin that is all one color. As skin is exposed to the environment, defends itself against disease, and is affected by nutrition, health habits, exposure, and time, it begins to change.

Scrapes and accidents we receive as children inevitably leave scar tissue, which develops from injuries. At puberty, the hormonal system begins functioning in a new way. Suddenly pores begin to enlarge, skin becomes oilier, apocrine glands start functioning differently, and the skin's appearance changes. Pimples form from impacted follicles and sometimes leave scars, particularly from the more severe forms of acne. Body hair begins growing, and skin texture changes as well.

Most teenagers are more concerned with the zit on their cheek than with how they will look at age 35 or 55. Many take their good skin for granted.

During the early 20s is when most people notice the beginnings of changes associated with aging skin. They begin to notice small lines and wrinkles around the eyes and sometimes other areas.

If you look closely and carefully at a square inch of skin on a baby's face and compare it with a square inch of skin on the face of someone in their 20s, you will notice many differences. The skin will look rougher; the texture will be coarser to the touch. The skin will no longer be all one color, but multicolored due to melanin deposits.

If you again compare this square inch of skin with that of someone in their 40s or 50s, you will notice even more dramatic changes. Many of these changes are due to sun exposure, which we will discuss much more completely in the chapter on sun and sun damage.

However, some of these changes happen naturally as years go by. The natural aging process of the skin is called intrinsic aging. In other words, these changes happen within the body and are not directly associated with external factors such as sun or weather (Figure 18-1).

## HEREDITY

Some intrinsic aging factors are hereditary. Family history and ethnic background do govern skin aging. For example, red-headed, thin-skinned, and fair-skinned individuals develop the skin characteristics of aging much more rapidly than thicker, darker skin, such as black or Hispanic skin. Although it is true that darker skins produce

**Extrinsic** aging factors are the effect of outside influences on the skin's health.

**Intrinsic** aging is the part of the aging process that is due to the actual passing of the years, wearing out of the body, and hereditary factors.

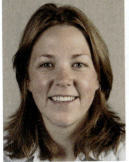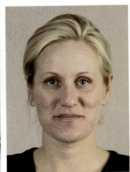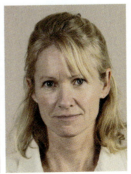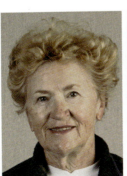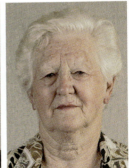

**Figure 18-1** Each decade may add more signs of aging skin

more melanin and therefore ward off more solar damage, the skin itself is very different between different ethnic groups.

In general, the darker the skin, the less visible aging will take place, depending on the amount of sun exposure an individual experiences. Thicker skin does not show signs of aging as fast as thinner, fragile skin types.

This is certainly not to say that dark skin types cannot or do not age. It is just that they are less likely to look aged as fast. A lot of this depends on how the skin is cared for.

## WHAT CAUSES AGING?

We will discuss several factors that influence aging. Gravity is certainly a factor. The gravity of the earth constantly pulls on our bodies, including the facial skin. This gravity is one factor that causes skin and muscle to sag. Even an individual who takes immaculate care of both skin and body will have some sagging of the face over a period of years. Even persons who have never exposed their faces to the sun will have some sagging. This sagging is referred to clinically as **elastosis**, which means loss of elasticity. Although facial treatments and good products can help the surface appearance temporarily, the appearance of sagging skin is best corrected on a long-term basis by plastic surgery (Figure 18-2).

Let's look at an example of elastosis. If you purchase a new pair of underwear, it has an elastic waistband. If you wear this underwear many, many times, the elastic will begin to wear out. At some point the elastic waistband will no longer "snap back" the way it did when the underwear was brand new. Skin is the same way—aging causes a wearing down of the elastin fibrils in the dermis that give skin its elasticity. If you pinch the skin of a 50-year-old person's cheek, it will not "snap back" as fast as that of a 20-year-old.

**Elastosis** means loss of elasticity of the skin.

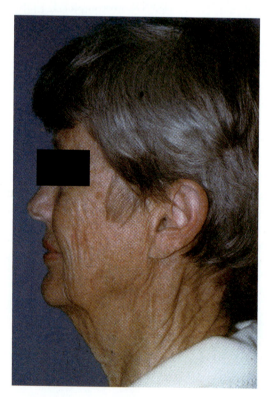

**Figure 18-2** Elastosis (Photograph courtesy David Rapaport, M.D., plastic surgeon, Park Avenue, New York)

Gravity also causes the nose to droop downwards and the ears to become larger over a period of years. In addition, cartilage in both the nose and ears can grow after age 40, making the nose and ears larger.

## Expression Lines

Expression lines are another symptom of intrinsic aging. Individuals will develop lines from consistent and repetitive facial movements. "Smile" lines occur in the nasolabial area. "Frown" lines may also occur in the forehead, eye, and chin areas. Any repetitive movement of a facial expression such as raising the eyebrows, frowning, smiling, scowling, or any other facial movement will eventually cause a crease to occur, just as pants will wrinkle more the more you wear them. "Eye smilers" smile and squint at the same time, creating additional eyelines. Squint lines also occur around the eyes from squinting due to sun exposure, light exposure, or facial expression. It is important to wear ultraviolet protective sunglasses while outside to provide protection against both ultraviolet light exposure and the tendency to squint when exposed to light.

Smokers will inevitably get "smoker's lines" around the mouth and eyes from continually moving these areas during smoking activities. Smoking also causes thousands of free radicals to invade the body and is known to interfere with proper collagen production.

Sleep habits, such as sleeping on one side or directly on the face, will eventually create lines and elasticity problems. Advise clients to sleep on their backs as much as possible, helping to avoid "sleep creases," which when they happen repetitively have a strong effect on the aging symptoms of the face.

## The "Wearing Out" of the Foundation

As time progresses, the muscles, fat, and skin on our faces undergo structural changes. The amount of fat in the subcutaneous layer decreases with age, providing less cushion and plumpness to the skin, resulting in less support. People who are overweight often do not have as many noticeable wrinkles on the face as thin people or people of normal weight. This does not mean that the skin has not aged; it simply means that there is more fat to "plump out" the skin, creating a smoother looking appearance. The skin is stretched back and forth over a lifetime, causing an "enlargening" of the skin, and gravity pulls down on the skin. The muscles have partially receded, causing the effect of more elastosis.

## Wrinkles versus Sagging

Wrinkles and skin sagging are characteristics of both intrinsic and extrinsic aging. Wrinkles are usually seen before sagging or elastosis. Clients usually express concern about wrinkles as early as age 30, and they express concern about sagging about 10 years later.

Wrinkles associated with intrinsic aging are primarily expression lines. Sagging associated with intrinsic aging is relatively minor and is attributable to gravity and intrinsic physiological changes.

Criss-cross wrinkling, wrinkles not in the normal facial expression, and severe elastosis are all symptoms of sun damage and will be discussed further in the chapters on sun and sun damage and the new science of aging skin treatment.

## PREVENTION OF AGING SKIN

Each year we learn more and more about prevention of aging of both the body and the skin. One of the newest theories is that the symptoms that we think of as "aging" are actually only an accumulation of tissue damage that has occurred over a number of years. In other words, the signs of aging may be a lot more related to damage of tissue than the actual passing of the years.

Although there is really very little anyone can do to completely prevent inevitable intrinsic aging of the skin, one can develop certain health habits that will help delay the onset and possibly lessen the severity of intrinsic aging symptoms. Prevention of sun exposure is the biggest preventable factor. Sun exposure is, of course, an example of extrinsic aging, which will be covered in great detail in the chapter on sun and sun damage.

## Diet and Exercise

Again, this will not prevent all intrinsic aging, but good health habits will help the body nourish the skin better and therefore help to fight aging. Avoiding excessive alcohol will also help the body function better. A regular aerobic exercise program and a well-balanced, healthy diet can certainly help an individual live longer and better and help the skin function in a more healthy manner.

Many scientists believe that a diet rich in antioxidant foods or use of antioxidant supplements, such as vitamins C and E and grapeseed and green tea extracts, may help protect body tissues, including the skin, from free radical damage, reducing the signs of aging. Smoking is known to severely affect health and function of all cells within the body. Smoking and exposure to second-hand smoke should be avoided for a healthy body or skin.

We learn more and more each day about nutrition and its relation to health. Although we will not focus on nutrition in this book, many estheticians find it helpful to receive a good nutrition education. Although it is not the role of the esthetician to give nutritional advice and counseling (this is the role of the physician and registered dietician), the esthetician should have a working knowledge of the elements of nutrition to better understand skin function and health and to be able to refer clients with nutritional or eating disorders to the proper qualified professionals. Investigate taking courses in nutrition and wellness through the departments of health or home economics at your local community college or university.

## Weight Gain and Loss

People who are overweight have problems with skin stretching to accommodate the extra fat. This can occur anywhere on the body, but it is especially noticeable in the face. Extra skin below the chin and on the neck is a good example.

When people lose weight, sometimes the skin has been overstretched and does not return to its original contour. This is especially true if the client is morbidly obese, has been overweight for a long time, or is older than 40 years of age. Again, this can occur anywhere on the body, but it is especially common in the facial skin.

## Good Skin Care

**Dehydration** is the decreasing ability of the skin to hold water.

Using good skin-care products and developing a routine facial skin-care program will obviously help the skin look better. As the skin ages, production of intercellular cement decreases, which decreases the skin's ability to hold water. This is **dehydration**, and it results in a rough-textured appearance. Many theories support the use of hydrating agents in lessening the signs of aging. Many researchers believe that good skin care with proper conditioners, free-radical scavengers, stimulating chemicals, hydrating agents, and sunscreens may help lessen the physical aging of the skin. It is obvious that many of these conditioning treatment agents help the skin look better, regardless of any long-term positive effects. Research continues in the use of these many agents to help lessen the symptoms of skin aging.

## Plenty of Sleep

Getting plenty of sleep is another good health habit, giving the body time to regenerate its tissues and repair damaged cells. Lack of sleep can cause eye circles and puffiness and contribute to stress that can have a debilitating effect on both the mind and the body.

## Stress

Each day medical researchers are learning more and more about stress and its effect on health, nutrition, and aging. Avoiding high amounts of stress certainly will help avoid premature aging signs of not only the skin, but of the other organs of the body.

Many resort spas, as well as day spas, now offer stress management, yoga, and other body treatments designed to reduce and manage stress. Massage services, aromatherapy services, and a soothing environment within the spa can help reduce daily services for you and your clients! Again, although estheticians cannot permanently change their clients' lifestyles, they should be abreast of the newest research regarding stress and health to help give their clients the best esthetic care possible. Estheticians should also be aware of referral services to qualified professionals who handle stress, such as psychologists.

## THE BEGINNING OF AGING

Many clients will notice signs of aging and occasionally "freak out" at the first wrinkle. Be understanding and give them the best advice you can, teaching them realistic preventative techniques. The word *realistic* should be emphasized, because ethical estheticians do not endorse "miracle" treatments; they advise clients about the best proper realistic skin-care program.

The key word here is program. Treatment of the aging skin must address the many factors of aging. One cannot apply a hydrator and expect to revive the skin from 40 years of sun damage and bad habits.

Good skin-care habits are most effective if started early in life to prevent problems, but many clients do not start using proper home care or develop good skin-care habits until they notice the first signs of aging.

A combination of good skin-care products, including daily-use sunscreens, hydrators, topical antioxidants, peptide serums and creams, collagen stimulant products, lipids, and alphahydroxy acids, along with regular salon treatments and alphahydroxy acid treatments can help the client manage and significantly reduce the visible signs of aging.

We will discuss sun damage and sunscreen usage more in detail in another chapter, but it certainly cannot be repeated enough that daily use of broad-spectrum sunscreen is by far the most effective method for prevention of premature aging.

Hydrators help add water to the skin surface, cosmetically smoothing the surface of the aging skin. Hydration ingredients include sodium PCA, sorbitol, glycerin, hyaluronic acid, or sodium hyaluronate.

Decrease in cell turnover occurs as the skin ages, resulting in uneven skin texture and a dull look to the skin. The decrease in cell turnover also results in a decrease of lipid production by the epidermal cells, decreasing barrier function and resulting in an uneven skin surface, making the skin look dull and rough textured. Lack of intercellular lipids causes the skin to become dehydrated, causing the skin to look less smooth and less firm, as well as interfering with other cellular functions.

Regular use of exfoliants such as alphahydroxy acids remove dried-out, dead, dull, crusty cells, helping the skin surface look much smoother. Mild daily exfoliation helps to stimulate the cell renewal process, increasing lipid production, relayering surface cells, and improving hydration as well as cellular and barrier function. Long-term results are much younger and healthier-looking skin.

Use of mechanical exfoliants at home several times a week can also help remove dead cells loosened by daily use of alphahydroxy acids. Mechanical exfoliating ingredients include polyethylene granules, corn meal, ground almonds, or hydrogenated jojoba oil beads. These products literally "bump off" dead cells and can produce a boost to the look of tired or neglected skin.

Enzymes such as bromelain, papain, or pancreatin or professional alphahydroxy acid products can be used in the salon to freshen dull-looking, aging skin.

Be careful, as with all skins, not to overexfoliate, which can be very irritating and damaging to the skin. Aging skin may be more vulnerable to mechanical or chemical damage because it is thinner or may have impaired barrier function.

Combining all of these modalities with state-of-the-art ingredient technology, such as the use of palmitoyl pentapeptide-3, other peptides, and collagen stimulant complexes, is the best program for avoiding or delaying the visible signs of aging.

For more information on all of these concepts, see the chapters on sun and sun damage and the new science of aging skin treatment.

## DERMAL AND EPIDERMAL STRUCTURAL CHANGES

Several histological changes take place within the dermis and the epidermis as the skin ages. These changes are often associated with sun damage and chronic sun exposure, but some of this occurs through the natural intrinsic aging process.

The epidermis slowly becomes thinner with age, and the dermis increases in thickness. Breakdown of the network of collagen and elastin fibrils within the dermis also occurs. Blood vessels tend to fragment, causing redness—telangiectasias, known to many estheticians as couperose. Because of this fragmented blood vessel formation the blood supply is also fragmented, resulting in poorer blood distribution than in younger skin.

Older skin, as we previously discussed, tends to be thinner than younger skin. Clients must be careful not to overexfoliate, use harsh abrasives, or use too much pressure. Hot water and extremely cold water should be avoided on skin with couperose or capillary fragility. Avoid using hot masks or steaming the face too closely. Clients who have extreme redness should be told to avoid alcoholic beverages, tobacco, and spicy foods, because all of these are **vasodilators**, which means they cause dilation of the blood vessels and sudden surges of blood flow in the already fragile vessels.

**Vasodilators** dilate the blood vessels, making more blood flow through the arterial system.

## "AGE SPOTS"

"Age spots," or dark splotches of hyperpigmentation, are one of the first signs of what we think of as skin aging. Hyperpigmentation of this type is virtually completely caused by sun damage and overexposure. It has nothing to do with age, only how much sun damage has occurred over time. Hence, we will discuss this further in the chapter on sun and sun damage.

## PSYCHOLOGICAL EFFECTS OF AGING

Clients may experience psychological effects when they realize that the aging process has begun. They may seek "immediate result" treatments, which do not exist. Work with these clients to establish a good, solid home care program, coupled with good salon treatments. The more often the client comes into the salon, the better the program will be, because this client needs lots of encouragement and "coaching."

Try to steer the client away from unrealistic "nonsurgical face-lift" approaches to skin care. Stress using sunscreen, avoiding sun exposure, using good hydrators designed for the client's skin type, and using specialty products, such as conditioners containing glycolic acid.

This type of client will also sometimes have a tendency to "drown" in heavy moisturizers, often causing comedogenic or acnegenic results. Explain to the client that aging is not a lack of oil. Only clients who are truly alipidic (oil-dry) need to be using heavy oily products, and then they need to contain the right kind of emollient.

## HOME CARE FOR THE AGING CLIENT

Home care should be adapted to help the client's aging signs, whatever their severity. Begin by thoroughly analyzing the skin. Always adapt the entire program to the skin type. Treatment conditioners for aging skin will not be useful if they are for the wrong skin type. Aging clients will still be predominantly dry or oily. For oily clients, stick to noncomedogenic fluids, lotions, or gels. For more oil-dry skin, you can use heavier emollients.

Stick to very gentle cleansers with little or no detergents. Remember, the aging skin already has fewer intercellular lipids. You do not want to strip these essential lipids by using too aggressive a cleanser. Low-foaming washes and cleansing milks are best to use for the aging skin.

Toners should be alcohol-free and should contain a humectant such as propylene glycol or glycerin. Toners should not have a strong astringent action.

Specialty products for aging skin may include alphahydroxy gels or creams, peptide and collagen stimulant serums and other products, antioxidant serums, and lipid-based serums. These are special functional products that help protect the skin from free-radical damage, and help exfoliate or hydrate the skin. These serum-type products are often layered under or over other products.

Day creams should contain a broad-spectrum sunscreen and a sealant agent such as dimethicone, mineral oil, or cyclomethicone. These agents will help the skin retain water better in the surface layers. The consistency of the day cream will vary depending on the oiliness or dryness of the skin. "Poreless" skin with poor sebum production will need more emollients, and the cream should generally be heavier. Oily skin should be treated with a noncomedogenic day cream containing less emollient and more hydration agents.

Night treatment will vary, again depending on the skin type. Hydrators such as lecithin (liposomes), sorbitol, sodium PCA, glycerin, and hyaluronic acid are appropriate.

Special treatment products for the eye and neck areas are very helpful to the aging skin. The skin of the eyes and the neck is much thinner than the rest of the facial skin, and is therefore very likely to show signs of aging. Heavier emollients are often used for these areas, with the exception of some of the newer liposome gels. The client should use eye and neck care products 24 hours a day for best results.

Many estheticians vary the night treatment for clients, alternating different types of night treatments. The theory here is that the change in night treatment will help stimulate sluggish skin.

## FACIAL TREATMENTS FOR AGING SKIN

Salon facial treatments for aging skin must be administered frequently. You should begin by treating the skin weekly or biweekly for six to twelve treatments, slowly decreasing to once every two to four weeks. Although it is normal to administer salon treatments monthly, aging skin often needs treatment more often. It is certainly advisable to perform facial treatments weekly or biweekly on drier, aging skin, if this is affordable for the client.

You should always design the facial based on skin type and conditions. Aging skin often will be thin, so be careful with harsh exfoliants, brushing, and suction machines. As skin gets older, it tends to become more oil-dry, particularly after age 50. Keep this in mind when treating the skin. Occasionally, you will see an oily or, more often, a combination aging skin. Because many treatment products designed for aging skin contain larger percentages of emollients and fats, be careful not to use creams that are too oily or heavy for combination and oily skin types.

## Microcurrent Treatment

**Microcurrent** is a low-level current application used to stimulate and improve the elasticity of aging and sun-damaged skin.

The use of **microcurrent**, a gentle treatment using an ultra-small amount of galvanic current is showing great promise to help both the signs of extrinsic and intrinsic aging (Figure 18-3). Regular use of microcurrent improves elasticity, skin texture, and can be combined with other modalities like AHA exfoliation, antioxidants, and peptide technology. For more on this method of treatment, see the chapter on the new science of aging skin treatment.

## Exfoliation

Mild exfoliation is good for aging skin. It gently stimulates the skin and removes dead, dry cells on the surface, helping the skin look and feel smoother and softer, and also helping to minimize the appearance of rough textures and wrinkles. Mild enzyme peeling treatments are effective in helping to remove this dead cell buildup. Mild alphahydroxy acid exfoliation treatments also are very helpful in improving aging skin symptoms. For more information on peeling treatments, see Chapter 21, Chemical Peeling and Exfoliation Procedures.

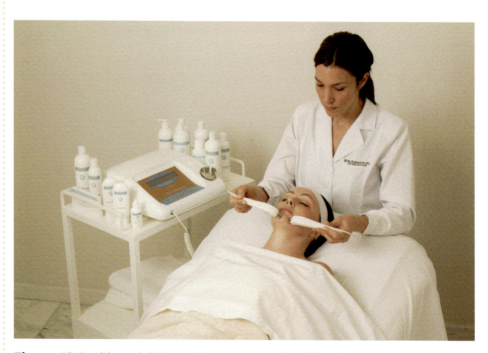

**Figure 18-3** Although it is not the same as a facelift, microcurrent, when applied correctly, has been shown in university studies to improve elasticity, collagen content, and elastin content (Courtesy Bio-therapeutic, Inc.)

Massage helps to soothe and hydrate aging skin by stimulating blood flow. Be careful not to overmassage or use rough massage techniques on fragile, thin, aging skin with distended capillaries.

## Treatment for Aging Skin

1. Remove makeup by gently massaging a cleansing milk into the skin and then removing the makeup and cleanser with damp, soft, facial cloths, sponges, or cotton pads. Follow with gentle toner on cool wet pads or a soft cloth.

2. After cleansing and toning, carefully examine the skin for elasticity, dryness, dehydration, couperose or distended capillaries, hyperpigmentation, and sun damage symptoms. See the chapter on sun and sun damage.

3. Apply a very lightweight hydrating fluid during steam treatment. Steam the skin at a distance of 14 to 20 inches with the hydrating fluid on the skin. This will help soften the skin and attract the steam. Do not use oil-based fluid or heavier creams. This will repel water instead of attracting it. As an alternative treatment, a gentle enzyme mask may be applied during steam instead of a hydrating fluid.

4. If the skin is not too fragile, you may use the brushing machine over a thick coat of hydrating fluid. (Do not use the brushing machine after enzyme or alphahydroxy acid treatment.) Avoid brushing if the skin is thin, red, or couperose.

5. Gently extract any clogged pores or comedones.

6. Use cold spray with a mild toner solution after extraction.

7. Apply a hydrating fluid, ampoule, or cream to the skin, designed for both the aging skin and the individual skin type. Gently massage the skin. Massage should last about 10 minutes. If using an ampoule, you may want to use electrical treatment before continuing massage.

8. Apply high frequency treatment at a low setting or ionization rollers over the ampoule, hydrating fluid, or specialty cream. Make sure to check all health precautions and contraindications before using electrical therapy.

9. Apply masks appropriate for the particular skin types. Most masks for aging skin are creamy and soft setting or are the gel variety. Clay masks may be used on oily or clogged areas.

10. Allow the mask to sit for 15 to 20 minutes. For extra dry skin, you may apply extra hydrating fluid or cream in lieu of a mask.

11. After 15 to 20 minutes, spray the mask with an atomized cold spray of diluted toner or conditioning water. This will help soften and loosen the mask. Apply strips of cool, wet cotton or soft facial cloths in a compress technique, gently molding the compresses to the face. Remove the strips one at a time, wiping the mask off the skin as you remove the compress.

12. Finish by applying an appropriate day cream with sunscreen.

Aging skin can be stimulated, cleansed, softened, firmed, and hydrated. With careful management, aging skin can be made to look much softer and smoother. However, no one can actually turn back the clock. Avoid using "miraculous" treatments. Explain sensible care to your client, emphasizing the importance of careful, consistent, diligent care both in the salon and at home.

## TOPICS FOR DISCUSSION

1. What changes occur in the skin from birth, to the 20s, to the 40s and 50s?
2. Discuss hereditary characteristics and aging.

3. What is the difference between intrinsic and extrinsic aging?
4. Discuss other factors related to aging.
5. Discuss home care procedures for aging skin.
6. Discuss salon treatment for aging skin.

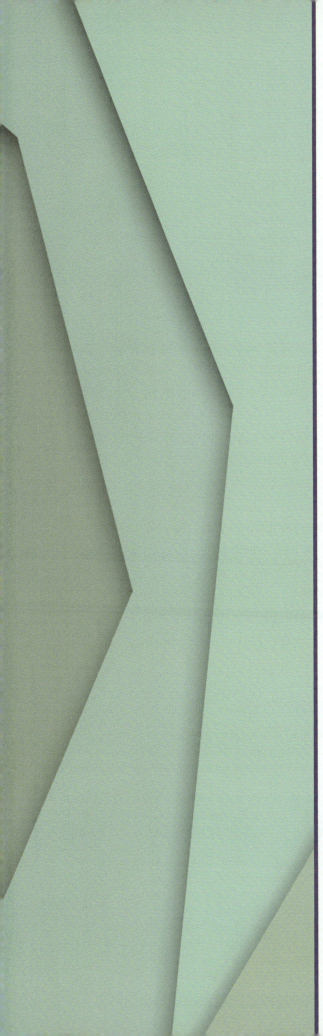

# CHAPTER 19

# Sun and Sun Damage

## OBJECTIVES. . .

The sun is a phenomenal structure that helps plants convert carbon dioxide to pure oxygen. We cannot live without oxygen, and we cannot live without sun. Yet the sun is, by far, the worst enemy of the skin. The sun creates free radicals, which cause cell damage. Cell damage eventually results in the destruction of collagen and elastin and possibly alters the DNA, eventually resulting in skin cancers. Repetitive exposure to the sun causes severe skin damage, premature aging, and skin cancer. Yet many people continue to bask in the sun's rays, achieving a golden tan but also accumulating terrible damage to the skin. In this chapter we will learn all about the way the sun affects the skin, in both the long and short term. We will learn about the best ways to prevent sun damage and skin cancer and how to detect skin cancer.

The sun projects three basic kinds of **ultraviolet rays**, or UV rays (Figure 19-1). **UVC rays** are short rays that are blocked by the ozone layer. They have germicidal properties, and in large doses are deadly to live creatures.

**Ultraviolet B rays** (UVB) are the next longest ultraviolet ray. UVB rays cause most skin cancers and are responsible for sunburns. They penetrate the epidermis to the basal layer. Some UVB rays penetrate the dermis, but most stop at the basal layer. UVB are much stronger than UVA rays, even though **UVA rays** are longer and penetrate the dermis.

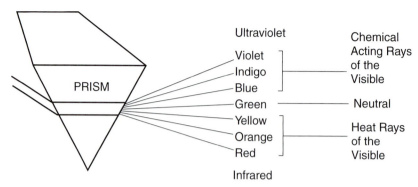

**Figure 19-1** Dispersion of light rays by a prism

**Ultraviolet rays** are short rays that are blocked by the ozone layer.

**UVC rays** are short sunrays blocked by the ozone layer.

**Ultraviolet B rays** are sunrays that cause sunburn and the majority of skin cancers.

**UVA rays** are longer, deep-penetrating rays that affect the dermis of the skin. These rays are responsible for most premature aging symptoms.

**Melanocytes** are cells that are "pigment factories" for the skin.

**Melanin** is the pigment of the skin.

Within the basal layer and upper dermis are the **melanocytes**, the pigment-producing cells. These cells are stimulated by exposure to ultraviolet rays and manufacture **melanin**, the skin pigment that is the body's natural sunscreen. Although many people think a tan is healthy, a tan is actually a chemical reaction of the body defending itself from the damaging rays of the sun. A tan is actually the body and the skin saying "don't do this to me"—just like a warrior picking up a shield to ward off an enemy!

Again, UVA rays are longer rays, penetrating the dermis and the precious collagen and elastin fibrils. UVA only burns in large doses and is therefore the type of UV ray used in most tanning beds and booths. Although the tanning bed is unlikely to burn the skin, the damaging UVA rays penetrate the dermis, affecting the supportive structure of the collagen and elastin fibrils and causing other detrimental changes to the skin.

## SHORT-TERM SUN PROBLEMS

Most of us know that long-term sun exposure causes skin aging and skin cancer, but very few people are aware of the short-term damaging effects of ultraviolet and sun exposure. Sun exposure causes a variety of short-term skin and esthetic problems. These may affect both beauty and health.

Sunburns happen very frequently, especially in the summer months. They can be mild to severe. The skin becomes very red, sore, and sensitive to the touch, caused by dilation of blood vessels and stimulation of nerve endings in the skin. The skin will eventually peel due to the extreme dryness associated with the sunburn. The skin literally bakes to a very dehydrated condition, just as cookies will burn and become dry if cooked too long in the oven. Many of these sunburns happen because people are ignorant about sun protection. Whereas Floridians and Californians are very familiar with sun protection, tourists from areas where sunbathing is not popular due to the climate are especially vulnerable to sunburn. It is important that estheticians be very familiar with sun protection methods to help their clients protect themselves from sunburn as well as from long- and short-term sun damage.

A variety of remedies can ease the pain of a minor sunburn. These include taking cool baths with vinegar added to cool water, applying cool packs, applying plain yogurt to the area, and using local spray anesthetics. The latter must be used with caution. Although the spray anesthetics can provide temporary pain relief to the sunburned area, many people have allergies to localized skin anesthetics. Advise clients to be very careful if using these products. Sunburn is actually a medical condition and therefore is in the domain of the physician, not the esthetician. Severe sunburns can cause shock, fever, nausea, and even death. Any "bubbling" of the skin or severe blistering should always be referred to a medical doctor.

After the initial burn is relieved, your client may ask you for help with the remaining esthetic skin problems associated with a sunburn. The skin may be extremely dehydrated, flaking, and peeling. Occasionally, these discolorations may be long term. First and most important, strongly advise the client not to expose himself or herself to any more sun until all the symptoms of the sunburn are completely gone, especially peeling of the skin. Further sun exposure during the peeling process following a sunburn often results in further long-term skin damage and permanent solar lentigenes (freckles induced by the sun) and other skin discolorations.

You should not attempt to treat sunburned skin that is still red or sensitive. If the skin is no longer red or sensitive, you may use very gentle techniques to hydrate the skin. Use cool steam, fragrance-free hydrating fluids and lotions, nonhardening nonstimulating masks, and other products designed for super-sensitive skin. Avoid exfoliating or stimulating treatments, including brushing, galvanic desincrustation, or heavy massage. Advise the client to use similar procedures at home until all symptoms subside. Give the client good instruction about the proper use of sunscreens to avoid a reoccurrence of the situation.

## Other Short-Term Sun-Related Problems

**Hyperpigmentation** is both a long- and short-term cosmetic problem caused by the sun. Hyperpigmentation is dark splotching and is one of the first visible signs of what we think of as skin aging. Hyperpigmented literally means overpigmented.

Sun-induced skin discoloration begins in the late teens and early 20s and gets continually worse. Skin that has been repeatedly burned or has not healed from a sunburn before additional sun exposure is especially vulnerable. If you look at the skin of a 15-year-old and compare it with that of a 25-year-old, the biggest difference you will notice is in the skin pigmentation. The main noticeable difference between teenage skin and skin in the early 20s is discoloration caused by deposits of melanin. If you look carefully at makeover pictures, one of the biggest differences between the "before" and "after" photographs is the even coloring of the individual's skin in the "after" picture.

Almost completely caused by long-term sun exposure, **chloasma**, also known as "liver spots," have nothing to do with the liver and everything to do with cumulative sun exposure (Figure 19-2). These dark-brown patches primarily on the face and hands are areas of concentrated pigment. You may notice that many clients do not exhibit hyperpigmentation on the body as much as they do on the face, arms, and hands. Although there are exceptions to this rule, the face, hands, and arms are areas that have been chronically exposed to the sun for many years. Hence the pigmentation is much worse in these areas (Figure 19-3A, 19-3B).

Hyperpigmentation may appear suddenly, especially in women, after years of sun exposure. It may appear first as subtle splotching that you may notice when examining the skin under a magnifying lamp or especially a Wood's lamp. From this relatively mild splotching, darker, larger splotches may develop. Hyperpigmentation occurs in many patterns and is also associated with hormone fluctuations and pregnancy (see the chapter on hormones).

**Hyperpigmentation** refers to any condition that has more than a normal amount of melanin.

**Chloasma**, often called "liver spots," are dark brown patches of hyperpigmentation on the skin caused by sun overexposure.

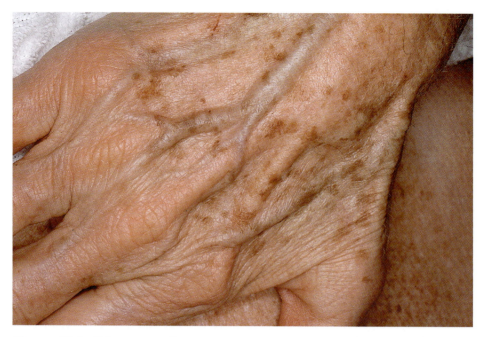

**Figure 19-2** Chloasma, or liver spots, are spots of concentrated melanin caused by sun damage

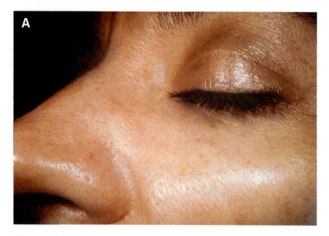 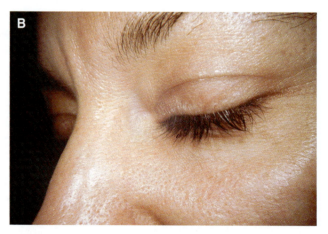

**Figure 19-3** Hyperpigmentation, often caused by cumulative sun exposure, can be improved with the use of alphahydroxy and betahydroxy acids, and lightening or brightening agents such as hydroquinone or magnesium ascorbyl phosphate. In this case study, a series of 30 percent alphahydroxy acid exfoliation treatments showed this improvement in three weeks (Courtesy Mark Lees Skin Care, Inc.)

**Melanin suppressant** is a substance that interferes with the skin's production of melanin pigment.

**Hydroquinone** is a drug ingredient in melanin suppressant.

Hyperpigmentation is treated by having the client apply a solution containing a **melanin suppressant**. These agents stop the chemical reactions occurring in the melanocytes at the basal cell level that lead to hyperpigmentation. **Hydroquinone** is the best known of these agents and the only one officially recognized by the U.S. Food and Drug Administration (FDA). Other unrecognized yet effective melanin suppressive ingredients include **kojic acid**, **magnesium ascorbyl phosphate** (also an antioxidant), **arbutin**, **bearberry** or **mulberry extract**, and **azelaic acid**.

Melanin suppressants are used in tandem with some sort of peeling agent like an alphahydroxy acid or prescriptive tretinoin. These keratolytic exfoliants help to remove already stained corneocytes and also help to increase the absorption of the melanin suppressant.

Clients being treated for any form of hyperpigmentation must agree to avoid sun exposure. Even hyperpigmentation caused by hormone imbalances can be made worse by sun exposure.

Explain to clients that wherever they have a hyperpigmented area, there is a concentration of active melanocytes in the lower epidermis and upper dermis, producing melanin and depositing it in epidermal cells that are drifting toward the corneum. This is the "factory" where melanin is produced. The melanin is the "product." Melanin suppressors, like the ones listed here, work by interfering with the chemical reactions that cause production of the melanin. They do not actually stop the "factory"; they just interfere with production. Because of this fact, the "factory"—the melanocyte—is still active, even when the hyperpigmentation has faded. This is why it is so important for the client to avoid the controllable factor that stimulates the melanocytes, namely sun exposure. As long as the client continues to expose himself or herself to the sun and not wear a broad-spectrum SPF-30 sunscreen or higher, melanin production will continue. There is mounting evidence that heat from the sun's infrared rays may play a big role in melanin production as well, and there is no screen for infrared heat waves.

Many clients concerned with hyperpigmentation are or have been active sun worshippers. It must be explained to these clients that sun exposure is what caused the pigmentation problem in the first place and that they must change this factor of their lifestyle to achieve any change in their skin.

**Tinea veriscolor** is what many refer to as sun "spots" or sun "fungus." These white splotches, which usually appear on the chest and back of avid sunbathers, are actually a fungal condition. The fungus interferes with the melanocytes' ability to make melanin, which causes the white splotches to appear when the body is tanned. If you have a client with this condition, refer the client to a dermatologist for treatment (Figure 19-4).

**Kojic acid** is a melanin suppressant "brightening" ingredient.

**Magnesium ascorbyl phosphate** is a stable form of vitamin C that also inhibits melanin production.

**Arbutin** is a melanin suppressant.

**Bearberry** or **mulberry extract** is a naturally occurring melanin suppressant.

**Azelaic acid** is a melanin suppressant, which is also used for acne and rosacea.

**Tinea versicolor** is what many refer to as sun "spots" or sun "fungus." These white splotches are a fungal condition.

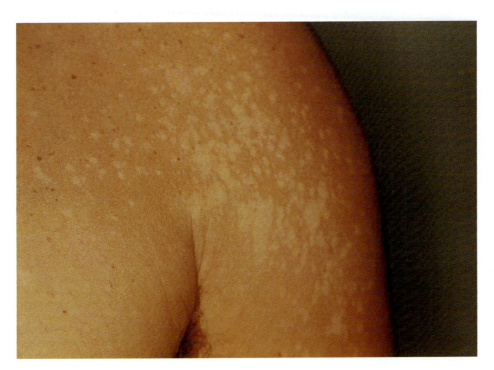

**Figure 19-4** Tinea versicolor (Courtesy Rube J. Pardo, M.D., Ph.D.)

## The Real Damage from the Sun

Continual exposure to sun results in the formation of more and more damaging free radicals. Although not visible at first, or even for years, the routine damage to the cells eventually accumulates, resulting in wrinkles, hyperpigmentation, elastosis, and rough-textured skin.

As we have previously discussed, the sun-exposed skin falls victim to the inflammation cascade, resulting in breakdown of collagen and elastin due to self-destruct enzymes manufactured through the immune system's defense against the sun exposure and damage to the cells of the skin. When enough damage occurs, it becomes visible in the skin's appearance.

## What You Don't Know about Short-Term Sun Exposure

We now know that sun exposure may actually suppress the immune functions of the skin. Exposure to sunlight "chases off" your protective macrophage "guard cells," allowing substances and organisms to enter the skin, increasing the chance of infection. A good example of this immune suppression is the flares of herpes simplex that occur in some individuals when they are exposed to sun. Many cases of lupus, an autoimmune disease, are diagnosed after a sunburn, when the immune system has overreacted to the injury.

It is so important that we teach young children to use sunscreen daily. We receive about 80 percent of the sun's damage to the skin before the age of 18. Sun freckles appearing on teenagers' faces represent problem areas in the future. Most sun exposure is not from sunbathing but from day-to-day exposure. Think about how many children play outdoors. Every time they go outside, they expose themselves to harmful ultraviolet rays. That's why every time they go outdoors, they should be protected with a good sunscreen. We tend to think about sunscreens during the summer months, but it should be a year-round consideration.

## LONG-TERM PHOTO DAMAGE

Almost every symptom we think of as aging is directly related to sun exposure. Even intrinsic aging symptoms, such as facial expression lines, are made worse because of sun damage. Hyperpigmentation, leathery texture, roughness, wrinkles, some forms of hypopigmentation, severe elastosis (sagging of the skin), chest and cleavage wrinkling, splotchiness, couperose and telangiectasias, flare of rosacea, neck texture problems, severe dehydration, and barrier function problems are all directly related to sun exposure.

**Dermatoheliosis** is the medical term coined to describe long-term damage to the skin caused by sun exposure. The skin is severely affected by long-term exposure.

Collagen and elastin fibrils in the dermis begin a process called **cross-linking**. In essence, collagen and elastin fibrils collapse due to cumulative effects of cell damage from repeated sun exposure, causing the support system for the skin also to collapse. Esthetically, this results in deep wrinkling of the skin, sagging, and elastosis.

Sun-damaged skin appears much more severely aged than skin that has aged solely from intrinsic factors. The wrinkling does not only appear in expression lines. Many, many lines develop, in all areas and in all directions. Wrinkles may be both horizontal and vertical. Normal expression lines are much deeper in sun-damaged skin.

The abnormal structure of the dermis and the epidermis give the skin a "leathery" appearance and feel. This type of skin is also severely discolored due to melanin deposits and hyperpigmentation.

**Dermatoheliosis** is the medical term coined to describe long-term damage to the skin caused by sun exposure.

**Cross-linking** is a process in which collagen and elastin fibrils in the dermis collapse, causing the support system for the skin also to collapse.

The skin of a person with sun damage is very rough to the touch, and the surface is actually uneven. This is caused by damage to the cells, which causes the corneum and other epidermal cells not to shed in a normal, even manner. This is due to the altering of the DNA from chronic sun exposure. The cells become "confused," divide unevenly, and no longer retain their normal shape. If you look at a cross-section of normal skin, you will notice that the cells in the epidermis form layers that look like layers of brick in a brick wall. In sun-damaged skin, the same structure looks like a brick wall that is collapsing, made with uneven bricks that are poorly made!

The epidermis of sun-damaged skin becomes progressively thinner, and the dermis slowly begins to atrophy, or collapse, and fall apart. This is how the sun eventually "zaps" the skin and destroys it.

Clients with sun-damage will have multiple wrinkles, not just around the eyes and neck, but all over the face. There will be many more pronounced wrinkles than in other clients. Their skin is literally a multitude of uneven colors, very freckled. This skin will have a leathery feel and look. There may be patches of dryness frequently, and clients may often complain about how "dry" their skin is. The truth is that as the skin cells become disfigured, they also fail to produce sufficient amounts of intercellular cement causing an impaired barrier function and making proper hydration of the skin practically impossible.

Use of lipid replacement ingredients such as ceramides, cholesterol, and phospholipids, along with the routine use of an 8 to 10 percent, pH 3.5, alphahydroxy acid serum or cream and the use of a good hydrator such as hyaluronic acid, glycerin, or sodium PCA can help this damaged skin retain more moisture.

Sun-damaged skin may also have many telangiectasias or couperose areas. Sun damage also causes collapse of some of the blood vessels and decreased blood flow. The small capillaries look like tributaries of a river. These vessels may be very fragile, and bruises may appear easily. You may notice how easily some of your older clients bruise. Although this may be due to many medical factors, sun-damaged skin bruises much more easily than normal, healthy, nondamaged skin. You will also notice that these clients who bruise easily have very thin-looking, dry, hyperpigmented skin. This is because the skin is almost always severely sun damaged.

## SKIN CANCERS AND OTHER SUN-RELATED SKIN GROWTHS

Skin cancer is caused by the damage to the DNA that we have been discussing. The cells begin dividing unevenly and rapidly, but the genetic material in the DNA is damaged from the sun. This rapid dividing of the cells may take the form of small tumors, which we know as skin cancer.

There are three major kinds of skin cancer. **Basal cell carcinomas** are the most common. They are almost always found on the sun-exposed areas, typically on the face, hands, legs, back, and chest. They look like small pearls. Sometimes they have a small blood vessel running through them. They are not usually perfectly round like a milium. On older hyperpigmented skin, they may be hard to differentiate from milia. You must look carefully to tell the difference (Figure 19-5).

Estheticians are not in the business of diagnosing skin cancer. However, you should know the signs of the major forms of skin cancer and be able to refer suspicious-looking lesions and areas to a dermatologist.

Basal cell carcinomas are very often curable. In fact, 95 percent of these cancers are cured. They rarely spread to the internal parts of the body, but can grow, and if they are not treated they can affect large areas of the skin. Basal cell carcinomas are sometimes removed surgically, sometimes frozen, and sometimes treated with laser or other means.

**Basal cell carcinomas** are the most common forms of skin cancer; lesions have a pearl-like appearance with small blood vessels running through.

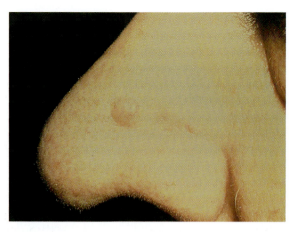

**Figure 19-5** Basal cell carcinoma (Courtesy Rube J. Pardo, M.D., Ph.D.)

**Squamous cell carcinomas** is a common form of skin cancer characterized by unexplained skin bleeding or a small red or pink, sometimes ulcerated, lesion.

**Mohs' surgery** is a specialized form of surgery for very precise removal of skin cancer cells.

**Melanoma** is characterized by moles or mole-like lesions that are dark in color.

**Squamous cell carcinomas** are the second most frequently diagnosed form of skin cancer. They may look like red or pink solid bumps on the skin. They may appear as open sores or ulcers that do not seem to heal. They may look crusty, or the client may notice a crusty area that bleeds easily (Figure 19-6). Many clients notice this when washing or cleansing the face. Again, these lesions appear on chronically sun-exposed areas. Treatment is similar to treatment for basal cell carcinoma, but squamous cell carcinoma may sometimes spread to other areas of the body. **Mohs' surgery** is a specialized surgical technique, named after its developer, Frederic Mohs, M.D. In Mohs' surgery, the dermatologist trims more and more tissue from the cancer lesion, carefully checking each sample of tissue for cancerous cells using a microscope, until all the cancerous tissue is removed.

The least frequently seen form of the three major kinds of skin cancer is also the most deadly. **Melanoma** is characterized by moles or mole-like lesions that are dark in color. The Skin Cancer Foundation has coined an expression that is easy to remember when looking at suspicious lesions (Figure 19-7). They call this the "ABCDEs of Melanoma." "A" stands for asymmetric. The melanoma lesion is usually growing to one side of the lesion and is uneven. "B" stands for border. The borders of melanomas are uneven and not smooth. "C" is for color. Melanomas often have dark brown and black colors and are usually splotchy and not all one color. "D" stands for

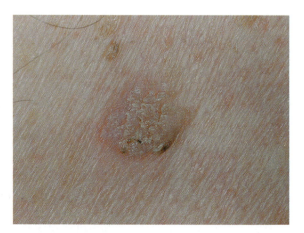

**Figure 19-6** Squamous cell carcinoma (Courtesy Michael J. Bond, M.D.)

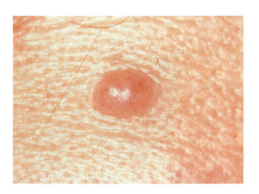

**Figure 19-7A1** Benign mole—symmetrical. Common moles are usually round and symmetrical (Images Courtesy of The Skin Cancer Foundation, www.skincancer.org)

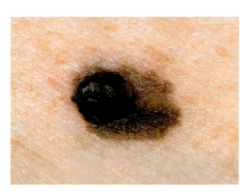

**Figure 19-7A2** Melanoma—asymmetrical. Most early melanomas are asymmetrical; a line drawn through the middle will not create matching halves (Images Courtesy of The Skin Cancer Foundation, www.skincancer.org)

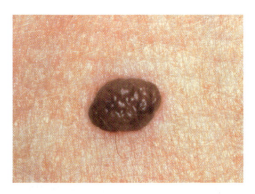

**Figure 19-7B1** Benign mole—even edges. Common moles usually have smooth, even borders (Images Courtesy of The Skin Cancer Foundation, www.skincancer.org)

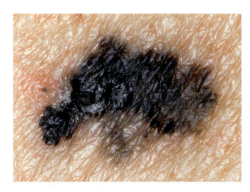

**Figure 19-7B2** Melanoma—uneven edges. The borders of early melanomas are frequently uneven, often containing scalloped or notched edges (Images Courtesy of The Skin Cancer Foundation, www.skincancer.org)

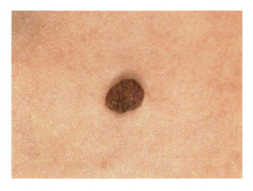

**Figure 19-7C1** Benign mole—one shade. Common moles usually are a single shade of brown (Images Courtesy of The Skin Cancer Foundation, www.skincancer.org)

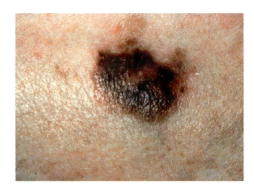

**Figure 19-7C2** Melanoma—two or more shades. Varied shades of brown, tan, or black are often the first sign of melanoma. As melanomas progress, the colors red, white, and blue may appear (Images Courtesy of The Skin Cancer Foundation, www.skincancer.org)

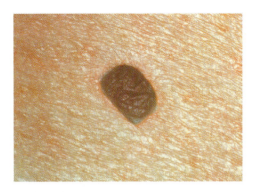

**Figure 19-7D1** Benign mole—6 mm or smaller. Common moles are usuaully 6 mm (1/4 inch) or smaller, but they can sometimes be larger (Images Courtesy of The Skin Cancer Foundation, www.skincancer.org)

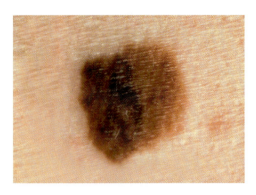

**Figure 19-7D2** Melanomas usually have larger diameters than benign moles. Typically, they are bigger than the size of the eraser on your pencil (1/4 inch or 6 mm). However, they may sometimes be smaller when first detected (Images Courtesy of The Skin Cancer Foundation, www.skincancer.org)

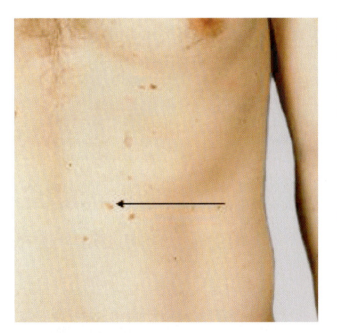

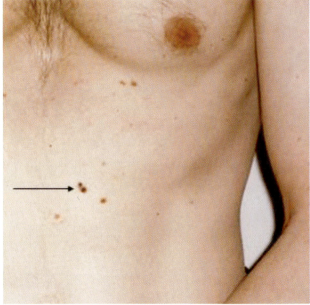

**Figure 19-7E1 and E2** Common, benign moles look the sam e over time. Be on the alert when a mole starts to evolve or change in any way. When a mole is evolving, see a doctor. Any change—in size, shape, color, elevation, or another trait, or any new symptom such as bleeding, itching or crusting—points to danger (Images Courtesy of The Skin Cancer Foundation, www.skincancer.org)

diameter. Melanomas are usually at least the size of a pencil eraser or bigger. Regular moles are usually smaller than this. "E" stands for evolving. You must watch for changes and "evolving" moles. Changes may include darkening or variations in color, moles that itch or hurt, and changes in the shape or growth of the mole.

Melanomas can be found on any area of the body but are most likely, again, to be found on areas that have had repeated sun exposure. They are most typically found on individuals with a history of sunburn and light-skinned individuals.

# Other Sun-Related Growths

**Actinic keratoses** are rough areas of sun-damaged skin, indicated by dysplastic cell growth. **Dysplastic** means abnormal growth. Actinic keratoses are frequently found on the faces of individuals who have had chronic sun exposure. They are also prevalent in light-skinned individuals. They are rough patches of skin and can be crusty, scaly, and rough to the touch. Sometimes they feel like small needles or splinters sticking out of the skin when they are touched with the fingers. They frequently occur in small groups or patches. Because they are dysplastic cells, they can become cancerous, and are often referred to as **pre-cancers** (Figure 19-8A and B).

Actinic keratoses may be treated surgically, with **cryosurgery** (freezing with liquid nitrogen), or with chemical therapy with a chemical called **fluorouracil** (also commercially known as Efudex®).

Unusual looking moles or moles that are changing should be checked by a dermatologist. If you or your client notices changes in a wart or mole, refer the client to a dermatologist for diagnosis and treatment.

**Sebaceous hyperplasias** are small, donut-shaped lesions that look like large, open comedones surrounded by a ridge of skin. Sebaceous hyperplasia actually means "overgrown oil glands." They are frequently seen on oily skins that have had repeated sun exposure, but they can appear on any skin, usually in someone 25-years-old and older. You will frequently find them on the forehead and temples, although they may appear anywhere on the face (Figure 19-9). Sebaceous hyperplasias are benign lesions that rarely cause any problems, except esthetically. They are rarely removed surgically, because the scar from excision is usually worse than the appearance of the lesion. Sebaceous hyperplasia can be treated with electrodessication with an electric needle or sometimes, cryosurgery. This helps flatten the lesion, but may need to be re-treated periodically, because the oil glands are deep within the skin and can still keep growing. Sebaceous hyperplasias are seen very frequently by estheticians, and clients are often concerned about them. Clients who have them also may have other symptoms of sun damage.

**Seborrheic keratoses** are large, flat, crusty-looking, brown, black, yellowish, or gray lesions that are often found on the faces of older, sun-damaged clients. They are

**Actinic keratoses**, or pre-cancers, are rough areas of sun-damaged skin, indicating dysplastic cell growth.

**Dysplastic** means abnormal growth.

**Pre-cancers** are conditions in cells that may become cancerous.

**Cryosurgery** is the dermatological removal of lesions by freezing, usually with liquid nitrogen.

**Fluorouracil** is a topical prescription drug used to remove multiple actinic keratoses.

**Sebaceous hyperplasias** are small, donut-shaped lesions that look like large, open comedones surrounded by a ridge of skin.

**Seborrheic keratoses** are large, flat, crusty-looking, brown, black, yellowish, or gray lesions that are often found on the faces of older, sun-damaged clients.

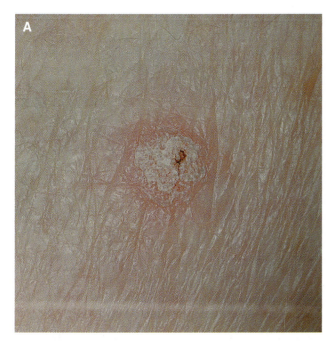
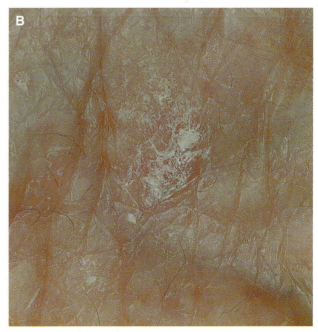

**Figure 19-8** Actinic keratosis is frequently seen in sun-damaged clients (Courtesy Michael J. Bond, M.D.)

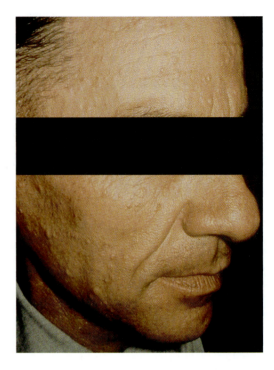

**Figure 19-9** Multiple sebaceous hyperplasia in an adult male with oily skin and sun damage. Sebaceous hyperplasias are typically found on the forehead, temple, and upper cheeks, but can appear anywhere on the face (Courtesy George Fisher, M.D.)

frequently found on the temples or cheekbones, although they can appear anywhere on the skin. They look almost like a scab, and clients will sometimes pick at them, which they obviously should not do. They are usually harmless growths but can occasionally turn into other more serious lesions, such as basal cell carcinomas. They are treated by the dermatologist, usually by curettage, in which a curette, a small, scoop-like instrument, is used to "scoop" the lesion off the face. Seborrheic keratoses are more of a cosmetic nuisance than anything in most cases. Nevertheless, they should be referred to a dermatologist for treatment. Also, they may indicate other areas or other forms of sun damage that may require treatment.

After a dermatologist treats skin cancer, the doctor may suggest that the client not have skin-care treatments until the lesion is healed completely. As a general rule, clients should not have facial treatment if there are still **sutures**, or "stitches," present in a treated lesion. Clients treated with fluorouracil should not have facial treatment until the therapy is completed, unless approved by the dermatologist, who may occasionally refer such a client for help with side effects. Make sure you have been properly trained by the doctor before treating these clients.

Other forms of growth treatment, such as electrosurgery or cryosurgery, generally do not cause any problem for treatment, except that facial treatment should not be performed until the lesion is healed or unless the doctor advises otherwise. Avoid these areas completely, and simply treat the rest of the untreated areas of the face. If you have any questions, contact the dermatologist, and remember always—when it doubt, don't!

**Solar freckles**, also known as "liver spots," are clumps of hyperpigmentation caused by sun exposure. They can appear on any area but frequently appear on the face and hands. These can be treated by the esthetician, and more severe cases can be treated by the dermatologist. More on treating hyperpigmentation will be covered in the chapter on the new science of aging skin treatment.

## PREVENTION OF SUN DAMAGE

Without question, the most effective treatment for sun damage is prevention. This involves routine use of sunscreen products. Sunscreen products are designed to filter, reflect, or absorb UVA and/or UVB rays emitted by the sun. Sunscreen products are

**Sutures** are materials used in reconnecting areas of surgical incisions.

**Solar freckles**, also known as "liver spots," are clumps of hyperpigmentation caused by sun exposure.

regulated as over-the-counter drugs by the FDA. There are sunscreen ingredients that absorb and neutralize ultraviolet light, and there are materials that reflect ultraviolet light.

**Chemical absorbing sunscreen** ingredients include the most popular sunscreen ingredient, **octinoxate** (formerly called octyl methoxycinnimate), **octisalate** (formerly called octyl salicylate), **oxybenzone** (formerly called benzophenone), and **avobenzone** (also known as Parsol 1789). These ingredients absorb and chemically neutralize ultraviolet light rays. They are often used in combination. As octinoxate and octisalate, they screen parts of the UVB spectrum; oxybenzone screens some of UVB and some of UVA; and avobenzone screens all UVA rays. When several sunscreen ingredients are combined to screen both UVA and UVB spectrums of light rays, this is known as a **broad-spectrum sunscreen**.

The advantages of the absorbing sunscreen ingredients are that they cannot be seen when worn, and are easier to formulate in higher SPFs. Their main disadvantage is that they are more reactive with the skin, particularly sensitive skin. Absorbing sunscreens can be one of the primary causes of skin allergy and irritation.

**Physical sunscreen** ingredients work by reflecting the light off the skin. There are only two approved for use by the FDA: titanium dioxide and zinc oxide. Physical sunscreens are sometimes referred to as sunblocks, although this term is no longer allowed by the FDA. They are excellent sunscreens, blocking out large portions of both UVB and UVA light. For many years, these took the form of opaque creams, such as the white cream that surfers wore on their noses (some still do). Micronized versions are now available, which are less noticeable. Unfortunately, the micronization process still leaves particles big enough to see, particularly on dark skin. These finely ground minerals sit on the skin, and literally bounce the light off. Physical sunscreens are much less likely to react with the skin than the absorbing screens, making them good choices for sensitive or allergy-prone skin. In high SPF numbers, however, they are hard to formulate without looking white or pasty on the skin or being sticky. Just like the absorbing screens can be combined to provide a broader spectrum of protection, the physical screens can also be mixed with the absorbing sunscreen agents. This works very well in many cases, producing cosmetically acceptable, higher SPF sunscreens, with broad-spectrum protection.

Because sunscreen is so important in skin treatment and sun damage prevention, broad-spectrum sunscreens are now included in most better day creams, along with moisturizing, conditioning, and other functional cosmetic ingredients. Sunscreens can be mixed into lotion or cream forms, with different weights and different amounts of emollient for different skin types.

**SPF** stands for **sun protection factor**. SPF is a number that represents how long a person can stay out in the sun without burning while using the product. It is a measurement of the **minimal erythemal dose (MED)**, which means how much time passes without the skin turning red from irritation. If a person normally burns in one hour without sunscreen, an SPF-2 sunscreen theoretically will allow the person to stay out in the sun two times as long, or two hours, without burning. An SPF-4 would allow the skin to be exposed four times as long, or four hours without burning. SPFs are really designed to prevent sunburns. They do not measure how much light is actually being blocked from the skin or how much UVA and UVB rays are being screened, which is actually more important in terms of sun damage prevention. An SPF-15 sunscreen blocks about 94 percent of UVB light, whereas an SPF-30 blocks about 98 percent. However, for sensitive skin, the higher the SPF, the more potentially irritating sunscreen chemical is used.

As a general rule, most dermatologists, pharmacists, and estheticians consider an SPF-15 sunscreen product to be a good protection against sun damage. It does not guarantee no sun damage. It simply means that an SPF-15 screen provides a fairly high amount of protection. Results will vary depending on the individual's heredity, method of application, frequency of application, his or her own skin, weather and climate conditions, and other factors.

**Chemical absorbing sunscreen** contains ingredients that absorb and neutralize ultraviolet rays.

**Octinoxate** is a UVB-absorbing sunscreen ingredient.

**Octisalate** is a UVB-absorbing sunscreen ingredient.

**Oxybenzone** is a UVB- and UVA-absorbing sunscreen ingredient.

**Avobenzone** is a UVA-absorbing sunscreen ingredient.

**Broad-spectrum sunscreens** protect against both ultraviolet A and B rays.

**Physical sunscreen** contains an ingredient that works by reflecting ultraviolet rays off the skin.

**Sun protection factor (SPF)** is a number that represents how long a person can stay out in the sun without burning while using the product.

**Minimal erythemal dose (MED)** means how much time passes without the skin turning red from irritation.

## SUN SKIN TYPES

There is a universal system of classifying skin types when discussing sun exposure. This typing system is generally accepted by the scientific community, and is referred to as **Fitzpatrick Skin Typing**, named after its originator, Dr. Thomas Fitzpatrick (Figure 19-10). The following is an excerpt from a brochure provided by the Skin Cancer Foundation.

◆ Type 1: Always burns; never tans. Very fair, with red or blond hair and freckles.
◆ Type 2: Burns easily; tans minimally. Usually fair skinned.
◆ Type 3: Sometimes burns; gradually tans.
◆ Type 4: Minimum burning; always tans. Usually white with medium pigmentation.

**Fitzpatrick Skin Typing** is a way of classifying skin by its tendency to sunburn or tan; indicates how susceptible a person is to sun damage and erythema.

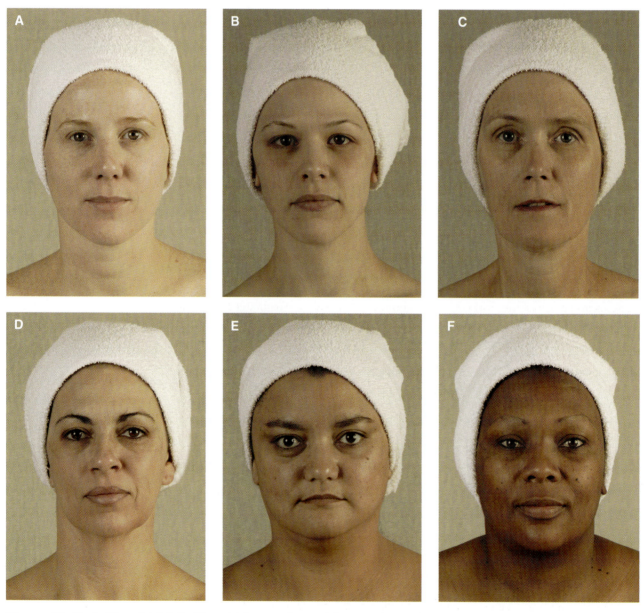

**Figure 19-10** *A*, Fitzpatrick I; *B*, Fitzpatrick II; *C*, Fitzpatrick III; *D*, Fitzpatrick IV; *E*, Fitzpatrick V; *F*, Fitzpatrick VI

◆ Type 5: Very seldom burns; always tans. Medium to heavy pigmentation.

◆ Type 6: Never burns, but tans darkly. Blacks as well as others with heavy pigmentation.

As you can see, the scale has a lot to do with hereditary and genetic skin characteristics. According to the Skin Cancer Foundation, your choice, or your client's choice, of a sunscreen should be based on the sun skin type, the amount of time you plan to spend in the sun, the intensity of the sun in your geographic region, and the preference of the formulation.

The geographic location does affect the intensity of the sun. As a general rule, the closer to the equator you live, the more intense the sun's rays.

## TYPES OF SUNSCREENS

Water-resistant screens are designed for individuals who participate in water sports, or who are outdoors in hot environments, or who plan on staying out in the sun for long periods of time. These products are often used by fishermen, athletes, and people who work outdoors. They usually contain a fairly large amount of oil, petrolatum, or fat, which makes them highly water-resistant. These products sometimes cause problems for oily-skinned individuals, and often the water-proofing ingredients are comedogenic or acnegenic.

Sunscreens that are made for oily skin are often in an alcohol gel. They are lighter weight and generally noncomedogenic. Unfortunately, they are also usually not very water-resistant and therefore should be applied more frequently.

Sunscreens are also available in oils, creams, and lotions. These are choices that are really a matter of personal preference and individualized skin type. Many cosmetics companies make a variety of products that vary in SPF strength, vehicles, and usage directions.

## TIME OF DAY AND THE SUN

Because the earth revolves, during certain times of the day the sun is closer and more intense and more ultraviolet rays reach the earth's surface. Most estheticians and dermatologists agree that the sun is at its most powerful between 10 A.M. and 3 P.M. Advise your clients not to go in the sun during these hours.

## FREQUENT MISCONCEPTIONS ABOUT SUN DAMAGE AND SUNBATHING

Consumers have many misconceptions about sunbathing and the way the sun damages the skin. It is the duty of the esthetician to dispel these wrong ideas. Some of these misconceptions are as follows:

1. *You cannot tan or burn if the weather is cloudy or rainy.* This, of course, is completely false. Clouds do filter a small amount of UV light but not enough to affect damage to the skin. It is certainly possible to tan or burn even in cloudy, overcast weather, particularly without using sunscreen.

2. *You cannot burn if you are in the water.* This too is false. Water may feel cool to hot skin that has been basking in the sun, but it has no effect on the sun's burning and damage potential. The heat from the sun is caused by infrared rays, not ultraviolet rays. Swimming and going into the pool or ocean may indeed remove some or a large amount of the sunscreen applied earlier. If your client plans on swimming or participating in water sports, advise him or her to use a

water-resistant sunscreen product. Sunscreens should be reapplied when swimming every time the client gets out of the water, or about once an hour.

3. *Umbrellas or large hats will prevent sun damage.* The real truth is that although these are a help, they do not prevent much sun from reaching the fragile skin and certainly do not replace a good sunscreen. They primarily cut down on glare so that the person does not squint as much, helping to prevent worsening of the expression lines. It's a good idea to wear lightweight but sun-resistant clothes, which also help filter light, but ultraviolet rays can burn the skin right through a lightweight shirt. Sun-filtering clothing is now available in sports and department stores. This clothing has been tested and actually has an SPF rating. Advise your clients to wear a hat and other proper attire and sit in the shade as much as possible but still wear a good sunscreen.

4. *Baby or mineral oil accelerates tanning.* This is simply not true. In fact, because these do not contain sunscreen, they may accelerate burning, and they do not provide protection against sun damage.

5. *Applying moisturizer after sunbathing will prevent peeling.* This is completely false! If the skin has burned, it will peel no matter what is done to the skin. Applying moisturizer to well-protected skin may help replace some of the water in the dehydrated, exposed skin, or it may lubricate peeling areas, making the skin look better, but it will not stop the sun-damaged skin from peeling.

6. *Applying lots of moisturizer will counter the damage the sun causes.* False again. Hydrating fluids do help replace some of the water that is also being robbed from the surface cells during sun exposure, but ultraviolet rays cut right through the skin. Remember, the UVA rays penetrate right through the dermis, destroying collagen and elastin fibrils and causing dysplastic cell growth and other horrifying effects we have already discussed. Esthetically, you should administer good, soothing, hydrating facial treatments to your sun-worshipping clients, but this will not treat or prevent the damage the sun causes to these clients.

7. *Wearing sunglasses helps prevent sun damage.* True, only if the sunglasses contain UV filters and only if they are worn constantly while out. When purchasing sunglasses, make sure to check if the glasses contain UV filters. The larger the glasses, the more area they will help protect.

## THE QUEST FOR THE GOLDEN TAN

In medieval and Elizabethan times, a suntan was considered a sign of poverty. A suntan meant that the person worked outdoors on a farm or less prestigious job. White skin was considered fashionable and a mark of success and sophistication.

However, in the 20th century, as leisure time increased, many people considered a tan a mark of success, because the person was successful enough to afford leisure time spent in the sun. Some clients will always value this "beautiful tan." Unfortunately, golden brown skin at age 20 translates to wrinkled, leathery, ugly, splotchy, old-looking skin at age 40 or 50. Although some clients will never listen to reason about tanning, you should always make an effort to inform, educate, and save them from the ugly, long-term ravages of sun exposure!

Tell your clients the following:

1. Sun exposure is the number one cause of premature aging and skin cancer. The best way to prevent sun damage is to stay out of the sun.

2. They should wear sunscreen every day, not just when sunbathing. We do not spend the majority of time at the beach. Hour for hour, most people receive more sun damage going to work, walking outside, and sitting by a window than we do basking in the sun. Sunbathing certainly makes the damage worse, but clients should use a good sunscreen moisturizer, for their skin type, daily.

3. As we discussed before, it is best not to go in the sun between 10 A.M. and 3 P.M.

4. Sunscreen should be applied 30 minutes before sun exposure. This provides better protection and allows the product to distribute itself more evenly.

5. Reapply sunscreen often if you are in direct light. Although sunscreen applications are not cumulative (two applications of SPF-15 sunscreen do not make an SPF-30 sunscreen), they are at least reapplying protection to these areas where the screen may have rinsed off due to sweating or water exposure.

6. Consider using self-tanning milk instead of sunbathing. These products cause keratin in the corneocytes to darken. Used on a regular basis, they can produce a beautiful golden color. Spray-tanning has gained popularity as a salon service. These booths are designed to spray an even layer of self-tanning lotion on the body. Two words of caution: Self-tanning products generally work better and more evenly on the body than on the face. A "tan" produced by a self-tanning product provides no additional resistance to sunburning!

7. A tanning booth is not a safe alternative. These machines still use rays that promote long-term damage, which can cause premature aging.

The sun is the number one enemy of the skin. Educate, teach, and warn your clients about its effects!

## Self-Tanning Products

Self-tanning lotions are becoming more and more popular. These safe alternatives to the tanning impart a tan color without exposure to the sun. These products contain **dihydroxyacetone (DHA)**, a chemical derived from sugar cane or beets that turns brown when exposed to alkaline environments. Self-tanning products stain the very surface cells in the stratum corneum and therefore shed in a few days to a few weeks. A darker color can be obtained by more frequent applications. Products containing more DHA will produce a darker tan (Figure 19-11).

**Dihydroxyacetone (DHA)** is an ingredient used in self-tanning agents that causes keratin to turn brown when applied.

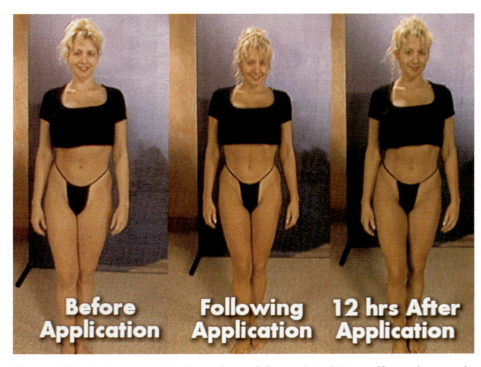

**Figure 19-11** Proper application of a well-formulated DHA self-tanning product produces beautiful results in a short period of time and is the only safe way to "tan" (Courtesy of St. Tropez Tanning Essentials.)

Self-tanning lotions will provide the best results when applied to healthy, hydrated skin. Skin that needs exfoliating or is very dehydrated will tend to "grab" the lotion, producing a splotchy result.

Some tips for good results with self-tanning are the following:

1. Carefully follow the manufacturer's directions. Self-tanning products do vary in spreading agent or DHA concentration.

2. Exfoliate with a mechanical scrub product before using the products. Loofahs tend to leave uneven texture, creating streaking. Continue to exfoliate at least twice a week.

3. Daily moisturization will help the self-tan look better.

4. Even application is extremely important. Uneven application will produce a muddy, splotchy result.

5. Make sure to wash your hands well immediately after application. Otherwise, your palms will turn dark, especially in the crevices between your fingers.

6. Make sure your feet are well exfoliated for an even application.

7. Do not shave immediately prior to application.

8. Generally speaking, self-tanning produces better results on the legs and arms than on the face. Facial skin renews faster and is therefore more likely to look splotchy or muddy.

Most importantly, make sure your clients understand that this is a fake tan. Many people have made the mistake of going to the beach, thinking they are "tan" and not using sunscreen. The result—a terrible, painful, and damaging sunburn!

## Tanning "Pills"

There is a chemical called canthaxanthin that appears on the "health food" market every few years as a "tanning pill." What this chemical does is accumulate in the skin *and the eyes*, turning them a yellowish-brown color. This product has not been proved safe. Avoid any pill that promotes tanning!

## TOPICS FOR DISCUSSION

1. Why is the sun the worst enemy of the skin?

2. Discuss what happens to the skin histologically after long-term sun exposure.

3. Discuss esthetic problems caused by long-term sun damage.

4. What are the ABCDEs of melanoma?

5. Discuss some rules for sun exposure and some common misconceptions about sun exposure.

6. What are UVA and UVB rays? What are the differences?

7. Explain what SPF means. What is broad-spectrum and why is it important?

8. What are some precautions for using self-tanning lotions?

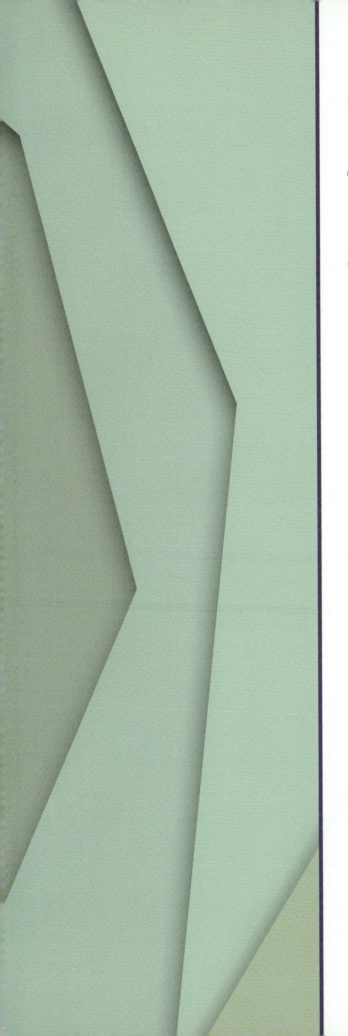

CHAPTER 20

# The New Science of Aging Skin Treatment

## OBJECTIVES. . .

Only in the past two decades have we discovered that there are many topical agents that can cause significant changes in the behavior and the appearance of aging and photo-damaged skin. In this chapter, you will learn about various agents and new technology that can really improve the appearance of aging and, specifically, sun-damaged skin.

# PHOTO DAMAGE

As we have previously discussed, aging skin does not look like it does because of the passing of years. The skin looks bad because of accumulated damage, most of which is from sun exposure, also known as photoaging or photo damage.

We have already touched on the long-term damage that cumulative sun exposure does to the skin. We have also already defined the difference between intrinsic aging, or aging of the skin that appears normally over time, and extrinsic aging, aging of the skin that occurs from induced or environmental causes, such as sun damage from exposure. These signs of aging skin from extrinsic sources do not show up for years. We know that the signs of extrinsic aging and sun damage are caused by free radicals and reactive oxygen species, unstable molecules that attack cell membranes and wreak havoc within the skin and the body. These unstable molecules interfere with normal functioning of the skin and cause the formation of different reactive molecules, creating a series of biochemical reactions called the **inflammation cascade**. These reactions eventually cause the breakdown of collagen and elastin fibrils and other support structures of the skin. We know that these reactions are primarily set into motion by exposure to the sun, and that the effects of these reactions are cumulative. Even though damage is occurring during a sunburn at age 4, it may not show up until a wrinkle appears at age 30, or a skin cancer at age 40. It is the cumulative effects of these inflammatory reactions that cause the symptoms that we think of as skin aging, which technically should be referred to as skin damage.

Sun-damaged skin is significantly more leathery, with deeper and more numerous wrinkles and severe loss of elasticity. Sun-damaged skin also has significant discolorations, splotching, and hyperpigmentation. Intrinsically aged skin does not have nearly as great a problem with hyperpigmentation and demarcation, nor does it have as many wrinkles or as pronounced elastosis.

Histologically, sun-damaged skin shows very large differences from normally aging skin. The epidermis of photoaged skin is remarkably thicker. There is a large increase in elastic tissue in sun-damaged skin, but it takes on the form of a disorganized "blob," with little apparent organized structure. The fibroblasts in the thickened dermis of sun-damaged skin are considerably more numerous and are overactive, producing more collagen, but obviously in a disorganized fashion. There are also significant decreases in the vascular system of sun-damaged skin, which carries much-needed blood to various areas of the skin.

In short, the skin has obviously desperately tried to repair itself, producing an overabundance of tissue fibrils, but in a panicked and dysfunctional manner.

# THE NEW SCIENCE OF AGING SKIN TREATMENT

Only in the past few years have we understood more about photo damage and discovered methods of effective treatment for photoaging. Although prevention and daily use of broad-spectrum sunscreens are still the best treatment, we now have at our disposal new and promising techniques and ingredients to help reduce the esthetic effects of photo damage and to help protect and maintain healthy skin.

Although the esthetician primarily treats the appearance of the skin, there is mounting scientific evidence that many of the new techniques and ingredients likely have a positive effect on skin health as well as sun-damage prevention.

# ANALYSIS OF PHOTOAGING SKIN

You will notice many symptoms of photoaging skin. Some of these symptoms may show up as early as the 20s. Severely sun-damaged skin will appear thick and leathery;

**Inflammation cascade** describes a series of biochemical reactions triggered by inflammation (often sun exposure) resulting in skin damage and breakdown; also sometimes called the free radical cascade.

will be rough to the touch; and will have many wrinkles, which may be both vertical and horizontal. Severe and multiple wrinkling in the nonintrinsic aging areas may be present. In other words, wrinkles around the eyes and nasolabial folds is normal, intrinsic skin aging. Severe wrinkling and surface roughness in the neck, cheek, chest, and other areas are usually not the result of intrinsic aging. These areas show cumulative effects of repeated sun exposure. Severe telangiectasias (couperose) are also often present. The skin is muddy looking, with diverse dark coloration, lentigines, and general brown splotchiness.

Redness on the sides of the neck in a horseshoe pattern may be a definite sign of photoaging. These red areas may be accompanied by hyperpigmentation and telangiectasias. This is known as **poikiloderma of cevattes** (Figure 20-1).

In younger clients, you may notice all of the previously mentioned symptoms in lesser amounts. The first sign may be hyperpigmentation, or dark blotchiness of the skin. Other signs might include rough, patchy skin and the beginning of "chicken neck," in which the skin of the neck has constant "goose pimples," which is reflected by small, pinpoint, noncolored elevation of the follicles on the sides of the neck, like a plucked chicken. Wrinkles around the eyes and mouth may be especially severe for

**Poikiloderma of cevattes** is a condition in sun-damaged skin resulting in horseshoe-shaped pigment and red splotching on the neck.

---

The treatment of the photo-damaged or photoaging skin is a program, not a magic bullet. There are many treatment methods that contribute to a successful age-/sun-damage management program. This combination topical skin-care program for photo-damaged skin can be summarized into six basic concepts:

◆ Prevention, using daily sunscreen protection

◆ Use of topical alphahydroxy acid (AHA) or other exfoliating agents

◆ Daily use of topical antioxidants

◆ Use of topical peptides and collagen stimulants

◆ Use of lipid-based products to repair or improve barrier function in ultradry skin

◆ Regular use of hydrators that help attract and bind essential moisture to the skin

---

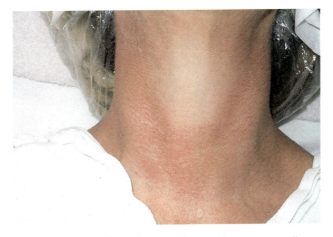

**Figure 20-1** Poikiloderma of cevattes is a condition of the neck skin with hyperpigmentation and telegiectasias caused by years of cumulative sun exposure (Courtesy Mark Lees Skin Care, Inc.)

the client's age. However, brown splotchiness is the most evident sign of premature aging due to sun damage. The use of a Wood's lamp will indicate even more hyperpigmentation beneath the skin's surface. Lack of pigmentation will also be observable.

# THE TREATMENT OF PHOTOAGING SKIN

## Prevention—No Sun!

Daily use of broad-spectrum sunscreen is the very first step in photo-damage treatment. Even if the skin is already severely sun damaged, daily application of sunscreen will not only prevent more damage; it also will allow the skin to have a better chance for good effects from other topical treatments.

The use of sunscreen on a *daily* basis cannot be emphasized enough! Many clients erroneously only worry about sunburn. They think of sun damage occurring only from visible sunburn and irritation. They are often likely to apply sunscreen only when they know they will be exposed to direct sunlight for several hours.

The truth is that the majority of our sun damage occurs from day-to-day exposure. Driving to work, going to the mailbox, playing with our children, and taking a walk are examples of everyday sun exposure that becomes cumulative. Even sitting by a window exposes us to deep-penetrating (and aging) UVA rays, which go right through glass! This is why it is *so* important that we help our clients by advising a good sunscreen to be used daily.

Remember that broad-spectrum sunscreens are important to shield the skin from UVA and UVB rays. Look for active ingredient lists with ingredients that protect against both forms of UV light. Effective combinations include octinoxate with titanium dioxide or zinc oxide or combinations of absorbing octinoxate, oxybenzone, avobenzone, and octisalate.

In most cases, clients can wear a day cream with built-in sunscreen. Most scientists and dermatologists recommend an SPF-15 or higher with broad-spectrum protection. It is usually not necessary to wear a separate moisturizer cream, except in extremely dry skin or extremely cold, dry climates. Good day sunscreens are now available in a variety of weights, in lotion, gel, or cream forms, so they can be selected for the right skin type. Many contain hydrators like glycerin or hyaluronic acid, soothing ingredients like green tea extract, and other conditioners for specific skin types.

Having this variety of daily-use sunscreens available helps with client compliance in using a sunscreen everyday. Clients will use a product that is comfortable and meets their individual needs, such as a lightweight product, a product that works well under makeup, or one that is also a moisturizer.

The very first treatment should be a thorough discussion with the client of the harmful effects of sun. This author recommends a no-holds-barred lecture (in a friendly way!) about the ravages of cumulative sun damage. Emphasis should be placed on the cumulative nature of sun damage. Many clients will say, "I haven't had any sun in months!" The truth is that most of the sun damage you will see is from sunbathing that occurred twenty years ago and years of daily exposure.

Unless the client implements good sun habits, or better yet, stays out of the sun altogether, improvement will be minimal, if any improvement occurs. The first need of sun-damaged skin is to remove the source of damage.

## Exfoliation

The cell "turnover rate" slows down with aging anyway, but even more so in sun-damaged skin. Not only is the rate often slower, the cells are disorganized and are not in even layers. You must remember that sun damage causes abnormal cell growth and generally disorganizes normal cell patterns. This, of course, also affects the epidermis, piling dead cells on top of the skin in uneven patterns as they accumulate. Microscopic cross-section photographs of sun-damaged skin show severe disfigurations of the normal growth patterns of the strata of the epidermis. This can be both a medical and a cosmetic concern. Dysplastic cell growth can eventually cause skin cancer but esthetically causes a rough, dry, scaly appearance on the skin's surface and contributes to the appearance of wrinkles.

Production of intercellular lipids is diminished, interfering with barrier function, and reducing the ability of the skin to hold essential moisture. Clients who have this type of sun-damaged skin have a great deal of difficulty keeping their skin moisturized. Hydrators attract water to the skin, but there is not enough lipid to bind the moisture. By removing this conglomeration of dry, dead cells, the surface of the skin appears much smoother, and wrinkles appear less deep. Hydrators applied over the alphahydroxy treatments perform better because they do not have to moisturize the dead cell buildup. Instead they work to hydrate the skin more evenly, which results in a much smoother appearance of the skin.

Imagine a thick layer of cells lying on top of the skin. These cells are all dried up, like a thick layer of dust lying on top of a piece of furniture. This cell buildup makes the skin's surface look dull and flat, just as dust prevents light from reflecting from a piece of furniture. Surface mechanical exfoliation, which we have already discussed, helps to remove some of the "dust." Alphahydroxy acids, however, work by loosening the "glue" of lipids that hold the cells together, helping to continually shed off this sheath of cells. This removal of dead cells is also beneficial to acne-prone skin, helping to loosen both surface cell buildup and impacted dead cells inside the follicle, which, as we have previously discussed, can lead to comedones and, possibly, acne.

Use of a daily chemical exfoliant helps to rid skin of thick epidermal corneum that makes skin look dull. Cell buildup can make wrinkles look worse, dryness more uncomfortable, and splotchiness and hyperpigmentation more apparent. Daily use of an alphahydroxy and/or betahydroxy acid treatment product can significantly improve skin texture, color evenness, depth of surface wrinkles, and smoothness.

More importantly, regular use of AHAs helps to "re-layer" the epidermal cells, which improves barrier function, hydration, and intercellular lipid production. All of these changes not only help the appearance, but also result in healthier skin. Using chemical exfoliants like AHAs, BHAs, or retinoids make the daily use of broad-spectrum sunscreen even more important.

## Retinoids

The first real science that showed that topical agents could be used to improve photodamaged skin was performed in the 1980s. Women who had been using the prescription drug Retin-A for their acne noticed that their wrinkles were less noticeable and that their treated skin looked smoother. Studies of this drug followed for the treatment of photoaging skin. Retinoids are vitamin A-based chemicals that include prescription tretinoin or retinoic acid, better known as Retin-A or Renova®, and **tazarotene**, a chemical cousin of vitamin A, commercially known as **Tazorac®**.

These prescription drug chemicals have been shown to reduce wrinkles, roughness, solar freckles, and hyperpigmentation and generally improve the skin's appearance. Renova®, a more moisturizing version of tretinoin, is the first prescription drug ever approved to treat the symptoms of sun damage.

Histologically, tretinoin has been shown to "reorganize" the skin, reestablishing a more normal epidermis, increasing blood vessel formation, increasing collagen production, and generally improving the damaged skin.

With these positive changes, there are some side effects, including redness, irritation, flaking, dryness, and severe dehydration. Sun exposure should be avoided, because the drug makes the skin more sun sensitive. A broad-spectrum sunscreen, as with any skin, is even more important for the patient.

**Tazarotene**, commercially known as **Tazorac®**, is a vitamin A–derived topical prescription medication used to treat both acne and aging symptoms caused by sun damage.

Nonprescription retinoids used in skin-care products include retinol and retinyl palmitate, which are other forms of vitamin A. These are good antioxidant ingredients, but do not work by the same mechanism or show the same results as tretinoin. Retinol, combined or used with alphahydroxy acid, has been shown to improve sun-damaged skin.

## Alphahydroxy Acids

Alphahydroxy acid treatment is probably the most effective tool that the esthetician has to treat the photoaging skin. We have already discussed how alphahydroxy acids affect the skin. Alphahydroxy as well as beta hydroxy acids have a remarkable effect on photoaging. They are an integral part of any program for treating photoaged skin (Figure 20-2A–D).

The terms alphahydroxy acid and glycolic acid are often used interchangeably. However, technically, glycolic acid is an alphahydroxy acid, and treatments may involve both alphahydroxy and betahydroxy acids.

Alphahydroxy acids include glycolic acid, lactic acid, tartaric acid, and malic acid. These functional agents can be used in products as an individual acid or in special AHA blends. Although very different from retinoids, these agents also help to "reorganize" the epidermis. Regular use of an 8 to 10 percent alphahydroxy treatment product, with a pH of no less than 3.5, can reduce the appearance of wrinkles, smooth the skin surface, reduce uneven coloring, and improve hydration and firmness. It cannot completely rid the skin of sun-damage symptoms, especially advanced sun damage

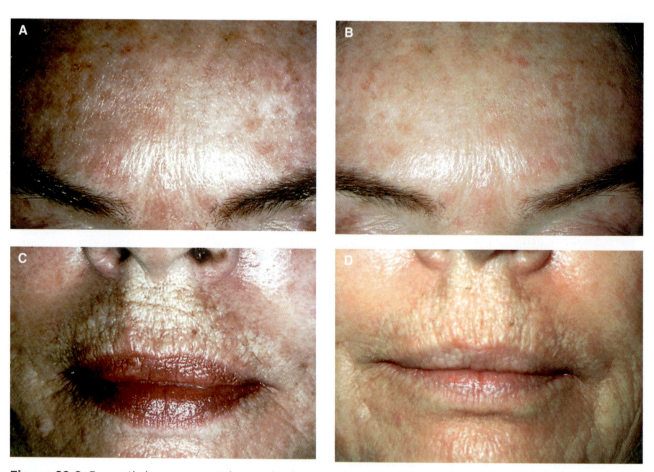

**Figure 20-2** Dramatic improvement is seen in the appearance of this skin, treated with alphahydroxy acids, peptides, collagen stimulants, and sunscreen (Courtesy Mark Lees Skin Care, Inc.)

### Rules for the Retinoid Client

1. Tretinoin and tazarotene and other prescribed retinoids are prescription drugs. The client must follow the advice of the dermatologist regarding usage procedures.

2. Cosmetic and skin-care product usage may be affected by the use of retinoids. Clients may find that they may be more sensitive to products that they normally and routinely use. The esthetician needs to help guide the client to choose products that can coexist with retinoids.

3. Facial treatments may need to be adapted for the patient using a retinoid. This includes discontinuing the use of any exfoliation treatment, using gentle, fragrance-free hydrators; and avoiding heat and any alcoholic or stimulating skin-care products.

4. Redness and peeling can be normal transitional side effects particularly when first using a prescription retinoid. These side effects can be minimized with the use of good hydrators and being careful with the amount and frequency of application of the retinoid. Some patients find it helpful to "phase in" retinoids, using the retinoid every second or third night and slowly switching to every night.

5. Sun should be completely avoided when using retinoids. Deliberate sun exposure is contraindicated and is counterproductive to any therapy for the improvement of photo-damaged skin.

6. Scented and fragranced products, alcohol-based lotions, stripping products, abrasive scrubs, microdermabrasion, alphahydroxy or betahydroxy acid products, benzoyl peroxide, sulfur–resorcinol, and other exfoliating agents should be avoided on clients using retinoids.

7. DO NOT WAX CLIENTS USING RETINOIDS! Electrolysis is usually acceptable after the transitional side effects have passed.

and elastosis, but it certainly improves the appearance of almost all sun-damage symptoms (Figure 20-3A–D).

Long-term use of alphahydroxy acids helps to replenish intercellular lipids that decrease with age and sun damage. The intercellular lipids, as discussed in previous chapters, make up the barrier function and are responsible for epidermal hydration.

Besides typical aging and wrinkles, alphahydroxy acids can help improve hand and foot calluses, general dry and dehydrated skin, and dry body skin.

## Stimulation

The circulation of sun-damaged skin is impaired by the malformation of blood vessels due to the sun damage. Therefore, the skin is not nourished properly through normal blood flow. The use of good but gentle massage techniques is helpful in improving the circulation.

Be careful when massaging skin that is being treated with a keratolytic such as glycolic acid or Retin-A. This skin can be treated, but be careful not to overstimulate.

## Alphahydroxy Home Treatments

Different products are formulated with individual vehicle ingredients, release symptoms, and different concentrations of alphahydroxy acid, depending on the type of problem treated. Preparations for acne, oily, and problem skin are usually in a gel

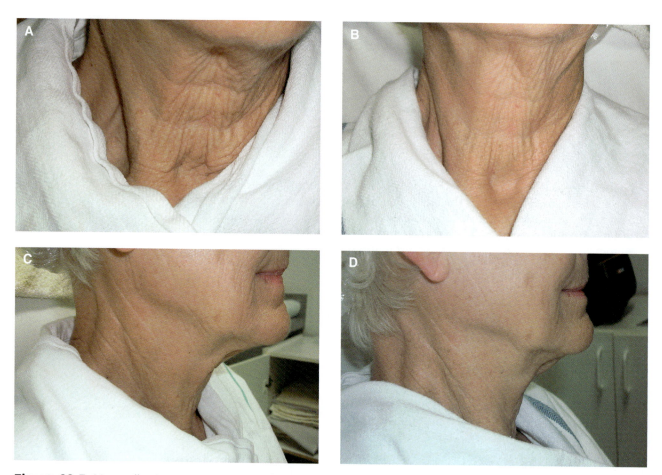

**Figure 20-3** Many clients are concerned about loss of elasticity. This client shows great improvement after using alphahydroxy acids, peptides, collagen stimulants, and sunscreen (Courtesy Mark Lees Skin Care, Inc.)

form, so designed to combat oily skin. They are very helpful when used in conjunction with other acne treatments. As a word of caution, be careful when combining peeling agents. Combining glycolic acid with benzoyl peroxide, salicylic acid, resorcinol, sulfur, or retinoic acid must be done very carefully, if at all. Check the manufacturer's instructions well before combining home keratolytic treatments. The alphahydroxy solution for oily and acne-prone skin should be applied to the face, usually twice daily, under a protective sunscreen moisturizer, or coupled with a light, noncomedogenic hydrating product at night. Some companies suggest treatments only once a day at home. Always check the manufacturer's instructions.

Alphahydroxy products for the body are usually made in lotion form, to be applied like a body lotion. These are almost always oil-in-water emulsions and sometimes are not designed for facial use. Again, check the instructions.

Alphahydroxy products for fading hyperpigmentation are in a gel or lotion form. The glycolic acid is mixed in the solution with a bleaching agent, hydroquinone or another melanin suppressant such as magnesium ascorbyl phosphate, licorice extract, kojic acid, bearberry extract, or arbutin. Alphahydroxy acid helps remove the buildup of dead cells, which helps the bleaching agent work better and faster. Age spots, sun freckles, pregnancy masks, and hyperpigmented areas from acne all can be helped with such a solution. As with any bleaching solution, the client should be instructed to use a good sunscreen and avoid sun exposure, which, of course, can result in recurrence of the hyperpigmentation.

In the treatment of wrinkles and the appearance of sun damage, alphahydroxy acid loosens the dead cell buildup, again helping make the skin look smoother and softer. The appearance of wrinkles can be greatly improved with continued use. The products available to help the appearance of aging skin are usually in a cream or lotion form. The cream form is for alipidic, dry, dehydrated, aging skin. Lotions are more appropriate for combination skin showing signs of aging including wrinkles, leathery texture, dull appearance, and uneven surfaces. The cream or lotion is applied under the moisturizer or sunscreen and under the night treatment. Most companies recommend twice daily application.

## Recommending Alphahydroxy Home Care

First, as always, carefully evaluate the appearance of the client's skin. You must also assess the client's current home care. If he or she is currently using home care that is inappropriate, such as strong soap for aging skin, this must first be corrected. Alphahydroxy treatment is most effective when used with a well-planned general home care program, designed for the skin type and conditions.

Explain how alphahydroxy acid works on aging skin and the importance of the "program." Best results cannot be expected if the client is using a hodgepodge of products along with the alphahydroxy acid. Be careful to find out if the client is using other peeling-type products or drugs. Heavily scented products or products that are extremely stimulating should also be avoided when alphahydroxy acid is being used. The client should also be instructed in the importance of regular use. No product will work if it is sitting in the medicine cabinet! Other problems such as hyperpigmented skin or problem oily areas should be addressed separately.

Alphahydroxy acid often produces a mild-to-moderate tingling sensation when applied to the skin. Usually the tingling feeling lasts only 10 or 20 seconds. The client should wait for a short amount of time (a few minutes) before applying other hydrating or conditioning products. When a client first starts using alphahydroxy acid, some slight cosmetic side effects might be experienced. In the case of dry or aging skin, the skin may show some flaking, which the client may misunderstand as dehydration. Explain that this is the dead cell layer coming off the surface, is a normal occurrence, and can be controlled by using the appropriate products along with the alphahydroxy acid cream. This is another reason why the "surrounding" products are so important. If the client uses the wrong treatment cream or a cleanser that is too harsh, side effects will be more intense. The client's skin may feel "crunchy," as if it is peeling. Again, this feeling can be alleviated by using a good hydrating fluid. In the case of clog-prone or combination skin, make sure that you recommend a moisturizer that is noncomedogenic.

If the client experiences severe peeling, tell the client to call you. Instruct the client to discontinue using the alphahydroxy solution temporarily until the peeling subsides. Then phase in the alphahydroxy product, starting once a day, and eventually working back into twice daily application.

Some clients with extremely thin skin may have problems with waxing. This is unusual, but it does occur sometimes. Waxing in these clients, or any other procedure that involves removing cells, should be discontinued. Allergic reactions to alphahydroxy acid are rare, but like with any other cosmetic ingredient, allergic reaction is possible. Allergic symptoms are the same as for any other reaction. These may include redness, itching, and general irritation. The client should, of course, discontinue the treatment.

Treatments with glycolic acid are also performed in the salon. For more information, please see the chapter on chemical peeling and exfoliation procedures.

## Microdermabrasion

**Microdermabrasion** is a technique using small crystals, usually aluminum oxide, to exfoliate the skin mechanically (Figure 20-4). A microdermabrasion machine uses pressure to spray the crystals onto the skin surface, physically removing dead cells

**Microdermabrasion** is a procedure using crystal particles that are pressure-sprayed onto the skin and then vacuumed. Microdermabrasion is a mechanical exfoliation technique that removes corneum cells.

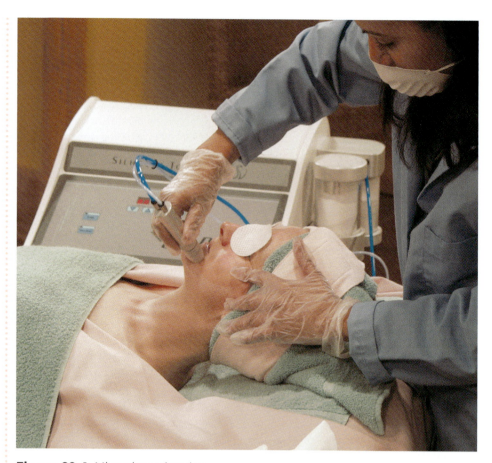

**Figure 20-4** Microdermabrasion

from the stratum corneum. Some companies also sell crystals in creams that can be applied with the hands.

Microdermabrasion is an alternate technique to forms of chemical exfoliation. Chemical and mechanical exfoliation should not be combined because the combination can overexfoliate the skin and cause barrier function damage if overused. Because microdermabrasion is mechanical, and its frequency of application, pressure of application, and number of passes (how many times the technique is applied to a certain area of skin) can vary with the esthetician's judgment, it can easily be overdone. Be very careful in assessing the sensitivity and thickness of the individual client before choosing the correct exfoliation technique.

## Antioxidant Therapy

There is growing evidence that the use of topical antioxidants reduces the visible signs of aging and makes the skin behave in a better way. We are now learning that antioxidants seem to work better when several different antioxidants are combined. We know that not all antioxidants work to squelch reactions at all levels of the inflammation cascade of chemical reactions. These combinations of antioxidants are referred to as **broad-spectrum antioxidants**. There are many types of antioxidants including vitamins like **vitamin C** as L-**ascorbic acid**, and **magnesium ascorbyl phosphate**, and **vitamin E** as **tocopherol** and **tocopheryl acetate**. Plant extract antioxidants include **green tea**, **white tea**, and **grapeseed extract** (known to be 50 times as strong an antioxidant as vitamin C). **Superoxide dismutase** is an enzyme that helps to squelch early reactions in the cascade of reactions. Some of the "newest"

**Broad-spectrum antioxidants** are a mix of various antioxidants that help to neutralize or stop various free radical reactions during the inflammation cascade.

powerful antioxidant ingredients include **alpha lipoic acid, idebenone,** and **stearyl glycyrrhizinate** (derived from licorice).

Antioxidants are believed to work by interfering or stopping reactions within the inflammation cascade, reducing production of damaging enzymes that can injure or destroy the collagen and elastin fibrils that keep the skin smooth and elastic. There is growing evidence and scientific acceptance that antioxidants are helpful in the prevention and the treatment of photo-damaged skin.

It is not enough to simply include these ingredients in a treatment product. The antioxidants must stay stable until they are used on the skin, and they must be delivered properly to where they are needed. Most antioxidants are unstable and must be formulated correctly so they are protected from oxidation. One sign that an antioxidant has been oxidized is that the product turns brown quickly when exposed to air, specifically oxygen.

Microencapsulated delivery systems such as liposomes provide good protection for the antioxidants. The lipid-based encapsulation protects the antioxidants from oxidation, and the lipid "shells" are readily accepted by the intercellular cement that comprises the barrier function, helping to penetrate into the epidermal layers easier.

Powerful broad-spectrum antioxidant complexes are often manufactured in serum form and should be applied before an alphahydroxy acid treatment product, sunscreen, or hydrator.

## Use of Lipid Products and Hydrators

Hydration is very important in improving the appearance of photo-damaged skin. Sun damage results in the skin losing its ability to hold water. Lipid ingredients, as previously discussed, are helpful in "patching" the "mortar" between the cells, helping to boost hydration, firmness, and smoothness and to reduce inflammation potential. These lipids include phospholipids, sphingolipids or glycosphingolipids (also known as ceramides), cholesterol, and fatty acids.

These lipid complexes can be included in sunscreens, hydrators, specialty creams, masks, or serums. They are extremely effective as a treatment for dry, alipidic, or extremely dry skin. The lipids work by helping hold essential hydration in the epidermis. They should be used with a hydrator to attract water to the skin.

Hydration ingredients include butylene glycol, hyaluronic acid or sodium hyaluronate, glycerin, sodium PCA, or sorbitol. These ingredients are also blended into the same products for sun-damaged skin as mentioned earlier.

Be careful to remember the skin type when you are choosing a hydrator or other cream. Aging oily or combination skin can become impacted and comedonal from exposure to too many fatty emollients. Gels, liquids, and lotions that are especially designed for oily or acne-prone oily skin should be recommended.

## Avoidance of Irritation

The symptoms of what we think of as aging is an accumulation of damage to skin tissue caused by chronic irritations, such as sun exposure. All clients should avoid irritating the skin at any age, but especially in already photo-damaged skin.

## A Typical Home Care Program for Photoaging Skin

Clients with photoaging skin should have the entire skin-care program explained to them in detail. It is important that they understand the function of all products prescribed and why each has importance in the success of their program. It should be emphasized that the client must be diligent about home care use for a successful program. Provide them with a step-by-step home care instruction sheet to follow, and use it to describe each step during the consultation.

---

**Vitamin C** is a water-soluble vitamin essential in the skin for helping to neutralize free radicals and needed in the production of collagen.

**L-ascorbic acid** is a water-soluble form of vitamin C.

**Magnesium ascorbyl phosphate** is a fat-soluble, more stable form of vitamin C ester.

**Vitamin E** is a fat-soluble vitamin that is a strong antioxidant.

**Tocopherol** is the chemical name for vitamin E.

**Tocopheryl acetate** is a more stable form of vitamin E often used in skin-care products.

**Green tea** is a very strong antioxidant, often used in soothing, anti-redness, and anti-aging products.

**White tea** is a strong antioxidant extract.

**Grapeseed extract** is a very powerful antioxidant extract, often used in soothing, anti-redness, and anti-aging products.

**Superoxide dismutase** is an enzyme that helps squelch reactions early in the cascade of reactions.

**Alpha lipoic acid** is a potent antioxidant.

**Idebenone** is a very powerful antioxidant.

**Stearyl glycyrrhizinate** is a potent soothing agent antioxidant derived from licorice.

---

### The Basics of Treating Sun-Damaged Skin

◆ Sun exposure must be carefully avoided, especially during the hours of 10 A.M. and 3 P.M.

◆ An SPF-15 broad-spectrum sunscreen should be worn on a *daily* basis, incorporated into a day cream or fluid.

◆ An 8 to 10 percent alphahydroxy acid product, with a pH no less than 3.5, should be used regularly.

◆ A daily stabilized antioxidant serum applied to the skin may help the skin against free radicals that can damage cells, resulting in wrinkles and elastosis.

◆ A serum or cream containing peptides, such as palmitoyl pentapeptide-3, should be used daily. Collagen stimulants may also be used, or combined into this type of product. Serums and creams are now available that contain a blend of liposomed antioxidants, collagen stimulants, and peptides.

◆ Avoid all irritation to the skin.

◆ Hydration helps improve moisture content in the skin, improving smoothness and elasticity.

◆ Lipid-based products are especially effective for dehydrated sun-damaged skin. Lipid products help improve hydration and barrier function.

---

Clients who are not used to a several-step program may wish to "phase in" to the program. This sometimes is helpful in getting clients accustomed to a home regimen, but you should insist to the client that the whole program must be followed to achieve the results they are expecting. In other words, be understanding of their need for simplicity, but also make them understand that all the products must be used to see the results they want.

Cleansing should be gentle and thorough, and the client must avoid any harsh cleanser, including bar soaps, which can be stripping and damaging to the barrier function. Cleansing milk or a light rinseable liquid cleanser is advised. This should be followed by a mild nonalcoholic toner, which helps to remove cleanser residue and also lower the pH of the skin.

After cleansing and toning, apply your antioxidant serum. It is important to follow manufacturers' instructions because products do vary in ingredients and product form, such as a serum versus a lotion.

Apply the alphahydroxy product, which could be a gel, lotion, or cream, depending on the skin type. During the day, this will be followed by an SPF-15 or higher broad-spectrum sunscreen, with built-in hydrator. For drier skin, make sure the sunscreen contains lipids to help support the barrier function and protect against daytime moisture loss. In the evening, the same basic steps are followed, but this may vary depending on the client's specific needs or differences in product type. For example, some clients may only be able to use an AHA once a day, depending on climate, skin thinness, or genetic characteristics. Some companies may prefer that the client use an AHA at night and an antioxidant during the day. Again, follow the instructions of your product manufacturer. In the evening, use a hydrating cream instead of sunscreen.

Supplemental products, such as eye creams, or specialty serums, such as a concentrated lipid serum, may be also advisable depending on the skin type. Concentrated lipid serums are very helpful for very dry, wrinkled skin or areas of extreme damage like the neck or wrinkles around the mouth or eyes. Lipid serum is applied after all other products, including sunscreen, but before makeup application.

## Salon Treatment Program

Begin by treating the skin with regular clinical facial treatments, emphasizing moisturization and light stimulation through massage techniques. Design the treatment for the skin type (oily, dry, etc.) and, if necessary, perform deep cleansing with extraction to any sun-damaged skin that is also oily or comedonal.

AHA exfoliations are extremely helpful in treating the sun-damaged skin. After the client has been using 8 to 10 percent AHA home care treatment for at least two weeks, administer 30 percent AHA applications in the salon, twice a week for three weeks; follow with weekly treatments if necessary. Discontinue or temporarily delay any treatment that is irritating or produces lasting redness. Long-term, regular monthly, or twice-monthly AHA exfoliation treatments are advisable, alternating with hydrating facial treatments.

## Microcurrent Treatments

The high-tech microcurrent treatments use extremely small amounts of galvanic current to improve both skin textures and elasticity. Microcurrent treatments are ideal for a client who is beginning to think about a facelift, but is not quite ready for surgery. Although it is not the same as a facelift, microcurrent, applied correctly, has been shown in university studies to improve elasticity, collagen content, and elastin content. Microcurrent stimulates the skin cells, increasing ATP (adenosine triphosphate) in the cells.

Sometimes referred to as "muscle re-education," microcurrent can help to tighten or relax muscle tissue, depending on the area.

The current used in microcurrent is so gentle that it does not cause visible muscle contraction. However, administered in the salon correctly in a treatment series, usually two to three times a week for 12 treatments, microcurrent can produce great improvement in elasticity and contour.

Microcurrent treatments must be routinely administered after the initial series to keep up the results. If the client quits coming for treatments, results will not be maintained. This should be explained to the client before ever beginning the series.

It is a great idea to have "before and after" pictures of clients' results to show to other clients considering the treatment. This is true for all types of aging skin treatment programs, including AHAs, peptides, and home care programs. You must, however, obtain written permission from the clients whose photographs you are presenting.

There are a few contraindications for microcurrent treatment. These are similar to those for galvanic current. Patients with heart problems or a pacemaker, persons who have seizure disorders, pregnant women, and any client that you feel might have questionable health conditions should not have treatment until they obtain written permission from their physician.

Well-made microcurrent machines can be expensive. As with all equipment and product lines, it is important to check out the qualifications of the company and their training programs.

## Light-Emitting Diode Treatments

We briefly discussed the use of light-emitting diode (LED) treatment earlier in this book when discussing treatments for redness. **LED treatment** devices are fast, flashing lights that emit energy to the skin. LED treatment has been shown to improve redness and improve collagen content in the skin (Figure 20-5).

LED treatments can be helpful in improving skin texture and diffuse redness in sun-damaged clients. These treatments are also administered in series and must be followed up to maintain results.

**LED treatment** emits energy on to the skin using fast, flashing light. It has been shown to improve redness and the collagen content of skin.

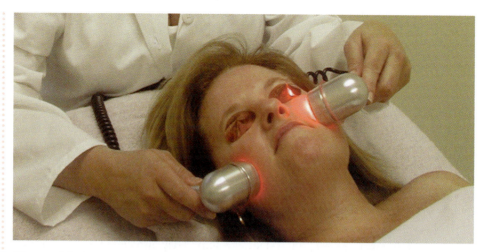

**Figure 20-5** LED treatment has been shown to improve redness and collagen content in the skin (Courtesy Mark Lees Skin Care, Inc.)

Contraindications for LED include epilepsy and seizure disorders. Other precautions such as using eye goggles for the client should be taken.

Again, carefully shop when purchasing an LED machine. There are differences among machines. Always work with a reputable manufacturer who can answer your many questions and who has documentation of results and safety.

## Which Treatment Is Right for My Client?

None of the treatment methods mentioned above are substitutes for one another. You should plan your client's treatment based on your skin analysis, and the client's desires. Many clients use all the methods mentioned. They are all different in what signs of aging they improve and treat.

Some estheticians tend to "drop" good treatment techniques, products, or ingredients because of trends. A new technique comes along, and they forget all the advantages of the classic treatment in favor of a new, trendy technique. This is not good scientific protocol. It is important to recognize the benefits or pitfalls of any treatment method and adapt the client's individual program to treat his or her specific needs.

The one rule of caution is not to overly exfoliate the skin. Overexfoliating can cause barrier function damage leading to inflammation, and the trauma can also cause postinflammatory hyperpigmentation. Never combine exfoliation procedures in the attempt to speed the results of the treatment. More is not necessarily better!

## Hyperpigmentation Treatment

One of the main symptoms of photoaging is hyperpigmentation. It is also one of the main concerns of sun-damaged clients and one of the most difficult disorders to manage. We have already discussed in other chapters how hyperpigmentation occurs during sun exposure. Long-term sun exposure, as well as hormonal activity, particularly in female clients, results in overproductive melanocytes in the skin.

The melanocytes, which are the cells that produce the melanin, are in the lower epidermis and upper dermis. They produce melanin when they are stimulated by sun exposure, but also can be stimulated by hormones, exposure to some chemicals (including overstimulating skin-care products), injuries to the skin (including laser surgery or some forms of chemical peeling), and many forms of inflammation. In some clients, melanocytes may actually be present in lower areas of the dermis. These clients will rarely be responsive to treatment.

When stimulated, the melanocytes produce melanin as a protective mechanism. Melanocytes have dendrites, which are small branches on the cells containing the melanin. The dendrites are "embraced" by the skin cells, which absorb the melanin, before they drift toward the surface of the skin. This process gives the cell a characteristic melanin color, which is seen as hyperpigmentation when concentrated areas of cells contain melanin.

There are three types of products and therapy that are effective in reducing skin pigment: chemical exfoliation, melanin suppressive agents, and sunscreens. Normally, all three are used in treating hyperpigmented photo-damaged skin.

Chemical exfoliants include alphahydroxy acid (usually glycolic or a blend), betahydroxy acid (salicylic acid), *or* tretinoin (Retin-A or Renova®). Use of both is not advised because this may produce unnecessary irritation. Chemical exfoliants remove cells containing melanin, helping to fade the skin. They also clear hyperkeratinized areas of cell buildup on the skin surface, enabling better treatment of the skin.

Melanin suppressive agents interfere with the chemical process of melanin production. Many inhibit tyrosinase, an enzyme used to convert the amino acid tyrosine, which is very instrumental in the production of melanin. The only FDA-approved skin-lightening agent at the time of this writing is hydroquinone, available in over-the-counter products at 2 percent and 4 percent prescription strengths. Other non-approved so-called "brightening" ingredients, which are all basically melanin suppressants, include kojic acid, arbutin, asafetida extract, bearberry extract, magnesium ascorbyl phosphate (also an antioxidant), and azelaic acid. There are two drawbacks to melanin suppressants, particularly hydroquinone. Many clients are allergic to hydroquinone, and it is a strong oxidant, which means it neutralizes and turns darker fairly quickly on exposure to air (oxygen). It is best to patch test clients for hydroquinone use before dispensing the product. It is also advisable to explain that hydroquinone solutions are fairly easily ruined and should be kept in a cool, dark place; also, they should always be securely closed after each use.

Daily use of broad-spectrum sunscreens (as all sunscreens really should be) and avoidance of sun exposure are imperative if the client with hyperpigmention wants to see results. Unfortunately, many of these clients are "sun addicted" and it is hard for them to give up tanning. Nevertheless, the esthetician should insist that for any pigment-evening treatment to work, sun must be avoided.

It should be mentioned here that hyperactive melanocytes do not just react to ultraviolet rays. They also react to heat from the infrared rays from the sun. There is no sunscreen available, or on the immediate forefront, that blocks infrared heat. So, the bottom line is that sun and heat must be avoided for these clients. A very thorough consultation with each client explaining all the facts about hyperpigmentation treatment as well as a handout is advisable.

Most companies recommend that an AHA product be used before application of melanin suppressant, then followed by sunscreen or a night hydrator. Some companies recommend AHA during the day and the melanin suppressant at night. It is best to check with the individual manufacturer and to remember that clients' skin types vary; twice-a-day application of both treatments may be too much for some.

## PREVENTION IS STILL THE BEST TREATMENT

Avoiding sun exposure and using sunscreens are still the best and most viable treatments for sun damage. Clients should always be instructed in the proper use of sunscreens to help prevent this terrible insult to the skin.

# TOPICS FOR DISCUSSION

1. What are some signs of the beginning of sun damage?

2. Discuss the research on the use of retinoids for photoaging skin.

3. What would you say when discussing sun damage with a client?

4. What precautions would you take to avoid overstimulating photoaged skin?

5. Discuss alphahydroxy acids and their effect on the appearance of photoaged skin.

6. How does alphahydroxy acid improve the surface of aging skin?

7. Explain the treatment for hyperpigmentation, and why it is important to have a thorough consultation with the client who is hyperpigmented.

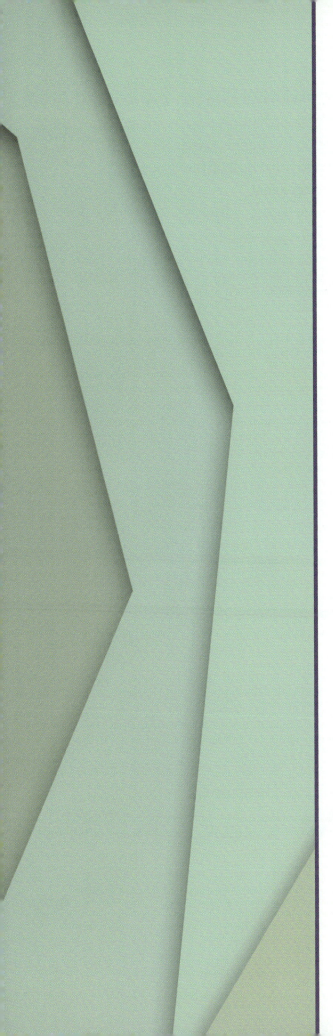

# CHAPTER 21

# Chemical Peeling and Exfoliation Procedures

## OBJECTIVES. . .

Many different types of peeling and exfoliation treatments are available, ranging from brushing treatment and light enzyme peels to strong surgical peels that are administered by dermatologists and plastic surgeons. This chapter discusses the various types of peeling treatments, both cosmetic and medical, and the various conditions that can benefit from different types of peeling treatments. This chapter is not a substitute for hands-on training in the use of superficial salon chemical peelings. The esthetician should always receive hands-on training before attempting any of the procedures discussed in this chapter.

The process of peeling the surface of the skin dates back to the 19th century in Europe. Chemical peeling was actually brought to America by a young esthetician, the daughter of a European doctor, who immigrated to America. The process of peeling the skin can take place in varying degrees, ranging from scrubs to salicylic creams to surgical-level phenol peeling. Removing cell layers from the surface of the skin can be used to treat a variety of both cosmetic and medical problems.

The esthetician's domain is the superficial epidermis. It is important to note that the esthetician should not perform treatments that involve live layers of the skin. This is medical peeling and is the domain of the dermatologist or plastic surgeon. Removal of dead cells by chemical means is chemical or esthetic exfoliation. It is preferred terminology that estheticians perform exfoliation treatments rather than "peels." However, we must be realistic and say that both estheticians and consumers alike use the terms interchangeably.

## SURFACE EXFOLIATION

There are basically two types of exfoliation treatments. Mechanical exfoliation uses some method of physical contact to literally scrape or bump cells off the skin. Granular scrubs, such as honey and almond scrubs; preparations with polyethylene granules or jojoba beads; the use of a brushing machine or microdermabrasion are all examples of mechanical peeling treatments. When the granules of these products or the bristles of a brushing machine come in contact with the surface corneum cells, the movement of the product or the brush literally "bumps off" cells from the surface of the corneum.

Many skin-care companies include brushing as a standard part of their salon treatments. The brushing machine is used over a layer of cleanser or moisturizer, which helps to buffer contact with the skin. The skin should be thoroughly cleansed, toned, and steamed before the brushing machine is used. Applying a noncomedogenic hydrating fluid before steaming the face is helpful in hydrating the dry surface cells, also helping to loosen dead cell buildup on the surface. This makes removal of the dead cells much easier, and gentler pressure can be used.

Removing the surface cells help the skin in the following ways:

1. The procedure helps remove uneven buildup of dead cells, so the skin appears much smoother.
2. It helps clear away dead cells and debris from the pore openings, making extraction and other treatment of clogged pores much easier.
3. By removing the dead cell layer, the lower-level cells are moved to the surface more quickly, improving the moisture content of the surface.
4. Mechanical treatment stimulates blood flow to the surface of the skin.
5. Removing the dry, dead cell buildup helps deliver moisturizers and other treatment deeper into the epidermis.

All of these advantages generally help to smooth the skin's surface, which makes makeup apply more evenly. The dead cells will eventually build back up on the surface, making this procedure only a temporary appearance change. However, regular use of mechanical exfoliators such as granular scrubs or alphahydroxy acid home treatment products helps maintain this appearance. Granular scrubs for normal to dry skin are usually recommended two to three times per week.

## Disadvantages of Mechanical Treatment

There are many circumstances when mechanical treatment is not appropriate. Do not use brushing machines, microdermabrasion, or any harsh mechanical peeling techniques on the following skin types and conditions:

1. Couperose skin, or telangiectatic skin, with many visible capillaries and blood vessels. The blood vessels in these skin types are very fragile and should not be subject to brushing treatment.
2. Fragile, thin skin that reddens easily. The epidermis of this skin is considerably thinner than other skin types. Brushing or abrasive treatment may redden and irritate this skin easily.

3. Older skin that is thin and bruises easily.

4. Severely sun-damaged skin. This skin also will often have many distended capillaries and redness.

5. Skin that is being medically treated with any prescription keratolytic drug, including tretinoin (retinoic acid or Retin-A), azelaic acid, adapalene (Differin®), alphahydroxy acid, or fluorouracil. (See the chapter on the new science of aging skin treatment.)

6. Acne-prone skin types, particularly those with inflamed acne, papules, and pustules.

7. Patients taking Accutane®.

8. Any skin that is red, irritated, thin, or extremely fair.

9. Skin that has a history of being easily irritated.

## Other Mechanical Exfoliation Techniques

As an alternative to using a brushing machine, you may choose to use a granular scrub, such as honey and almond scrub, after steaming. Apply the scrub with your fingertips and gently massage in upward, outward circular movements. Do not scrub the face for more than one or two minutes. Be extremely gentle with the pressure you apply. For thinner skin types, you may dilute the scrub with cleanser or moisturizer before applying the preparation. This dilution helps to provide a buffer between the skin's surface and the scrub, which cuts down on irritation potential.

For oilier skins, you may apply a granular scrub made with fine polyethylene beads or granules. These preparations often contain a small amount of sulfur or salicylic acid as additional chemical exfoliators and antiseptics. These scrubs are generally excellent for oily, problem skin and will help clear the surface of dead cells and other debris, making extraction easier.

One of the most recent techniques in mechanical exfoliation is the technique known as **microdermabrasion**. This process involves "shooting" aluminum oxide (corundum) crystals at the skin with a special apparatus. The crystals, after hitting the skin and exfoliating dead cells, are then picked up by a vacuum attached to the same handheld apparatus. This technique must be learned hands-on, under the supervision of an expert in the procedure.

Microdermabrasion is used to treat superficial symptoms of aging, similar to those treated with an alphahydroxy acid product and salon exfoliations. It is generally administered in a series of treatments.

Microdermabrasion is favored by many estheticians because it shows fairly quick results in improving skin texture. Microdermabrasion should be used with extreme care, especially in clients prone to hyperpigmentation. Overuse can cause increased pigmentation in some clients.

It would appear that even though alphahydroxy treatments do produce visible improvements in skin texture, the ongoing and long-range improvements in skin moisture, lipid content, and barrier function are likely due to daily applications of AHAs, which does not happen with microdermabrasion. Microdermabrasion should not be performed with alphahydroxy treatments, unless the two treatments are spaced well apart. Most estheticians recommend that clients not use AHA home products for up to two weeks after having had a microdermabrasion treatment.

## Home Care Using Mechanical Exfoliation

For dry to normal skin, recommend a light scrub such as honey and almond scrub two or three times per week. The client should apply the scrub after cleansing with a milk-type cleanser. Instruct the client to be very gentle with the scrub. Home care scrubs

**Microdermabrasion** is a procedure using crystal particles that are pressure-sprayed onto the skin and then vacuumed. Microdermabrasion is a mechanical exfoliation technique, that removes corneum cells.

should not be recommended for extremely thin skin or skin that is being treated with the therapies already listed in the precautions.

For oily and problem skin, granular scrubs are sometimes recommended on a daily or twice-daily basis. This, of course, will depend on the skin type, contraindications previously discussed, and what other drug or esthetic therapies are being used to treat this skin type. Exfoliation and removal of dead cells usually are very helpful in treating problem oily and clog-prone skin.

## SALON EXFOLIATION TREATMENTS

Salon exfoliation treatments are actually a type of chemical exfoliation, but they are extremely gentle. They are sometimes appropriate to use when mechanical exfoliation is not appropriate. These procedures involve the use of enzymes, specifically proteolytic enzymes. *Proteolytic* means "protein dissolving." The enzymes work to destroy the keratin in the dead cells on the surface of the skin. These are often referred to as enzyme peeling or enzyme treatments.

One enzyme often used in these treatments is papain, which is derived from the papaya fruit. Papain is also used in meat tenderizer for its ability to soften tissue and dissolve protein. In Europe, this type of treatment is known as a lysing or lysis. Another biological enzyme often used is pancreatin, which is derived from beef by-products.

There are two basic types of proteolytic enzyme peeling. One is a cream that is applied to the skin after steaming and initial preparation. This cream contains paraffin, which dries and forms a hardened crust. The cream dries in about ten minutes, and then is massaged or "rolled" off the skin. Treatments of this type are often called "vegetal" or "vegetable" peelings. This treatment is actually a combination of enzyme and mechanical peeling. The "rolling" provides friction that physically removes dead cells. The flakes coming off the skin are not dead cells but dried paraffin. The actual dead cells removed are not visible without a microscope. They can also be irritating for the skin types listed previously.

The second, and probably more popular, type of enzyme treatment uses a powdered form of enzyme. Mixed with warm water immediately before application, this treatment stays soft during application and does not dry. It is easily removed because it is soft and moist. This type of enzyme treatment generally produces a more even peeling of the cell buildup and helps to slightly dilate the follicle openings, which makes extraction much easier. Brushing the skin may miss some of the cells, whereas this type of enzyme treatment works evenly across the surface of the skin. Enzyme peelings are often available in varying strengths and suitable for the following conditions:

1. Oily, clogged skin with open and closed comedones and minor acne breakouts.
2. Dry or dehydrated skin with cell buildup, flaking, and tight dry surface.
3. Dull, lifeless looking skin. This skin condition actually has a tremendous buildup of dead cells that produces a slight gray color on the surface of the skin.
4. Skin with multiple milia.
5. Clients who desire a smoother appearance to their skin and a more even surface for makeup application.

Enzyme treatments are generally gentle enough to repeat even on an every-two-week schedule, although most clients have them with their regular monthly facial treatments. Most clients notice immediate softening of the skin after the very first application of the enzyme. Because enzyme treatment slightly dilates the pore openings, which helps with extraction, clients notice that extraction is more comfortable and that gentler pressure may be used to facilitate extraction of the clogged pores, comedones, and other impactions.

# Procedure for Enzyme Treatment

**Caution:** Always follow manufacturer's directions for using particular peeling treatments! The following is an example of typical treatment with enzymes, but these directions may vary with the manufacturer.

1. Remove all makeup and cleanse the skin well, using a milk cleanser appropriate for the skin type.

2. Apply a pre-peel lotion, usually furnished by the manufacturer. This solution is applied in a similar method as a toner. This solution is normally slightly alkaline, which helps remove excess oils on the surface of the skin, making the enzyme come in better contact with the dead surface dells.

3. Choose the appropriate strength of enzyme preparation for the particular skin type, thickness, and condition. Most companies make at least two strengths or furnish formulas to dilute the enzyme action of the product.

4. Mix the product with warm water in a small mixing cup or beaker. Most enzyme treatments have the consistency and thickness of mayonnaise when mixed with warm water. Stir the preparation until the treatment is smooth and free of powder lumps.

5. Apply the enzyme to the face with a soft mask brush. Stay clear of the eye area and other sensitive areas unless otherwise directed by manufacturer's instructions.

6. Many companies recommend steaming during the application of the treatment and during treatment setting time. The steam helps keep the treatment warm and also helps to keep the preparation from drying out on the surface. It is important to keep the preparation moist. If enzymes are allowed to dry on the face they can be irritating to the skin and are also hard to remove. Allow the treatment to set for about eight minutes. Remove with tepid, damp sponges or a damp, soft, facial cloth. Be careful to remove the enzyme treatment thoroughly. It is easy to leave remnants of the peeling, particularly around the perimeter of the face, such as under the chin, on the jawline, and in front of the ears. This leftover enzyme can be irritating if not removed after the appropriate amount of time.

7. Brushing is not necessary when using an enzyme treatment. In fact, it can be irritating. Do not use the brush during an enzyme treatment.

8. Because of the follicle dilation caused by the enzyme, desincrustation using galvanic current is usually not necessary. It can also be irritating to thin, sensitive, or dry skins when combined with enzyme treatment. Excessively oily skin; acne-prone skin; and thick, oily skin with multiple comedones may benefit from galvanic desincrustation after an enzyme treatment. Use your best judgment and remember, when in doubt, don't!

9. Proceed with extraction in a normal manner. You will probably find that you do not have to use nearly as much pressure during extraction. This will appeal to the client as well, because treatment is more comfortable.

10. Apply a toner to lower the pH of the skin immediately after extraction. It is important to lower the pH after the enzyme treatment.

11. Proceed with the rest of treatment as normal. You should not massage the skin before applying the enzyme. This may increase irritation potential. Any facial waxing should be done toward the end of the treatment session, not before the enzyme is applied. The waxing procedure will also physically remove dead cells. It is best to perform waxing after the enzyme is removed, or, on sensitive skin, suggest that the client make a separate appointment for a different day.

12. You may find that you do not need to use as aggressive a mask as usual after an enzyme treatment. Some masks also remove dead cell buildup. On dry or thin

skins, apply a gel mask, a cream mask, or simply apply a thick layer of hydrating fluid as a mask. These types of masks are nonhardening and are easier to remove from sensitive or thin skins.

Most skin-care salons charge an additional fee for enzyme treatments. You may want to allow the client to try the enzyme treatment once at no charge so that the client can see the nice results.

# ALPHAHYDROXY AND GLYCOLIC PEELING TREATMENTS

Before reading this section, review the section on alphahydroxy acid in the chapter The New Science of Aging Skin Treatment. Glycolic acid is available in a variety of strengths for salon use. The typical concentration of glycolic acid used in salon treatment is between 15 and 30 percent. Higher strengths are usually used only by dermatologists. It is strongly suggested that you not experiment with higher percentages of glycolic acid!

The Cosmetic Ingredient Review of the Cosmetics, Toiletries, and Fragrance Association has issued a recommendation that licensed estheticians use alphahydroxy acid salon exfoliation products that do not exceed 30 percent concentration and have a pH of 3.0 or above. Higher concentrations or lower pH can cause irritation.

Before administering alphahydroxy acid exfoliation, the client should have been using an 8 to 10 percent concentration gel, lotion, or cream at home for at least two weeks. Home use of the AHA before AHA exfoliation should be mandatory because it helps acclimate the skin for higher strength salon products. Failure to use AHA at home as described may result in increased discomfort during the procedure and increased chances of redness and irritation after the exfoliation treatment.

The standard treatment consists of a ten-minute application of 30 percent, pH 3.0 gel. This is administered twice a week for three weeks for a client beginning AHA treatments. Maintenance treatments are usually twice a month, but vary with client needs, budgets, and sensitivity levels. It is very important to pay attention to manufacturers' instructions, which may vary from product to product.

Alphahydroxy exfoliation works by dissolving surface binding lipids that hold the cells of the corneum together. AHA treatments can be used to help the same conditions listed for enzyme exfoliation but will also improve hyperpigmentation, fine lines and wrinkles, and surface roughness. Continual use refines pore appearance and helps achieve even texture and coloration.

Mild glycolic treatment may be influenced by the cleansing procedure that takes place before extraction. The cleansing procedure determines how much surface oil is removed before applying the glycolic peeling treatment. The following is a typical procedure for glycolic treatment, but read the instructions of the particular product you are using and follow them.

## Procedure for Glycolic Exfoliation

1. Cleanse the skin with a mild cleansing milk, removing makeup.
2. Apply a compress to the eyes to avoid accidentally spilling the solution into the eyes.
3. Set a timer for ten minutes, or the length of time suggested by the manufacturer. Apply the glycolic acid gel with two cotton swabs held together. Begin with the forehead, and apply the gel using small, circular motions with the cotton swabs. Proceed to other areas in a precise clockwise pattern. It is important to follow a precise pattern to ensure even application of the gel.

The glycolic treatment is allowed to stay on the skin for the prescribed amount of time, as recommended by the manufacturer. A typical time for a low-strength solution is ten minutes. After ten minutes remove the gel from the face with cool, wet, gauze pads. Rinse the face well with the wet gauze. You may follow this with a cool spray of plain water in an atomizer and another cleanup with wet gauze. Finish by applying a sunscreen moisturizer (Figure 21-1).

This treatment is normally performed twice a week for the first three weeks. The pretreatment before application of the glycolic acid gel can influence the strength of the treatment. The strength of the cleansing products used will determine the amount of surface oils and corneum cells removed before application of the gel.

You should, during the first treatment, cleanse with a very mild cleansing milk. If the first treatment does not produce any redness or irritation, the second treatment may be preceded by a slightly stronger milk cleanser. For the third visit, again assuming there is no irritation, you may add a mild toner to complete the cleansing. The fourth treatment may be strengthened by using a slightly stronger milk cleanser with a slightly stronger toner. The cleansers and toners used should never be extremely strong or alcoholic.

It is strongly recommended that a minimum of six treatments be given before assessing the results. Results will not be particularly dramatic after one treatment. It takes several applications of 30 percent alphahydroxy acid, over several weeks, to see appreciable results in many cases (Figure 21-2A and B).

After the initial treatment, you may decide to repeat the treatment weekly, biweekly, or monthly, depending on the results. You should reassess the condition of the skin after the first few applications to determine a further treatment course.

## Precautions to Take When Administering Glycolic Peelings

1. Always make sure the skin has been pretreated with lower strength alphahydroxy acid at home for at least two weeks before administering salon-strength

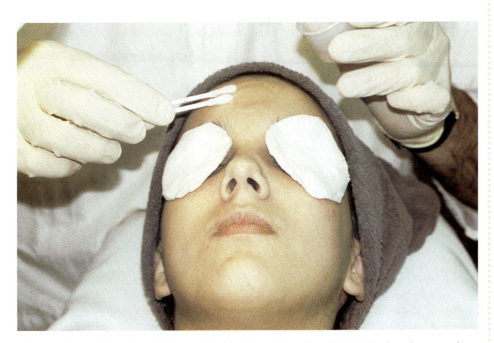

**Figure 21-1** Glycolic acid is applied to the skin of a client who has been using a lower strength glycolic treatment product for at least two weeks at home. This treatment is applied with cotton swabs and carefully monitored according to manufacturer's directions (Courtesy Mark Lees Skin Care, Inc.)

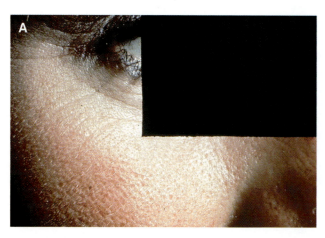 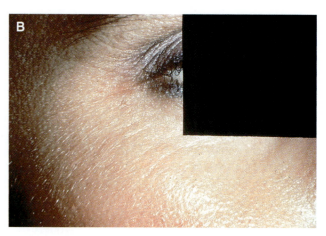

**Figure 21-2** Glycolic treatment is popular for lessening the appearance of facial wrinkles. Shown here are before and after photos of the eye area (Courtesy Murad Skin Research Laboratories, Inc.)

treatment. Failure to do this may cause irritation. For instructions on home care AHA treatment, see the chapter, The New Science of Aging Skin Treatment.

2. Do not use the alphahydroxy acid treatment if the client is currently using prescription keratolytic drugs including tazarotene (Tazorac®), tretinoin (Retin-A or Renova®), adapalene (Differin®), or azelaic acid (Azelex®), or other prescription peeling agents. Treatment with any of these drugs should be discontinued for several weeks before using salon alphahydroxy exfoliation treatments.

3. Do not use glycolic or alphahydroxy acid on patients taking Accutane®.

4. Do not administer AHA treatments if the client is under a dermatologist's care for any skin disorders, without first obtaining approval from the dermatologist.

5. Be careful to use eyepads, and avoid getting the alphahydroxy acid close to the eyes.

6. Do not use the peeling gel on a male client immediately after he has shaved. It is best to wait several hours after shaving to apply glycolic salon treatment.

7. Check with the client before each successive treatment to make sure the client has not experienced any irritation from the previous treatment. If irritation developed after the previous treatment, do not add precleansing steps as discussed earlier. Avoid any area that is peeling, red, or irritated, or wait a few days before resuming treatment.

8. Do not administer AHA treatments to any skin that is already irritated. This includes rosacea flares, seborrheic dermatitis, eczema, windburned or sunburned skin, or skin that is irritated from a previous treatment of any type. Never double-exfoliate skin, or use other keratolytics at the same time, chemical or mechanical, especially microdermabrasion.

9. A broad-spectrum sunscreen of SPF-15 or higher, appropriate for the skin type, should be applied after any AHA exfoliation treatment and should be used daily by the client at home.

10. Do not use AHA treatment or any other form of chemical exfoliation if the client has a history of herpes simplex (cold sore) breakouts. The client should be referred to their doctor for prophylactic treatment for herpes simplex before administering any chemical exfoliation treatments. Always remember, when in doubt, don't!

You should not combine professional alphahydroxy acid application with other salon facial treatments when first beginning AHA treatment. After the initial series

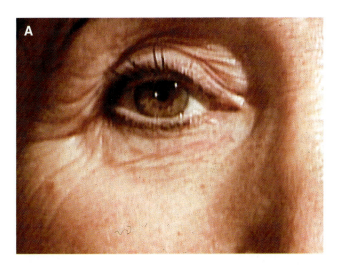
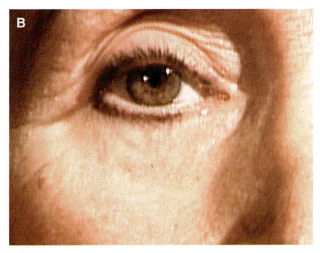

**Figure 21-3** Routine use of home alphahydroxy acid products along with a series of alphahydroxy professional treatments can produce dramatic effects on the appearance of wrinkles in aging skin (Courtesy of Murad Medical Group)

of AHA salon applications, you may administer glycolic treatment during facial treatments, depending on the client. As always, check manufacturer's instructions for instruction regarding combining AHA treatment with other types of salon skin-care treatments.

The skin should never be exfoliated before AHA application. Avoid pretreatment with any technique or product that is stimulating, heating, or irritating.

AHA treatment with low-strength gel can be administered indefinitely on a weekly, biweekly, or monthly basis, depending on the client and the skin type (Figure 21-3A and B).

## Using AHA Treatment for Acne

The procedure is essentially the same as we have just discussed. You may notice an apparent increase in comedones and blackheads during the first few treatments. Because AHA is an exfoliating treatment, it uncovers closed comedones and loosens open comedones while exfoliating the dead-cell layer on the surface of the skin, which can be fairly heavy on oily, problem skin. You should explain the possibility to the client that the skin may seem to get worse before it gets better. Continued treatment, along with alternating extraction treatments on different days, will help loosen the acne impactions (Figure 21-4A and B, Figure 21-5A and B).

## Treatment for Hyperpigmented Skin

Again, the treatment method is essentially the same. The client should, as always, be pretreated at home for several weeks before starting salon treatment. The client should use home care products that include a melanin suppressant such as hydroquinone, kojic acid, magnesium ascorbyl phosphate, arbutin, asafetida extract, or a combination of these agents. There are premixed solutions available that include combinations of the above with alphahydroxy acids. The theory here is to remove already stained corneum cells while suppressing melanin production in the melanocytes. Needless to say, hyperpigmented clients should wear a daily broad-spectrum sunscreen of SPF-15 or 30, and should avoid sun exposure completely. Infrared rays, which are not blocked by sunscreen products, cause heat in the skin, resulting in melanin production (Figure 21-6A and B, Figure 21-7A and B).

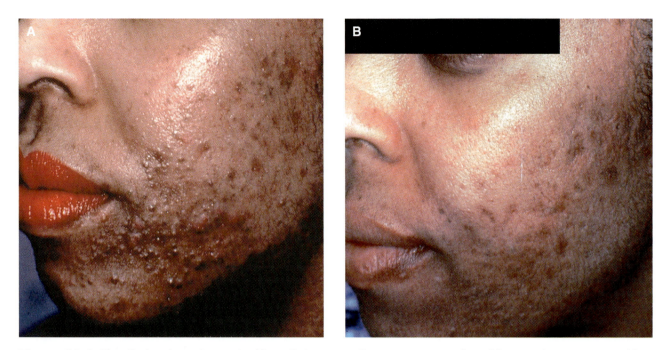

**Figure 21-4** Glycolic treatment can significantly improve the appearance of problem and acne-prone skin (before and after) (Courtesy Murad Skin Research Laboratories, Inc.)

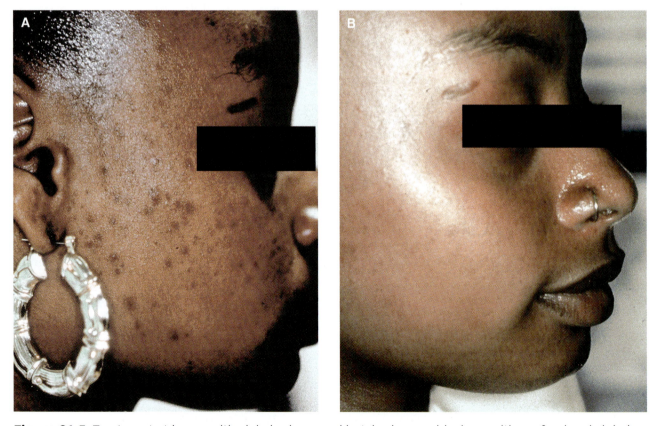

**Figure 21-5** Treatment at home with alphahydroxy and betahydroxy acid, along with professional alphahydroxy acid and extraction treatments, can help to clear blemishes and improve hyperpigmentation in the skin of color (Courtesy Murad Medical Group)

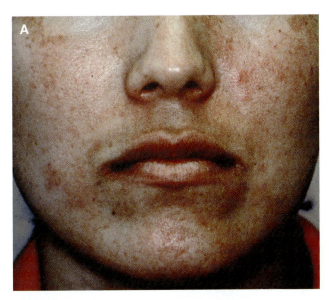
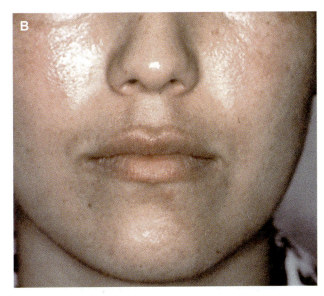

**Figure 21-6** Glycolic treatment can help the appearance of hyperpigmented skin conditions (Courtesy Murad Skin Research Laboratories, Inc.)

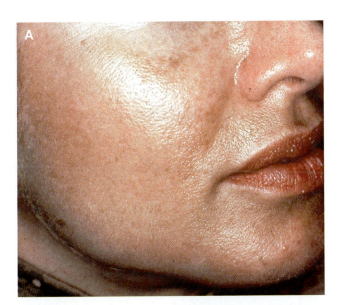
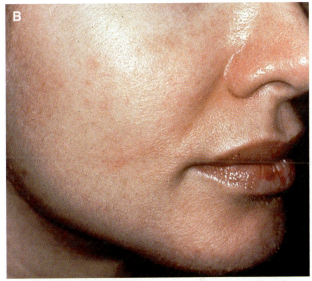

**Figure 21-7** Hyperpigmentation can be improved by the daily use of alphahydroxy acids and hydroquinone, and of course, daily sunscreen at home, as well as professional alphahydroxy treatments in the salon or clinic (Courtesy Murad Medical Group)

## Stronger Glycolic Peeling

Stronger solutions are available for salon use, but with added strength comes added risk. They should be used conservatively and should never be left on the skin for more than two minutes. The amount of time glycolic acid is allowed to contact the skin is directly related to the strength and depth of the treatment. Do not experiment! Stick to manufacturer's directions at all times!

## Medical AHA Treatment

Dermatologists and plastic surgeons may use glycolic acid solutions in concentrations of 50 to 70 percent. These are medical grade strengths and should never be used by estheticians unless they are working under the direct supervision of a dermatologist or plastic surgeon. High strengths are used to treat deeper wrinkles, solar lentigines, and actinic keratoses.

## STRONGER PEELING TREATMENTS

The treatments we have been discussing using 20 to 30 percent alphahydroxy acid are generally very safe and helpful for cosmetic effects. This level of alphahydroxy acid is acceptable for almost all skin types and produces a good cosmetic effect with a very low amount of potential irritation. One company calls their treatment "rapid exfoliation," indicating that it is actually a "high-tech exfoliator," rather than a "chemical peel."

The stronger peels are of three types and three levels.

**Surgical phenol peeling** is a deep peeling procedure that should only be administered by a dermatologist or a plastic surgeon. This procedure involves applying a very strong solution of a very strong chemical called phenol. Phenol peeling must be administered in a doctor's office or surgical unit. Phenol, in large amounts, can be absorbed into the bloodstream and rarely can cause heart fluctuations. The heart is monitored during this procedure to ensure safety. The phenol peel penetrates to the aged, severely wrinkled skin, and can also be used to treat skin growths such as repeated instances of skin cancers and actinic keratoses (Figure 21-8A and B). It may produce hypopigmentation of the skin and a ruddy surface to the face (Figure 21-9A and B). For further information on phenol peeling, please read the chapter, Treating the Plastic Surgery Patient.

**Surgical phenol peeling** is a very deep peeling procedure performed by a plastic surgeon or dermatologist. The peel affects the dermis and has considerable risks.

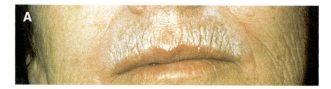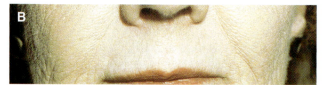

**Figure 21-8** *A*, Phenol solution is used on the wrinkled lip of this patient. Shown here is the "frosting" effect after application of the phenol solution. *B*, Several months after the peel, the lip is much smoother (Courtesy Kirk Smith, M.D.)

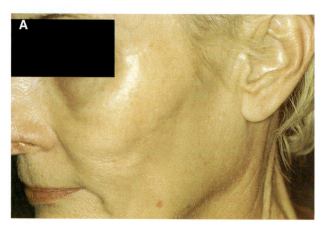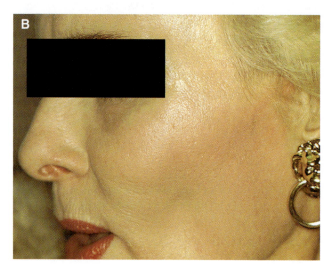

**Figure 21-9** In-depth phenol peel (before and after) (Courtesy Melvin L. Elson, MD.)

Laser resurfacing is a surgical technique of using a laser to reduce wrinkles and skin texture imperfections. Laser resurfacing uses a **carbon dioxide (CO₂) laser** to remove skin layers. In most cases, the entire epidermis and some of the dermis is **ablated** or evaporated through laser application. $CO_2$ and erbium lasers are **ablative** lasers, meaning they remove or destroy tissue.

Deep wrinkles cannot be removed unless part of the dermis is removed. Deep wrinkles involve severe damage to the collagen and elastin network, which cannot be removed with weaker peeling techniques. Again, all procedures that peel living tissue are the domain of the dermatologist or plastic surgeon and should never be attempted by estheticians.

**Medium depth peels** include 50 to 70 percent glycolic acid applications and 40 to 50 percent trichloracetic acid, better known to the medical community as TCA. TCA at this strength penetrates to the layer of the dermis, and again is a procedure that should only be administered by a dermatologist or a plastic surgeon. Combinations of TCA and glycolic acid are sometimes used by doctors to treat deeper wrinkles.

TCA does not have the potential for absorption into the bloodstream like high concentrations of phenol. Lighter peelings can be given with TCA at concentrations of 15 to 35 percent, but they do not have the dramatic results of the deeper phenol peels. Some doctors will use repeated treatments with these smaller concentrations of TCA. TCA in general also does not have as great a potential for scarring as phenol peeling.

Some companies sell low-percentage TCA to estheticians. It is the opinion of this author that TCA belongs in the hands of dermatologists and plastic surgeons only. TCA is too unpredictable and is beyond the scope of esthetic exfoliation.

**Superficial peeling** is the deepest type of chemical peeling performed by estheticians. Superficial peelings, unlike deep and medium medical peelings, only remove cells from the stratum corneum. The most frequently used type of chemical is known as Jessner's Solution, which is a mixture of salicylic acid, resorcinol, lactic acid, and ethanol. Some superficial peeling formulas also contain a small amount of phenol, usually 2 percent, and sometimes sulfur. Although Jessner's Solution is a liquid, some cream forms of peels are similar and produce similar effects on the skin.

One of the latest exfoliation treatments available to the esthetician is 20 percent salicylic acid in a special vehicle called a Microsponge®. With proper training, this liquid exfoliation treatment is a safe and effective procedure.

These superficial chemical peels are helpful for treating small, superficial wrinkles, dark spots, and other forms of hyperpigmentation, melasma, and acne-prone skin.

The superficial peel evens the surface skin pigment, smoothes the appearance of the skin, and dries the surface of acne and problem skin. Like AHA, superficial peeling may also increase the amount of surface acne lesions, because it loosens impactions and causes them to move toward the surface. In other words, it may cause acne to get worse before it gets better.

## Candidates for Salon Superficial Peelings

Clients who have sun-damaged skin, hyperpigmented skin, or other forms of melasma are the best candidates for superficial peeling. Technically, most adult clients can benefit from these peelings, because most adults do have some form of fine wrinkling or hyperpigmentation.

There are, of course, many other alternatives for treating these cosmetic problems. Glycolic acid, hydroquinone solutions, or a combination can be very effective for many forms of hyperpigmentation. Low-strength AHA peelings are also another alternative. Most estheticians will attempt to treat these cosmetic conditions with more conservative treatments, such as the ones listed before resorting to superficial chemical peeling.

Make sure that your client has started on home care before administering superficial chemical peeling. This pretreatment will ensure that the client's skin is in better

**Carbon dioxide (CO₂) laser** is a surgical laser used in resurfacing. It removes epidermal and dermal tissue to treat wrinkles in sun damaged skin.

**Ablated** is a medical term meaning "removed." Tissue ablated during laser resurfacing is removed by the laser.

**Ablative** is a term describing a laser that removes tissue.

**Medium depth peels** are performed by dermatologists or plastic surgeons. These trichloracetic acid (TCA) peels affect the dermis, but not as deeply as phenol.

**Superficial peeling** effects the epidermis and is performed by estheticians or physicians. These peels include alpha and beta hydroxy acids, Jessner's solution, and resorcinol peeling treatments.

shape before using chemical peelings. Many estheticians insist that a client have facial treatments for a period of time before administering a chemical peel. This is not a bad idea because it allows you to learn about the client, the client's skin, and the client's needs before using peelings.

Many clients will call the salon specifically asking about chemical peels. Information given out over the phone should be minimal, because you have not seen the client's skin. Ask the client to make an appointment for a consultation before you issue an opinion about her skin. Many clients have cosmetic problems that can be treated by other, simpler methods than chemical peels. Some clients are not using proper home care. Good home care and salon care may make the difference they need and establish a good, healthy program for their skin for a lifetime. Chemical peeling should not be looked at as a "band-aid" or a "magic bullet" for skin problems. The client needs to continually take care of the skin at home on a regular basis.

Other forms of lighter peelings such as enzyme or AHA may be sufficient for treating the client's problem.

Chemical peeling is probably the most drastic and dramatic treatment administered by an esthetician. There are some disadvantages to superficial peeling. These include discomfort, temporary discolorations, a small risk of allergic reaction, a bad appearance to the skin during the actual procedure, and a possibility of hyperpigmentation. All of these disadvantages should be explained to the client long before the procedure is administered. When the client agrees to have the superficial chemical peel, the client should be required to sign a release saying that the client has been informed of all the possible side effects and discomfort that may be associated with chemical peeling. Clients should also be shown pictures of what clients look like during the peel so that they know how they might look.

These few paragraphs are not meant to discourage the use of chemical peelings. They are meant to clarify that clients do not always fully understand chemical peeling or for what conditions it is intended. Clients who are not familiar with good skin care and do not use a regular skin-care program will generally not have as good or as long-lasting results as clients who have regular salon treatments and are good about home care.

You should also get to know a client's personality. Chemical peeling is uncomfortable, and during the procedure the skin looks terrible. A client who is nervous or who becomes hysterical easily should not have chemical peelings. You will save yourself a world of trouble by getting to know your client well before performing chemical peeling.

Other clients who should not have chemical peeling are the following:

1. Clients who are pregnant or are lactating.

2. Clients who have a history of heart problems.

3. Clients who have a history of medical problems. These clients should have written permission from their physician. Examples of these conditions include, but are not limited to, eczema, lupus, seborrhea, rosacea, psoriasis, bacterial skin infections, mental disorders, extremely sensitive or hyperallergic skin, and other systemic problems. Take a thorough health history, and refer the client to a medical doctor if you have any questions.

4. Clients who have a history of fever blisters or herpes simplex, which can be stimulated by chemical peeling. Clients should discuss this with a physician.

5. Clients using Accutane® or other dermatological drugs.

6. Clients using retinoic acid (Retin-A), which should be discontinued about three months before superficial peeling is administered.

7. Clients who have extremely thin telangiectatic or couperose skin.

# THE PRE-PEEL CONSULTATION

At least a week before the peeling is scheduled, you should have a consultation appointment with the client. Explain to the client what normally happens, step-by-step. Make sure the client understands the discomfort and how the client will look during the procedure. Explain that the client should not have any sun exposure for eight weeks after peeling and must use a broad-spectrum sunscreen at all times. Clients who are being treated for hyperpigmentation should always be especially careful about sun exposure.

Show the client pictures of what a normal peel looks like during the process. Take pictures of the client's skin before and after the procedure. This will allow you to show the client the improvement in the skin's appearance.

Have the client sign a release saying that the client has been fully informed about the possible disadvantages of peeling and the actual procedure that takes place. It is very important to be honest with the client.

Superficial peeling will not do the following:

- Remove deep wrinkles.
- Remove scarring or acne pocks.
- Repair severe sun damage to any appreciable degree.
- Cause a lifting effect on the skin.

Superficial peeling will do the following:

- Improve the skin's texture.
- Even the coloring.
- Help lighten hyperpigmentation.
- Improve fine lines and rough textures.

# THE SUPERFICIAL PEELING PROCEDURE

Several different procedures are used for superficial salon chemical peeling, which will vary according to the manufacturer. The following are two examples of typical procedures for liquid and cream peelings. These are meant to serve only as examples. *Always follow the manufacturer's direction for the preparation that you are using*.

## Liquid Peeling

The liquid type of peeling solution is normally Jessner's Solution. Another is a 20 percent solution of salicylic acid. Again, you should follow any specific directions furnished by the manufacturer. You should also have complete hands-on training on the treatment before attempting the procedure in the salon! The solution is applied with cotton swabs to the face. The following procedure is typical:

1. Complete all the pre-peel consultation procedures discussed.
2. Remove the client's makeup thoroughly with a cleansing milk.
3. Apply a "prep" lotion furnished by the manufacturer. This solution is usually acetone, which removes excess oils and surface dead cells.
4. Turn on a small fan and place it so it blows gently on the client's face. Do not turn the fan to high speed, because this may blow the liquid. Some companies do not recommend using a fan at all for this reason. Some fans are small enough for clients to hold them in their hands.
5. Put on a pair of latex gloves. Paint the liquid solution onto the face using two cotton swabs held closely together. Begin with the forehead and apply the solution in

**Frosting** describes a white appearance of the skin that appears after applying a strong exfoliation or peeling substance.

small, gentle, circular motions. Do not apply pressure with the swabs. Proceed from the forehead down the cheek and around the face. It is very important that the application be as even as possible. Do not apply the solution to the lips, ears, or upper lids. Lower lids may be treated, but it is strongly suggested to stay within ⅛-inch of the lower lid edge. Again, this depends on the manufacturer's recommendations. The client should keep the eyes shut during the procedure.

6. Allow this coat to "dry" for two minutes. If you notice any white areas forming on the face, this is known as **frosting**. Frosting occurs when the peel is complete. Some clients will frost after one coat, and some after two or three coats of solution. If frosting does not occur after the first coat, repeat the application procedure, and wait for another four minutes. Occasionally, areas of the face will frost when other areas will not. If this happens, reapply the solution to the unfrosted areas only.

7. Apply the solution at four-minute intervals until frosting occurs. Most clients will only require one to three coats.

The solution remains on the face, and the client should stay in the salon for about an hour.

A strong burning sensation will be felt when application starts. The intensity of the burning sensation will vary with the client. This is the reason for the fan, which helps cool the sensation. After about 15 minutes, this burning sensation will stop, and the skin feels numb and slightly tingly (Figure 21-10, Figure 21-11A–F).

## The Cream Peel

The preparation procedure is the same as for the liquid peel. No prep solution is used with the cream peel.

1. With gloved hands apply the cream peel to the forehead, cheeks, nose, chin, and neck and finish with a very light application to the lower lids using a cotton

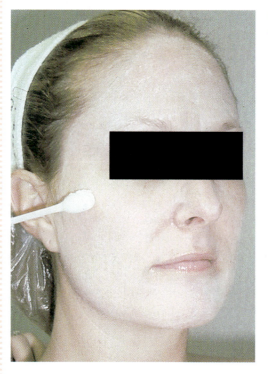

**Figure 21-10** Application of salicylic acid using a large swab

A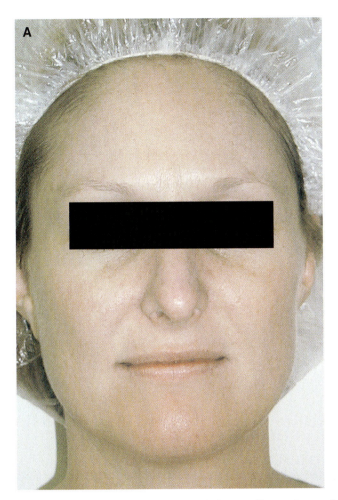

B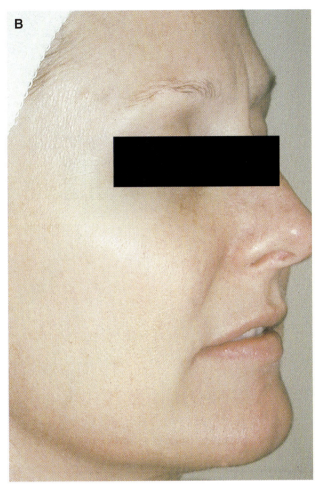

**Figure 21-11** *A, B* This series of photos illustrates exfoliation treatment using 20 percent salicylic acid. Notice the frosting on the skin where the treatment has been applied. Before any treatment, cumulative sun damage results in uneven pigmentation and hydration (Courtesy Mark Lees Skin Care, Inc.)

swab. Apply evenly. The face will begin to burn and sting. Again, this sensation can be lessened by the use of a fan and usually subsides after 15 to 20 minutes.

2. You do not have to watch for frosting with this treatment. It will happen automatically. There is no need for a second application until the next day. This thick treatment stays on the face for 1½ hours. After this time the cream is gently removed with a tongue depressor and then cleansed well with cool, wet, cotton compresses.

3. After removing the treatment, apply the thick moisturizing cream furnished in the peeling kit. The client will continue to apply this emollient cream to the face at home. The skin should be well lubricated with the emollient at all times.

4. On the second day, the same procedure is repeated in the salon with this cream peel. The client continues to keep the skin moist with the emollient cream.

Although these procedures sound fairly simple, you must be thoroughly trained and experienced to perform them correctly. You must have hands-on training to perform chemical peeling. Do not think you are qualified simply from reading this chapter or a manufacturer's handbook. You should observe several peeling procedures before attempting to perform peeling!

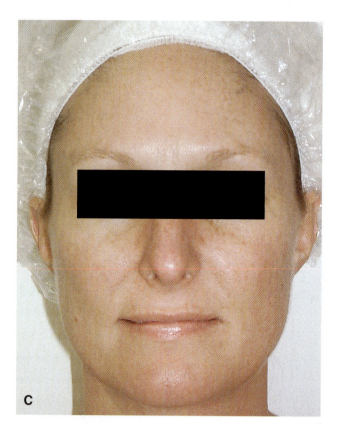

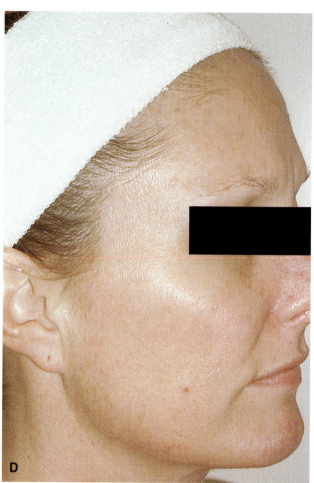

**Figure 21-11** *C, D* Note improvement after two treatments, six weeks apart (Courtesy Mark Lees Skin Care, Inc.)

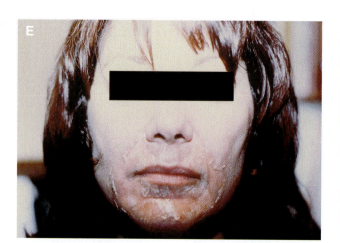

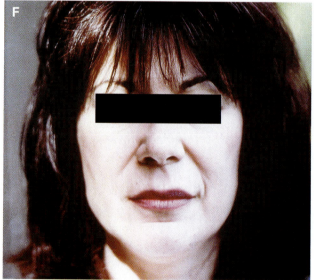

**Figure 21-11** *E, F* Temporary hyperpigmentation and discoloration can occur during the first one or two weeks following salicylic treatment. In this more extreme case, dark splotches exfoliate to reveal a smoother texture and tone (Courtesy Sothys, USA.)

# AFTER THE TREATMENT

Immediately after treatment the skin often looks slightly red and flushed. There is often little change in the first day. On the second day of either peel, the skin will become tan-looking, sometimes splotchy.

On the third day the skin becomes very dark and often splotchy and will feel very tight and dry. Peeling will begin around the mouth and chin first, then the cheeks, then the eyes. The neck and forehead are the last to peel. The skill will peel usually from the third through the sixth or seventh day. Occasionally, the peeling will continue for several more days. The client should be warned not to pull on the loose skin. This can cause infection and possible hyperpigmentation. It is best for the client to visit the salon daily for a quick check, and the esthetician can gently peel off areas that are ready.

Clients should not wash the face at all during the peeling procedure. They may use moisturizer, depending on the manufacturer's instructions. Cool water may be applied, but not cleanser.

Granular scrubs and other keratolyic preparations should be discontinued for at least the first two weeks after peeling. These include glycolic acid, benzoyl peroxide, sulfur, resorcinol, Retin-A, salicylic acid, lactic acid, or any other peeling or exfoliating agent.

The skin should be completely protected with a daily sunscreen for at least eight weeks after peeling. Direct sun exposure must be avoided.

# REACTIONS TO PEELING

Rarely, a client will have an allergic reaction to a chemical peeling. The symptoms may include severe itching, swelling, severe redness, and stinging. Refer this client to a dermatologist who is familiar with your services, particularly your peeling procedures. Normally, a steroid cream is prescribed, which quickly alleviates the problem.

Dark skin types sometimes have a tendency to hyperpigment after a peel. Many estheticians will not administer chemical peeling to darker or black skins. If the client pulls off skin that is not ready, splotchy hyperpigmentation can occur. Normally this fades within a few weeks, as long as the skin is protected with a sunscreen. Sometimes you may need to treat the skin with a mild bleaching cream, if the hyperpigmentation does not decrease within two or three weeks after peeling.

Your proficiency in chemical peeling will increase as you perform more and more peelings. This is why it so important that you thoroughly train with someone accomplished in the practice of superficial peeling and observe the actual peeling that takes place during the six or seven days after the procedure is performed. With this training you can become proficient at superficial chemical peeling.

# TOPICS FOR DISCUSSION

1. Discuss the difference between mechanical and chemical peeling.
2. What is the difference between "peeling" and "exfoliating"?
3. What are some skin conditions that can benefit from enzyme peeling?
4. What are the differences between deep, medium, and superficial peels?
5. Discuss the consultation procedures for superficial chemical peeling.
6. What conditions will not be improved with salon superficial peeling?
7. Discuss the procedures and possible problems associated with salon chemical peeling. Why is it so important to receive hands-on training?

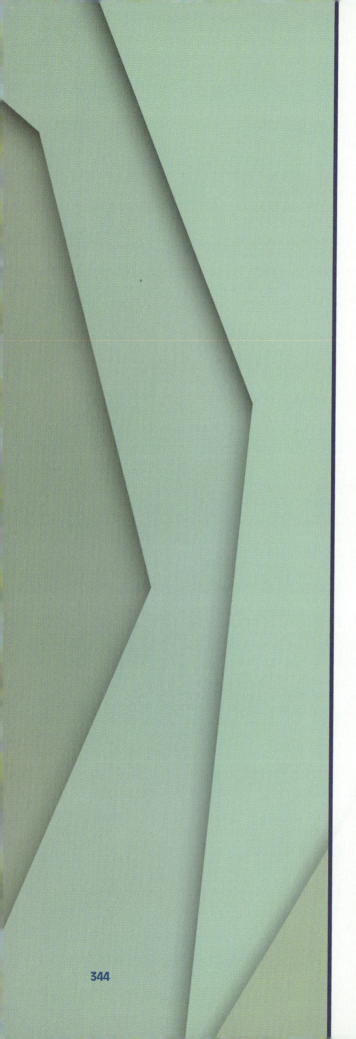

# CHAPTER 22

# Treating the Plastic and Cosmetic Surgery Patient

## OBJECTIVES. . .

More and more frequently, clients are having plastic surgery performed. In this chapter we will discuss the many types of plastic surgery procedures used and common problems of the plastic surgery patient. We will also discuss treatments for preparing the patient for plastic surgery, counseling the plastic surgery patient for referral, and how to treat cosmetic side effects of plastic surgery.

Management of postoperative skin-care and makeup needs by a licensed esthetician (skin-care specialist) can be beneficial to both the surgeon and the patient. An esthetician who is well-trained and experienced in clinical preoperative and postoperative care can help the postoperative patient by providing services in proper skin care, moisturization, control and mitigation of erythema and milia, camouflage makeup instruction for coverage of bruising, post-laser erythema, and contouring techniques for diminishing the look of swelling, not to mention providing health education and emotional support. The esthetician can be the patient's "lifeline," managing problems that may not be pathological but are of great concern to the patient.

# CONCERNS OF THE PATIENT

Postoperative patients are frequently referred to the esthetician and arrive at the esthetician's clinic or salon very concerned about their immediate appearance. Rarely are these problems pathological; they are usually purely cosmetic and self-limiting. However, they are of immediate concern to the patient who needs cosmetic help, relief of discomfort, and reassurance to make it through the postoperative period.

## Psychological Needs

The esthetician can play a significant role as a health educator and psychological support for the patient. An ear that understands the immediate concerns of the patient is sincerely appreciated by the patient. The esthetician should be well-versed and experienced in postoperative procedures in order to answer basic questions regarding cosmetic prognosis.

## Proper Esthetician Training

It is vitally important that the esthetician be adequately trained to assist in managing postoperative cosmetic surgery patients. This means that the esthetician should have hands-on experience with actual patients under the supervision of a cosmetic surgeon, dermatologist, or a very experienced postoperative trained esthetician. Estheticians should take all the classes and seminars they can on postoperative procedures and post-laser esthetic treatment.

# PLASTIC SURGERY

Years ago plastic surgery was considered by many to be a sign of vanity and reserved only for the rich and famous. Now plastic surgery is performed daily in every major American city. It is no longer considered unacceptable for people to want to look better. There are two basic types of plastic surgery—*cosmetic* surgery and *reconstructive* surgery.

**Cosmetic surgery** generally refers to surgical procedures used for cosmetic purposes only. These procedures include eyelid, face, and forehead lifts; dermabrasion; chemical peelings; liposuction; laser resurfacing; collagen injections; and other procedures. Body cosmetic surgery includes body sculpting contour surgery, body liposuction, tummy tucks, and breast augmentation or reduction.

**Reconstructive surgery** generally refers to surgical techniques used to correct noncosmetic abnormalities such as skin cancer removal, surgery needed due to accidental injury, and other physical deformities. These surgical procedures are often medically necessary, and in some cases, such as melanoma, can be treatment for serious, life-threatening diseases.

For the purposes of this discussion, we will primarily discuss facial cosmetic surgery, although we will briefly discuss reconstructive surgery.

# TYPES OF SURGEONS

Several different types of physicians perform plastic, reconstructive, and cosmetic surgery. All of these doctors receive four years of medical school training, followed by an internship and residency that takes four or more years to complete. These various specialists are then board certified by their particular specialty associations.

**General plastic surgeons** perform all types of plastic, reconstructive and cosmetic surgery. They often also perform hand surgery. They perform surgery on all areas of the face and body. They are board certified by the American Board of Plastic Surgery, which is associated with the American Society of Plastic and Reconstructive Surgeons (ASPRS). These doctors generally limit their practices to plastic surgery.

**Cosmetic surgery** generally refers to surgical procedures used for cosmetic purposes only.

**Reconstructive surgery** generally refers to surgical procedure techniques used to correct noncosmetic abnormalities such as skin cancer removal, surgery needed due to accidental injury, and other physical deformities.

**General plastic surgeons** perform all types of plastic, reconstructive, and cosmetic surgery.

**Facial plastic surgeons** specialize in plastic surgery of the face, head, and neck.

**Facial plastic surgeons** specialize in plastic surgery of the face, head, and neck. They generally do not perform body surgery. They are usually trained in otolaryngology, the specialty area of medicine that treats diseases of the ears, nose, and throat, and surgery of the head and neck. Their professional association is called the American Academy of Facial Plastic and Reconstructive Surgeons. They may perform facial cosmetic or reconstructive surgery, but they may also perform surgery on the sinuses, ears, nose, and throat.

**Ophthalmic surgeons** are medical doctors who treat eye diseases and perform eye surgery.

**Ophthalmic surgeons** are medical doctors who treat eye diseases and perform eye surgery. They perform eyelid surgery, or reconstructive surgery involving the eyes.

**Dermatological surgeons** are dermatologists who also perform plastic or cosmetic surgery.

**Dermatological surgeons** are dermatologists who also perform plastic or cosmetic surgery.

You should always work with surgeons who are board certified in their specialty areas.

# COMMON TYPES OF COSMETIC SURGERY

We will first discuss the various types of facial cosmetic surgery procedures. We will break these procedures into several subjects: symptoms of need for plastic surgery, discussion of the actual surgical procedure, suggestions for pre- and post-care treatment (salon treatment and home care recommendations for before and after surgery), makeup needs of the postoperative patient, and long-term needs of the patient.

*Warning: Do not perform services on any postoperative patient until the patient has been released and approved for esthetic treatment by the attending cosmetic surgeon or dermatologist! Treating a patient before or without the surgeon's approval or without proper training is dangerous and a tremendous legal risk.*

## Rhytidectomy

**Rhytidectomy** is the medical term for a face lift.

**Rhytidectomy** is the medical term for a face lift.

**Presurgical Facial Characteristics.** Presurgical facial characteristics include sagging skin with marked lack of elasticity, folds of skin in the jawline and neck area, jowls in the cheek and jawline area, and general lack of skin tone.

**Surgical Procedure.** Incisions are made in front of, or inside, the ears, following around the back of the ears, and into the hairline in the back of the head. After the incision is made, the face is literally "pulled up," and excess skin is clipped away. The underlying muscle structure may also be surgically altered, or excess fat may be removed. In some cases a small incision may have to be made under the chin. After the excess skin is removed, the skin is reconnected in the areas of the incisions and sewn together with materials called **sutures** (often called "stitches" by laypeople). In some cases surgical staples are used instead of suture material (Figure 21-1A–D).

**Sutures** are materials used in reconnecting areas of surgical incisions.

After surgery the face is very swollen and bruised. The head is wrapped in gauze dressing to provide support for the surgical area. The patient is instructed to keep the head elevated for several days, even when sleeping, to provide gravity for draining fluids. Skin discolorations, mainly due to bruising, are typical after surgery and may last for weeks. Some patients notice numbness in certain areas, particularly in front of the ears.

The sutures and dressings are removed a few days after surgery by the plastic surgeon. Most patients are pleasantly surprised by how little pain is associated with rhytidectomy, but any pain can be managed with medication. The skin may feel very tight at first, but generally feels better after a few weeks when the facial swelling has subsided.

**Mid-face lift** is a surgical procedure used to lift the middle section of the face.

A **mid-face lift** is a newer procedure that is usually performed at the same time as a regular face lift. Classic face lifting concentrates on affecting the jaw line and

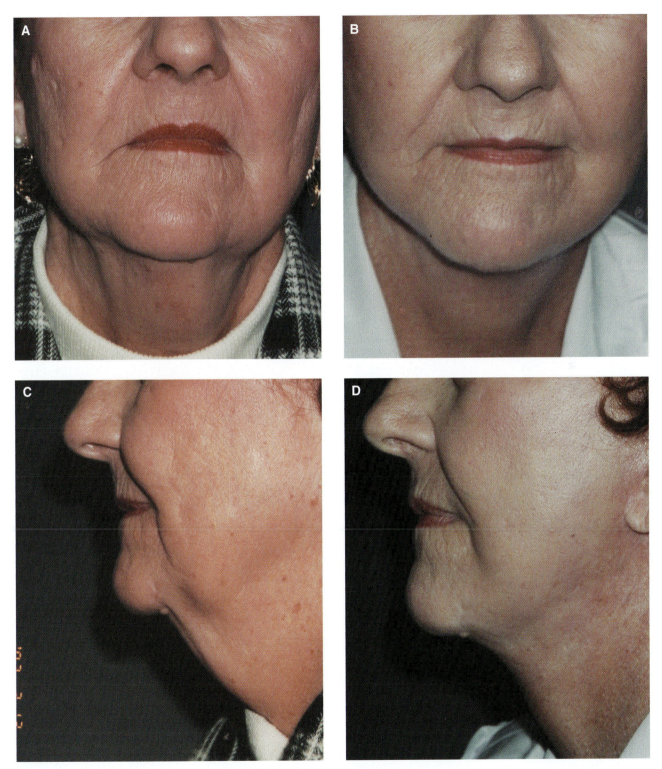

**Figure 22-1** Rhytidectomy, or face lifting, can dramatically improve the appearance of sagging facial skin and elastosis. A forehead lift has also been performed on this patient (Courtesy Samuel J. LaMonte, M.D.)

neck. The mid-face lift helps to give the patient a more uniform look after surgery by also altering the contour of the area just under the cheekbones and a lifting effect on the nasolabial folds.

The procedure for the mid-face lift involves the surgeon adjusting the muscle and skin from the cheekbone and repositioning the muscle in this area. This produces a more evenly distributed look to the lift procedure and in most cases looks more natural and is less likely to look "draped." Not only has the jaw line and neck been recontoured, the cheek area has been lifted as well. There is a little more down time and bruising associated with mid-face lifting as a result of the adjustment of the muscle and tissue around the cheekbones. Most patients, however, are very pleased with the results (Figure 22-2A–F).

**Pretreatment for the Lift Patient.** The same pretreatment procedures are followed for blepharoplasty, rhytidectomy, and forehead lift. Ideally, treatment should begin at least three months before surgery. Treatments should be administered weekly or biweekly for a minimum of six treatments. The purpose of these treatments is to thoroughly cleanse the skin, to improve circulation through massage and electrical treatment, and to have the skin in the best condition before surgery. Skin that is in prime condition before surgery will most often look better after surgery, and the good condition will aid healing.

Before starting the treatment program, you should talk to the client extensively about plans for the surgery, including the dates of the surgery. Plan your treatment schedule around the date of the actual surgery. You should explain all the benefits of skin treatment in general, as well as how important it is for the patient to take perfect care of the skin before and after the surgery, and emphasize the need for ongoing care after the surgery is completed. You should give the client realistic expectations of

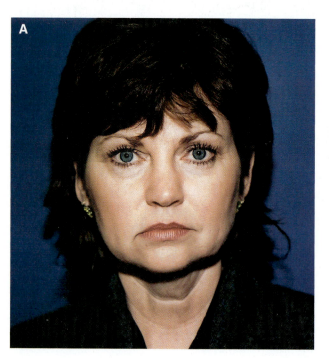
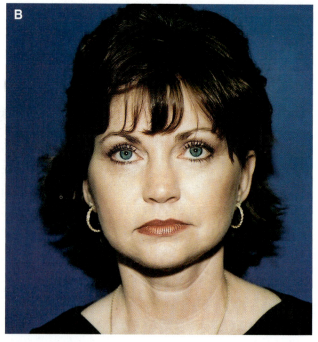

**Figure 22-2** This patient had a both a face lift and mid-face lift, upper and lower eyelift, facial liposuction, and an endoscopic forehead lift. She also had her neck muscles resculpted for a much more youthful look. This series of before and afters is a good example of how natural looking results in facial rejuvenation can be achieved with good plastic surgery (Courtesy Derek A. Jones, M.D., F.A.C.S.)

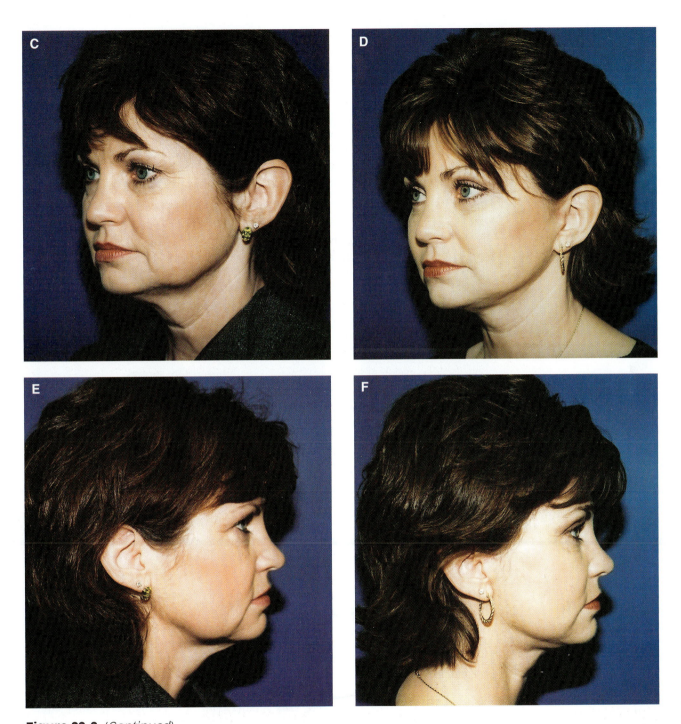

**Figure 22-2** (*Continued*)

what you will accomplish and the differences between what the surgeon and the esthetician will do to improve the appearance of the skin and face.

1. To begin treatment, thoroughly cleanse the face.
2. Thoroughly examine the face under a magnifying lamp, making notes of all problems, especially conditions that will not be improved by plastic surgery, such as comedones, milia, fine wrinkles, hyperpigmentation, rough, dehydrated areas, etc. Type the skin and write up a detailed analysis as you would for any new client.

Regardless of the surgery, you should treat the skin as you always would for the analyzed condition. Design treatment based on the examination. Client home care will also be directly related to the analysis, as always.

3. Begin the procedure by using the steamer on the skin for eight to ten minutes. During the steam you may apply an exfoliating treatment if necessary. Scrub creams are frequently helpful, provided the skin is suitable for scrubs. Brushing may be used over a layer of hydrating fluid. Using hydrating fluid during steam can greatly help to soften a rough-textured surface. If the skin is oily, apply a desincrustant pre-mask to the skin to help soften comedones and sebaceous filaments. Enzyme exfoliation may also be helpful to this type of skin.

4. After steaming, proceed with galvanic desincrustation (assuming there are no contraindications) to all areas with comedones, sebaceous filaments, or other impactions. Oil-dry (alipidic), poreless areas of the skin should not be treated with galvanic desincrustation.

5. Begin extraction of any impacted areas. Be thorough, but do not perform more than ten minutes of extraction in one visit.

6. After extraction, apply a toner with an antiseptic.

7. Apply a lightweight, noncomedogenic hydrating fluid to the face and begin a thorough massage appropriate for the skin type. Oily skin should not be excessively massaged, nor should areas that are still clogged. A good facial massage will be excellent for improving the circulation before surgery.

8. Apply more hydrating fluid and apply high frequency to the skin with the mushroom electrode for two to three minutes.

9. Apply a mask appropriate for the skin type. You may need to use more than one mask, such as a cleansing clay mask for the oily areas and a soft-setting gel or cream mask for dry areas. After the setting time has passed, remove the mask and apply a moisturizer with sunscreen.

**Home Pre-Care.** The main difference between this home care procedure and that of a regular client is that the client must be very diligent about performing home care daily. Not enough emphasis can be placed on good routine home care. You should mention that home care may need to be altered after surgery depending on the case and the surgeon's wishes.

**Bruising and Vitamin K.** Vitamin K is a fat-soluble vitamin necessary for proper clotting of the blood. Topical vitamin K creams are now available. These are used to treat bruising of all types on all body areas and telangiectasias and distended capillaries, and they are also used as a presurgical treatment to help prevent and reduce bruising from plastic surgery. These creams are available to the esthetician to sell and recommend to their clients.

For two weeks before facial surgery, the vitamin K cream should be applied daily or twice daily to all areas that will be affected by bruising during surgery. This includes surrounding areas as well as areas where incisions will be made. After surgery and with the surgeon's approval, vitamin K can continue to be used in areas of bruising, but should not be used on incisions until they are completely healed and approved for use by the surgeon.

**Postsurgical Skin Care.** Immediate post-care for the patient will be handled by the surgeon. The client should check with the surgeon to see when regular home care can resume.

After the client has been given the approval by the surgeon to continue home care, the client should be instructed to be extremely gentle with the skin, being careful not to pull on the skin or apply significant pressure to the suture areas. Light massage at home, always using a hydrating fluid, will help dissipate bruising. Instruct your client how to perform light effleurage and tapotement (piano massage) to the face nightly.

**Post-Care Salon Treatment.** Never begin treatment of a postsurgical client without the approval of a plastic surgeon. After you have established a good working relationship with a plastic surgeon, you should sit down and discuss both of your expectations for post-care of the patients he or she sends you. The plastic surgeon may establish a general set of rules for administering postsurgical treatment to patients. You will both be fully informed of each others' procedures and precautions. The patient should not have treatment while sutures are still in the skin, unless otherwise directed by the surgeon. Be extremely gentle with all facial procedures. The client may still be sensitive from the surgery, and you do not want to pull on the suture areas or apply firm pressure, especially immediately after surgery. Generally, salon treatment can resume about two to three weeks after surgery.

The main objectives of post-care are to help improve the circulation, reduce swelling, and dissipate any discolorations from bruising. Long-term goals of postsurgical treatment are to improve the texture and appearance of the surface of the skin, putting the "icing on the cake" by routinely providing care to improve the surface appearance.

Assuming the patient has approval from the surgeon, the following is a typical postsurgical treatment:

1. Apply liquid cleanser to the face with gloved hands, using very gentle application movements. Use very soft facial cloths, sponges, or cotton pads to remove the cleanser, being careful not to pull on the skin too much.

2. Apply a light hydrating fluid to the skin and allow it to be steamed for about eight minutes. Cool steam is a good choice if the client has redness present.

3. Remove the hydrating fluid and examine the skin under a magnifying lamp. Check for bruised areas and look carefully at the suture areas. In general, suture areas should be avoided during treatment.

4. If there is a lot of surface flaking, apply a diluted nondrying exfoliator, such as honey and almond scrub, and gently massage, removing the scrub with the same careful technique. Avoid using brushing or suction immediately after surgery. Wait about three months before using these techniques after rhytidectomy.

5. Any extraction should be very minimal. In general, unless there are large open comedones, extraction should be avoided at this particular time.

6. Apply a lightweight hydrating fluid and begin a thorough but gentle massage, using light effleurage and tapotement. Avoid petrissage, rolling, friction, or any rough type of massage. Plenty of hydrating fluid should be used to keep the skin slippery during the massage, which helps to avoid excessive pulling. Concentrate on the eyes and neck, using gentle, circular effleurage movements.

7. Apply more hydrating fluid and apply high frequency with the mushroom electrode set at a very low intensity. Move around the face in small, gentle, circular movements for about three to four minutes.

8. Apply a nonsetting, nonstimulating mask, or apply a thick coat of hydrating fluid. It is very important that whatever you put on the face is easy to remove. Setting masks and thicker creams may be more difficult to remove, causing you to pull on the face more than normal.

9. After the mask has processed for ten minutes, wet it well using a spray of cool toner to help loosen it for removal. Remove the mask gently using soft facial cloths, sponges, or cotton pads. Apply a moisturizer-protectant appropriate for the skin type with sunscreen.

10. Although it is best to avoid makeup immediately after treatment, this may be impossible for the plastic surgery patient. Be understanding and help her with

makeup after treatment. Do not start any "new" treatments on the client immediately after surgery. There is a rare possibility of allergic reaction, particularly with new products that the client has not tried. Do not recommend new products for home use at this point. Wait until the healing process is further along to start any new procedures.

**Makeup Needs.** The postsurgical rhytidectomy patient will likely experience extensive bruising. Many patients who undergo extensive presurgical skin care at home and in the salon seem to have less bruising and any bruising seems to dissipate faster.

Bruises are the main problem immediately after surgery. As soon as the surgeon approves, the esthetician may help the client with camouflage makeup for the bruising. You should make available to the client a heavy coverage camouflage makeup to help conceal the bruises. The bruising usually occurs under the eyes, on the lids, in a half-moon pattern on the upper cheeks, in front of the ears, and sometimes along the jawline and neck.

Prepare the skin in the normal manner. Yellow toner may help conceal purple bruises. You may wish to apply a layer of amber or yellow toner before applying the coverage.

Apply the coverage makeup with dabbing movements using a latex makeup sponge. Blend in the edges with the client's normal foundation. As the patient heals, bruises will start to change color as the blood is absorbed by the body. Bruising also tends to shift with gravity—that is, bruises that start on the jawline may slowly seem to move down the neck and decollete, and occasionally onto the chest. During this time there may be variation in color, ranging from normal black-purple bruising to yellow or green. Apply the proper color toner to help neutralize the colors.

After the bruising has totally subsided and the suture lines have healed completely, have a second makeup lesson with the client and teach her to cover the incision scars. Work with her hairstylist to establish a good hairstyle that will help conceal the scars from the incisions. This is particularly necessary in front of the ears. Occasionally, a plastic surgery patient will experience a small amount of hair loss in the surgical area, and sometimes hair areas from above the ears end up in back of the ears. Again, the skills of a good hairstylist are very important.

Within a few months of surgery, after all swelling has subsided, the client should have a new makeup lesson, teaching her how to best complement her new look, emphasizing the new contours that the surgeon has created.

**Long-Term Needs.** The main long-term need is great skin care! Clients will often be interested in new products and treatments to improve the look created by the surgery. Most patients are very interested in protecting their "investment" by taking good care of their skin.

## Blepharoplasty

**Blepharoplasty** is the surgical procedure for "lifting" the eyes and removing excess skin from the eye area.

**Presurgical Facial Characteristics.** These characteristics include puffiness, bags under the eyes, and drooping or flapping upper lids. Sometimes the drooping of the upper lids is so dramatic that it actually interferes with the patient's vision.

**Surgical Procedure.** The patient is anesthetized or sedated. Incisions are made in the normal fold of the upper lid, and excess skin is trimmed away. The suture line is made in the actual fold of the lid, rendering it practically invisible when it heals.

Lower lids are corrected by making an incision in the lower lash line. The fat pocket in a "bag" is removed, and, again, the excess skin is trimmed away and sutured

**Blepharoplasty** is the surgical procedure for "lifting" the eyes and removing excess skin from the eye area.

along the lower lash line. Newer procedures now often allow the lower lid to be corrected from the inside of the lid, completely eliminating outside incisions.

The brows are lifted by making an incision in the lower part of the browline. Excess skin and fat is removed from this area as well. More and more patients are having a **forehead lift** at the same time as their eyes are corrected. Much of the sagging of the upper lid may be attributed to elastosis in the forehead. In a forehead lift, an incision is made about an inch back into the hairline. The excess skin is removed from the hairline incision, simultaneously lifting the brow area. Forehead lifts may be a problem in persons with extremely high foreheads or in men who have receding hairlines or male pattern baldness, because the scars will not be concealable (Figure 22-3A–D).

**Endoscopic forehead lifting** is a newer procedure in which small incisions are made several inches back into the scalp and special suture materials are attached to the forehead; essentially the forehead is pulled up using these special suture "cords." The suture material is secured. The advantage to this procedure is that the hairline is not directly adjusted, and there is no suture scar in the forehead hairline, as there is in a traditional forehead lift. The only different possible side effect of endoscopic forehead lifting is numbness in the area of the incisions in the mid-scalp. This numbness usually subsides over time (Figure 22-4).

**Pretreatment.** The same basic procedure is followed as is already outlined in the pretreatment section for rhytidectomy.

**Home Pre-Care.** Use the same procedures as for rhytidectomy patients.

**Postsurgical Skin Care.** Follow the same post-treatment recommendations for post-rhytidectomy patients. Mild massage of the lids, after they have healed and with

**Forehead lift** is a surgical procedure that helps to correct elastosis of the forehead and lift the brows.

**Endoscopic forehead lifting** is a surgical procedure used to lift the forehead area by working from small incisions made farther back into the scalp.

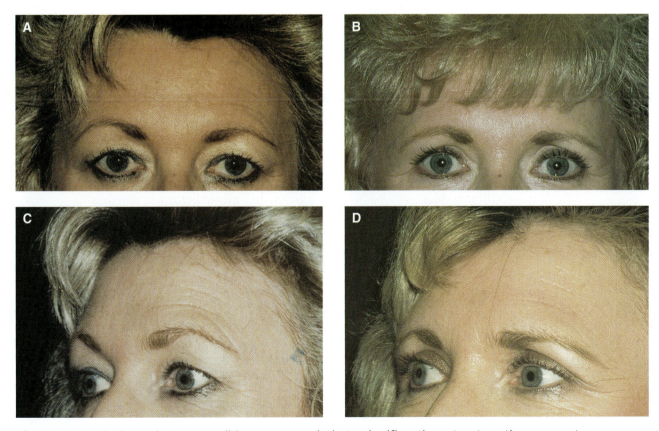

**Figure 22-3** Blepharoplasty, or eyelid surgery, can help to significantly restructure the eye contours, achieving a more alert, youthful look (Courtesy Samuel J. LaMonte, M.D.)

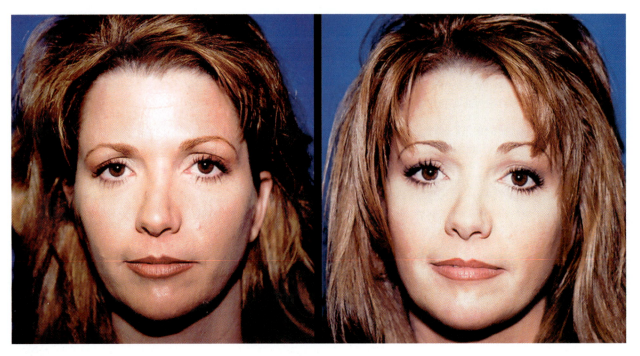

**Figure 22-4** This patient had an endoscopic forehead lift, with a blepharoplasty (eyelift), achieving more youthful contours in both the forehead and eye areas (Courtesy Derek A. Jones, M.D., F.A.C.S.)

the surgeon's approval, may help to dissipate discoloration from bruising and swelling. Makeup needs will be the same.

A patient may occasionally choose to have only a forehead and eye lift, without a general face lift. Although this is sometimes appropriate, particularly in young individuals who only have eyelid drooping and puffiness, in most cases, general face lifting is also necessary. Most plastic surgeons will encourage these clients to proceed with face lifting at the same time as the corrective procedure for the eyes.

**"Thread Lifting."** **Thread lifting** is a less invasive procedure for lifting the skin of the cheeks and jaw line and is sometimes used for the eye area. Commercially known as "contour threads" or "featherlifting," this procedure uses a needle to insert a barbed thread into the skin of the treated area. The barbs "anchor" the skin tissue, allowing the doctor to "pull up" the skin and attach it to a hidden base area with a suture.

The advantages of this procedure are that it is less invasive; requires very little downtime; is less expensive; and is a quick, usually in-office procedure. The disadvantages are that the procedure does not alter the muscles of the face, which normally need re-contouring in aged skin, and the results are relatively short-term. It also does not remove the excess skin (Figure 22-5A–F).

## Rhinoplasty

Rhinoplasty is the term for surgically altering the nose. Commonly called a "nose job," many clients of many different ages request this procedure. In an older individual, a rhinoplasty may make the entire face look younger, particularly if the nose is "drooping."

**Presurgical Facial Characteristics.** This will vary in the rhinoplasty procedure. The nose may be crooked, too long, too short, upturned, or drooping. In many cases rhinoplasty is medically necessary to correct internal blockages of the breathing passages caused by chronic sinus problems or a deviated septum (Figure 22-6A–D).

**Thread lifting** is a less invasive procedure for lifting the skin of the cheeks and jaw line.

**Surgical Procedure.** An incision is made inside the nostrils. The bones of the nose are reshaped using special surgical tools. The nose is then "redraped" over the new bone structure. Occasionally, excess skin and cartilage is removed, and any internal problem affecting breathing is corrected. After surgery a splint is placed on the nose, which is removed after a few days. The nose will be quite swollen immediately after the surgery. Swelling may last for weeks after surgery, and results cannot be assessed until the swelling has completely subsided.

**Pretreatment.** In the salon, the follicles of the nose should be cleaned routinely before surgery. It is advisable for the client to have about six weekly or biweekly treatments, concentrating on deep cleansing as well as general skin care. The same

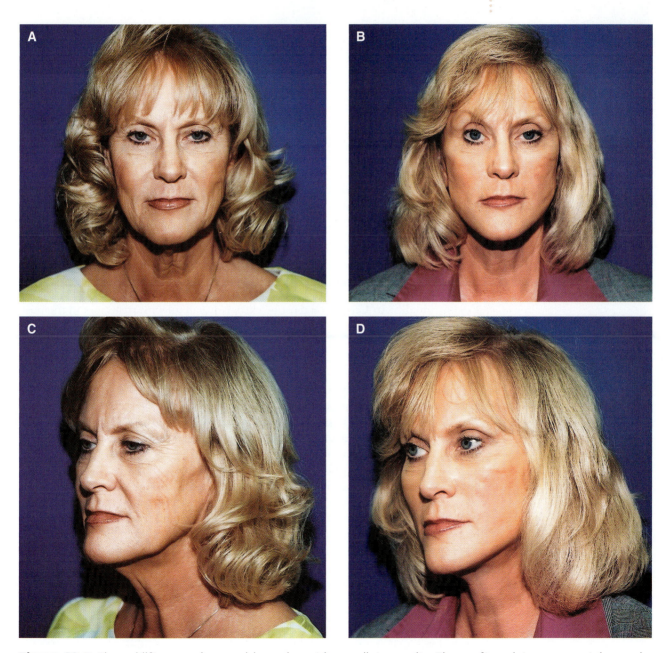

**Figure 22-5** Thread lift procedures achieve almost immediate results. These after pictures were taken only 3 days after the procedure. The patient had threads placed in the brows, cheeks, jowls, and neck (Courtesy Derek A. Jones, M.D. F.A.C.S.)

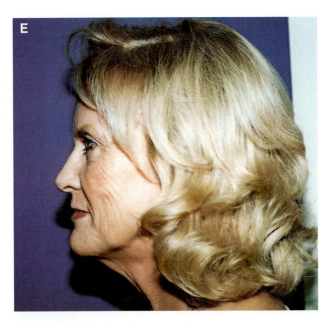
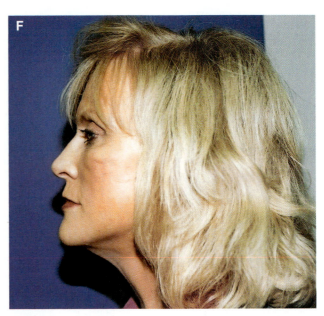

**Figure 22-5** *(Continued)*

procedure should be followed as for rhytidectomy, outlined earlier in this chapter. If the general skin of the face is in excellent shape, the skin in general will be in better condition for healing.

**Home Pre-Care.** Again, the procedure is the same used for rhytidectomy patients. You may recommend that the client apply a deep cleansing mask to the nose, especially clients with extremely oily skin, with many clogged follicles on the nose.

**Postsurgical Skin Care.** You must be extremely careful with treatment of the nose for several months after surgery. Remember, the bones have been reshaped, and no pressure should be applied. This is particularly important regarding extraction. Essentially, no extraction on the nose or on surrounding tissue should take place for several months after surgery.

In lieu of extraction, you may use enzyme treatment on the nose to help remove excess cell buildup. Comedones on the nose may be increased after surgery due to trauma, because of surgical dressings, and because cleaning the nose may be uncomfortable for the client. Use of enzyme peelings or desincrustant pre-masks on the nose will help to soften pore accumulations.

If this is followed by clay-based deep cleansing masks, improvement may be obtained without extraction on the nose area. The tissue around the nose and upper cheeks should be treated in the same manner. Use "wet" treatments—do not apply treatments that need to be rubbed or lifted off. Stick to fluid type treatments that can be easily removed. Clay-based masks should be thoroughly moistened before removal. After the clay mask dries, spray it with a cold spray of diluted toner to loosen and wet it before removal.

You may notice that the client is uncomfortable, even during massage and basic cleansing. Be very gentle when cleansing the nose area, and avoid any movements that pull upward on the nose.

Avoid the use of brushing or suction on the nose area. Galvanic desincrustation can be beneficial, but be careful with the amount of pressure used.

**Makeup Needs.** Because of swelling, clients may need help with contouring makeup to minimize the appearance of swelling, particularly during the first few weeks

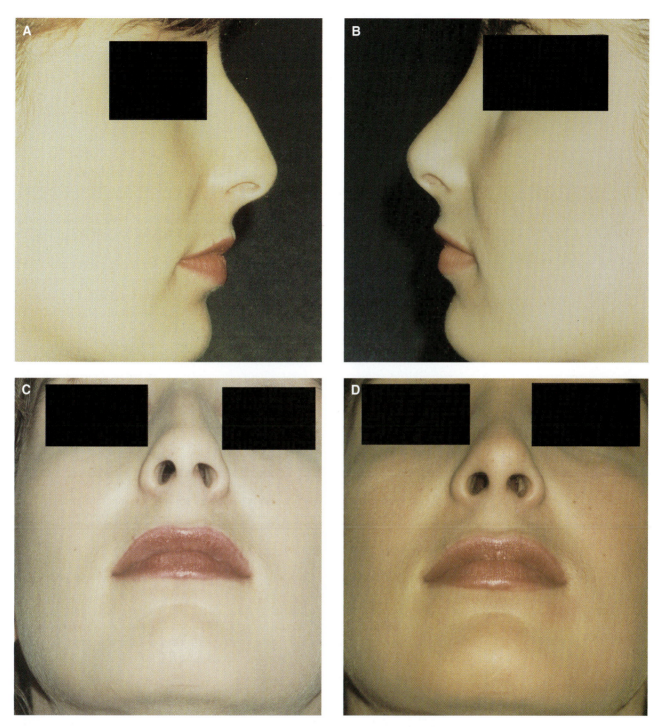

**Figure 22-6** These views feature the patient before and after a rhinoplasty. Note the reduction of the nasal bone protrusion, the straightening of the nostrils, and the softer look of the face in general after surgery (Courtesy Samuel J. LaMonte, M.D.)

after surgery. Bruising of the eyes and cheeks may occur. Use the same procedures outlined earlier in this chapter to help the client cover these areas.

**Long-Term Needs.** After several months have passed, you may proceed with extraction, being very careful and gentle. The client may need frequent treatments to help with clogged pores, especially while extraction is being avoided.

# Dermabrasion

**Dermabrasion** is the technique of reducing acne scarring; scar tissue; and, in some cases, wrinkles.

**Dermabrasion** is the technique of reducing acne scarring; scar tissue; and, in some cases, wrinkles (Figure 22-7A–D).

**Presurgical Facial Characteristics.** These characteristics are acne scarring, "icepick" scarring, "pock" marks from acne, hypertrophic (raised) scarring, and wrinkles in limited areas such as around the mouth.

**Surgical Procedure.** The patient is anesthetized or sedated. The surgeon uses a rotating attachment, similar to an esthetician's electric brush, except the attachment is an abrasive steel instrument. The skin is literally "sanded," and the tissue is "planed" to a low level, helping to smooth out imperfections.

Generally, only areas that are affected by the scarring are treated. Although the treatment sounds painful, most patients are surprised at how little pain is involved.

**Pretreatment.** This procedure probably requires the most intensive preoperative and postoperative salon treatment. Many dermabrasion patients are present or former acne sufferers, who often still have very oily, problem skin. If the acne has been or is cystic, the client should be seen by a dermatologist for treatment. It is vitally important to be sure that acne is not recurring before performing surgery. If the surgery is performed while cysts are still developing, the patient may risk more scarring after surgery.

Assuming the client has finished any dermatological treatment, treat the client as you would any acne or oily skinned client, using deep cleansing treatments routinely in the salon before the surgery. Frequent treatment, weekly or biweekly, before surgery is usually necessary. Follow the treatment program outlined in the chapter on acne. The ultimate goal is to have the skin completely clear, with oiliness under control, and as clean as possible before surgery.

**Home Pre-Care.** Again, follow the procedures outlined in the chapters on acne and comedogenicity. The client should use completely noncomedogenic products at home. Keratolytics such as salicylic acid, resorcinol, sulfur, glycolic acid, and benzoyl peroxide are useful before surgery. Because of the nature of the dermabrasion procedure, keratolytics must be discontinued after the surgery, until otherwise advised by the plastic surgeon or dermatologist.

**Postsurgical Skin Care.** During the dermabrasion procedure, the skin is traumatized, and this often results in multiple milia development. Sometimes dozens and dozens of milia appear after a dermabrasion. After the surgeon has approved your treatment of the skin, you may begin treatment of the milia. There is also a lot of redness usually present. Normally, treatment in the salon may resume three to four weeks after surgery. The following is a suggested treatment for post-dermabrasion clients with multiple milia:

1. Cleanse the face thoroughly with cleansing milk.
2. Steam the face with lukewarm steam over a layer of desincrustant pre-mask or solution. Do not use brushing, enzymes, or suction on the skin at this time.
3. Using a sterile lancet, begin extraction of the milia, which are usually very soft and easily removed. Do not perform this procedure unless you have been thoroughly trained in extraction of milia! Only extract for a few minutes, and discontinue immediately if redness seems to worsen. The skin is still erythemic from the surgery. You must be very careful not to traumatize the skin.
4. After extraction, spray the skin with an antiseptic toner solution.
5. Apply cold compresses to the extracted area. Allow to sit for 15 to 20 minutes.

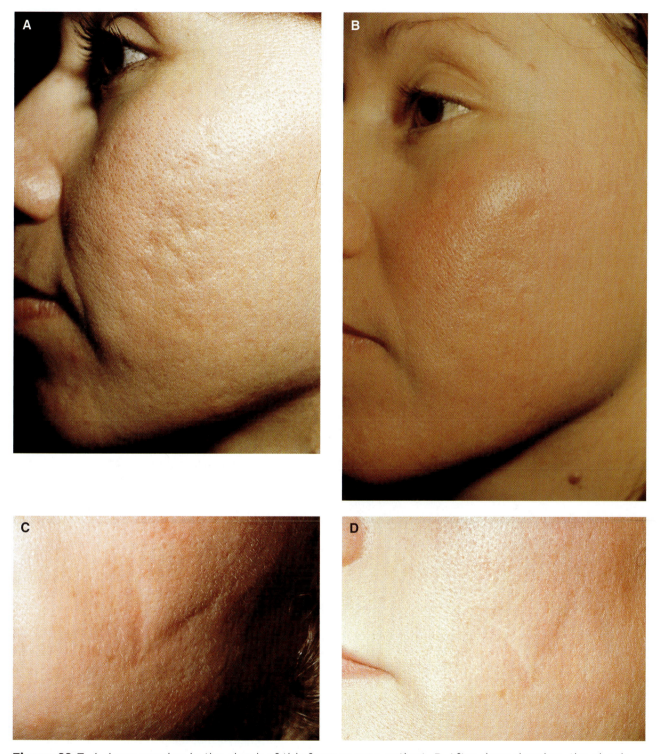

**Figure 22-7** *A*, Acne scarring in the cheek of this former acne patient. *B*, After dermabrasion, the cheek area is much smoother. *C*, This patient needed both dermabrasion and revision of this large surgical scar. *D*, Notice how much smoother the appearance

6. Do not apply tightening or abrasive masks to freshly dermabraded skin. The skin has already been exfoliated through the surgical procedure.

7. After compresses have set on the face for 15 to 20 minutes, remove them and apply a noncomedogenic moisturizer-protectant sunscreen.

Treatment for the milia may take several weeks. The client should visit for treatment either weekly or biweekly.

**Postsurgical Home Care.** Advise the client to use a rinseable cleanser, a mild toner, a protectant sunscreen, and a night hydrating fluid. Remember, you are still dealing with oily skin, but this oily skin has been severely exfoliated. Avoid the use of any keratolytic or peeling agents for at least the first eight or ten weeks, depending on the surgeon's recommendations. All home care should still be completely noncomedogenic, as it should be for any oily skin. You should explain the differences in home care to the client before the surgical procedure so that the client can anticipate and understand the need for the change of products.

**Makeup Needs.** The client will need help in concealing the redness caused by surgery. Using a green-colored toner and beige-based makeup is helpful in concealing the redness in the areas treated. The client's normal makeup can be blended into the outer nontreated areas. Remember to keep all makeup products noncomedogenic!

**Long-Term Needs.** After the initial post-treatment is completed, the milia have subsided, and the redness has diminished, the client generally has much smoother skin. The client should have a makeup lesson to learn to best complement the change in skin texture. The skin normally still has oily tendencies, and treatment should be adapted to the current conditions of the skin four to six months after surgery. At this time it may be appropriate to return to the keratolytic treatments previously used.

## Chemical Peeling

We have already discussed surgical chemical peeling. Here we will discuss only phenol-type peeling treatments administered by plastic surgeons or dermatologists.

**Presurgical Facial Characteristics.** These characteristics include multiple deep wrinkles and superficial lines in the areas to be treated. Treatment may be isolated to one or two areas, such as around the mouth. Many clients will often seek information about chemical peeling for acne scarring, but dermabrasion is the most commonly used procedure for acne scarring. Chemical peeling can also be used for medicinal purposes to treat recurring skin cancers and pre-cancers.

**Surgical Procedure.** After sedating the patient, the plastic surgeon paints the affected areas of the face with a phenol solution. The patient is closely monitored. The face may or may not be taped with adhesive-like tape strips. The tape, if used, is removed within a few days of the procedure. The skin looks very red and scabbed at this point. Patient discomfort is common and is controlled by prescribed medication. The doctor will often recommend a special ointment to keep the skin lubricated at this point.

**Pretreatment.** Salon pretreatment should begin about twelve weeks before the treatment. Treatment every two weeks is typical. Several layers of skin are actually "burned off" during phenol peeling. The main reason for treatment is to have the skin in the best shape possible before surgery. Postoperative care, and particularly makeup, is often more important in the phenol peeling patient.

**Home Pre-Care.** This procedure is designed for the sun-damaged, but sensitive skin.

**Postsurgical Skin Care.** Extensive redness is typical for several weeks after chemical phenol peeling. Treatment should not begin in the salon until approved by the surgeon, usually about three weeks after surgery. All keratolytic and exfoliating treatments should be completely avoided, unless otherwise recommended by the surgeon.

Use an extremely gentle, soothing treatment. Avoid the use of any scrubs, peels, or stimulating treatment. Cool aloe compresses are often used as a mask. The primary purpose of esthetic treatment for postoperative peel patients is to help with redness. Effleurage and very light tapotement are the only massage movements that should be used. Masks should be gels or liquid hydrating treatments that do not tighten and can be easily removed. Milia may form during healing, similarly to dermabrasion but usually not as severe. Patients who have received chemical peeling often need more emotional support than other plastic surgery patients. The skin may be red for weeks after surgery, and hypopigmentation is sometimes a side effect. The skin may appear grainy, and pores may appear larger than before surgery. The client will need esthetic help to minimize these problems with proper skin care or makeup.

See the upcoming section on treatment for post-laser patients for step-by-step treatment instructions.

**Post-Home Care.** The client, with the surgeon's approval, should use very mild cleansers, usually milks or liquid rinseable cleansers followed by a mild, nonalcoholic toner. Sunscreen must be used. Skin often no longer tans after a chemical peel, making routine use of sunscreen a must. Hydrating products that are fragrance-free are the best bet.

Creams with soothing ingredients such as dipotassium glycyrrhizinate, green tea extract, or bisabolol help minimize redness. The client, again, should avoid scrubs or any sort of peeling or exfoliating products!

Home care for post-chemical peel patients is similar to that for post-laser patients. See the upcoming section on post-laser home care for more information.

**Makeup Needs.** Plastic surgeons frequently refer chemical peel patients for makeup lessons to help conceal the redness after a chemical peel and to help the patient conceal any lines of demarcation that may be present as a result of the peel treatment. Application of a green-colored toner after proper skin preparation will help neutralize redness. Then apply a liquid foundation, carefully matching the patient's neck color. In some cases cream makeup may provide better coverage, but liquid generally looks more natural if it is feasible to cover with a liquid. Teach the client to carefully blend in any lines of demarcation, such as darker areas that have not been treated by the chemical peel. Makeup designs that focus attention on the eyes may help draw attention away from other treated areas of the face.

**Long-Term Needs.** Besides good general skin care, the chemical peel patient will need help with the aforementioned possible side effects of the peel.

Phenol peeling is most often recommended for seriously sun-damaged, wrinkled, and leathery skin. Although the peel procedure does seem to tighten the face, it is not a substitute for a face lift. The phenol peel is often reserved for patients who need serious help because of severe wrinkling and rough texture from sun damage. The possible side effects of phenol peelings must be considered acceptable risks for this sun-damaged skin.

# ESTHETIC MANAGEMENT OF THE POST-LASER PATIENT

The following information is condensed from an article written by the author for *Les Nouvelles Esthetiques—American Edition.* The author wishes to thank Les Nouvelles Esthetiques for its cooperation in reprinting this information (Figure 22-8).

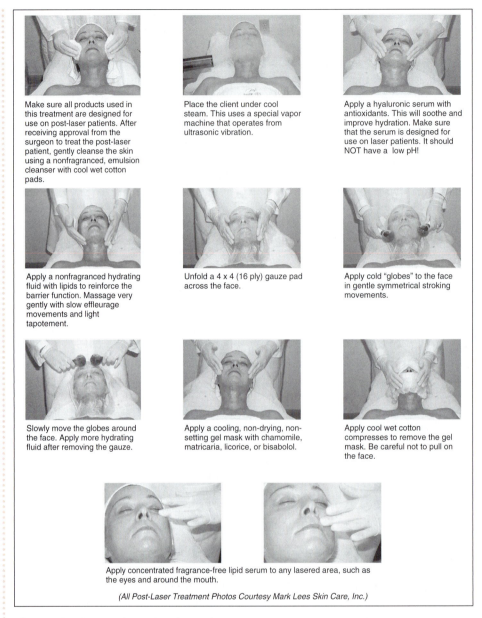

Make sure all products used in this treatment are designed for use on post-laser patients. After receiving approval from the surgeon to treat the post-laser patient, gently cleanse the skin using a nonfragranced, emulsion cleanser with cool wet cotton pads.

Place the client under cool steam. This uses a special vapor machine that operates from ultrasonic vibration.

Apply a hyaluronic serum with antioxidants. This will soothe and improve hydration. Make sure that the serum is designed for use on laser patients. It should NOT have a low pH!

Apply a nonfragranced hydrating fluid with lipids to reinforce the barrier function. Massage very gently with slow effleurage movements and light tapotement.

Unfold a 4 x 4 (16 ply) gauze pad across the face.

Apply cold "globes" to the face in gentle symmetrical stroking movements.

Slowly move the globes around the face. Apply more hydrating fluid after removing the gauze.

Apply a cooling, non-drying, non-setting gel mask with chamomile, matricaria, licorice, or bisabolol.

Apply cool wet cotton compresses to remove the gel mask. Be careful not to pull on the face.

Apply concentrated fragrance-free lipid serum to any lasered area, such as the eyes and around the mouth.

*(All Post-Laser Treatment Photos Courtesy Mark Lees Skin Care, Inc.)*

**Figure 22-8** Post-laser treatment

## Laser Surgical Procedures

Plastic surgery, like many other fields, is benefiting from advanced technology. The best current example is the popularity of lasers for skin resurfacing. Lasers are basically very concentrated stream forms of polarized light. In laser resurfacing, the laser is used to retexturize the surface of the skin, literally vaporizing layers of skin. This helps to "plane down" wrinkles and, if "full-face" laser is performed, it does have a slight firming effect on the face.

Lasers can be used for surface lines and wrinkles and minor scarring. For shallow imperfections, lasers are good alternatives to surgical chemical peeling, because the penetration level is easier to control. The depth of the procedure is controlled by how many "passes" the patient has, or basically how many times the surgeon passes across particular areas of the face.

There are two types of lasers currently being used for resurfacing: carbon dioxide ($CO_2$) and erbium. The $CO_2$ laser is generally stronger and is a better choice for deeper wrinkles and more severe sun damage. $CO_2$ cannot be used on the neck, however, because the skin on the neck is not as thick as facial skin. The erbium laser is primarily used for a "refreshening" procedure, in younger clients or clients with less severe wrinkling. The two types of laser are used in combination by some surgeons. Some surgeons also use a laser at the same time as when performing another procedure such as rhytidectomy or face lift. Lasers can also be used on particular areas such as around the mouth and eyes. Patients can experience many cosmetic side effects during recovery from laser surgery. The esthetician can play a significant role in the management and control of these esthetic side effects.

**Pretreatment.** The surgeon will generally meet with the patient several weeks before the surgery. Medical pre-care varies from doctor to doctor but generally consists of use of either Retin-A or an alphahydroxy acid home care product coupled with a melanin suppressant such as a 4 percent hydroquinone preparation.

# PROCEDURES FOR THE ESTHETICIAN

## Before Surgery

The esthetician should meet with the client and establish a plan of treatment. This may vary slightly with the particular individual needs of the patient and the procedures being performed. For example, laser resurfacing may accompany a blepharoplasty, or a partial resurfacing may be performed with a face lift. Some patients will elect to only have their perioral or periocular regions resurfaced.

Typically, the esthetician should perform at least one deep cleansing procedure, carefully removing impactions, comedones, or milia. Some patients will require more than one session for cleansing, again depending on individual needs.

A series of treatments performed weekly for six weeks before surgery can be very helpful in optimizing the health of the skin. This should consist primarily of light exfoliation using 30 percent alphahydroxy acid, which will help remove dead cell buildup and dislodge clogged follicles.

The mission of pre-care is to have the skin in top shape before the resurfacing, theorizing that skin that is in excellent condition will heal better and have fewer potential complications than skin that is in poor condition.

On the last visit before the resurfacing, the esthetician should consult with the client and instruct her in her step-by-step postoperative home care program, making sure that the client has all the products she needs. A camouflage makeup shade should be chosen and the client should have very basic instructions on how to use this product. As previously mentioned, a more involved makeup lesson should be performed two to three weeks after the resurfacing to individualize the technique for the particular case.

## After Surgery

**Laser Patient Referral.** The plastic or dermatological surgeon generally refers patients after any sutures are removed, usually around eleven to twelve days post-laser, and after the skin is sufficiently re-epithelialized and no longer raw, to reduce any risks of infection or poor healing. *It is only with the surgeon's approval that the esthetician should proceed with esthetic treatment.*

The esthetician will evaluate the individual case for skin type, age of the patient, amount of redness, dryness, discomfort, and areas of treatment. A good esthetician should also be trained to recognize conditions such as infection that should be referred back to the surgeon (Figure 22-9A–F).

## Case Studies in Post-Laser Care

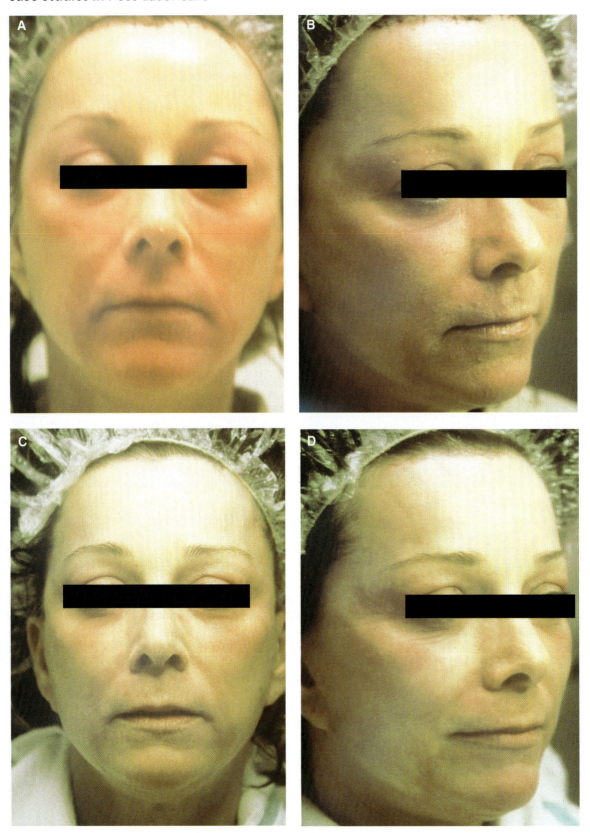

**Figure 22-9**

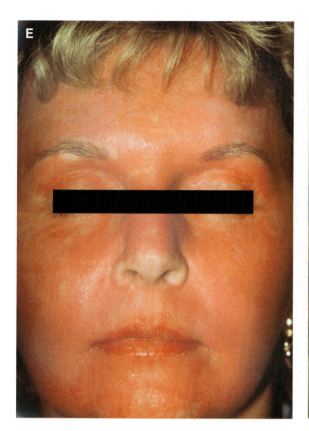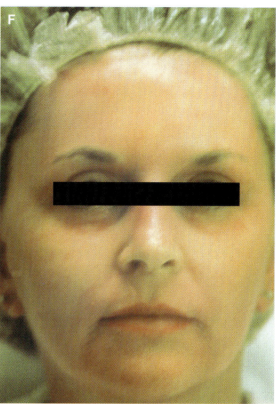

**Figure 22-9** *A,* The patient arrived 11 days post-CO$_2$ laser resurfacing, concerned with extreme redness and dry, tight skin. *B,* The patient complained of extreme tightness around the mouth, and dryness was evident from crusty flaking above the upper lip. The patient was instructed in the use of proper camouflage makeup and how to achieve as natural a look as possible. The patient was instructed to use a fragrance-free moisturizer along with a lipid-based serum to increase hydration. The patient was also instructed in proper cleansing of the skin, using a nonfoaming gentle cleanser. A facial treatment using a lipid-based hydrator with hyaluronic acid and sodium PCA and a gentle steam treatment to increase hydration were administered. Cool steam was applied over which high-frequency current was applied to provide a gentle massage. After this, cold cryogenic globes were applied over gauze. These are special glass or Pyrex® balls filled with cold refrigerant chemicals, like those used in chemical ice packs. Another layer of hydrator was applied over the entire face and allowed to sit for 20 minutes. After the treatment a lipid serum was applied. *C,* The patient experienced significantly lessened redness in five days. *D,* Flakiness and dryness were lessened and smoothness was achieved in five days. The patient reported ease of dryness and discomfort almost immediately. *E,* This patient had an extreme amount of redness after full-face CO$_2$ laser resurfacing and full face lift. She had an important engagement in only a few weeks and was very concerned about having a natural appearance for this event. Again, this patient was given the same hydrating cream, lipid serum, and gentle cleanser and was instructed in the use of camouflage makeup to cover the redness. *F,* The patient had tremendous improvement in only five days. Within a short period of time, she was able to discontinue the heavier camouflage makeup and return to the use of a lighter weight liquid makeup.

**Hyperpigmentation.** Hyperpigmentation is a problem for some patients following laser resurfacing. Generally, the lighter the skin of the patient, the less the hyperpigmentation problem or risk. Laser is not a good alternative for any patient who experiences hyperpigmentation easily.

Pre-care use of a prescribed 4 percent hydroquinone preparation helps reduce the likelihood of pigment problems after the procedure. Postoperative hyperpigmentation may also be avoided by the proper use of a broad-spectrum SPF-15 or higher daily-use sunscreen, which will be used routinely after the skin has healed. Management of any severe postoperative hyperpigmentation should be referred back to the surgeon.

**Redness.** Redness or erythema is typical of many resurfacing procedures, particularly laser resurfacing. This is one of the biggest, if not the biggest, concern of post-laser surgery patients and a side effect that the esthetician can help alleviate. Patients are anxious to get back to work and their normal lifestyle without appearing red and drawing attention to their situation.

Redness is easily covered with camouflage makeup for the short term, but in laser and chemical resurfacing patients, this redness can last for weeks, and in some cases, for months. Patients are very interested in reducing the redness, not just covering it up. The use of lipid-based products, antioxidant complexes, and effective hydrators can help reestablish the barrier function of the epidermis and minimize postoperative redness.

**Dryness.** The surgeon often prescribes an antibiotic ointment for the first few days after the laser procedure. Sometimes the surgeon will use a dressing such as Flexan® to protect the face.

After the dressing is removed, the surgeon will often recommend a heavy, occlusive, emollient, petrolatum-type product. This is to protect the skin with a barrier while the skin is reestablishing the epidermal tissue and the natural barrier function. Although these products definitely serve their purpose and are temporarily necessary, heavy, occlusive ointments are very sticky and oily and are not user-friendly. They cannot be used with makeup and are uncomfortable.

Dryness of the skin, particularly during the transitional period from the post-resurfacing patient's use of a heavier, occlusive emollient, and the return to a daily use moisturizer, can be aesthetically displeasing as well as uncomfortable for the patient. Patients frequently complain of tightness and discomfort, as well as unsightly flaking that can accentuate skin wrinkles or imperfections and add to difficulty in makeup application. Foundations tend to clump in areas of extreme dryness, adding to the patient's cosmetic problems, even with camouflage coverage makeups. This can actually draw attention to the area, rather than detract from it.

**Dehydration.** Because the surface layers have basically been removed, the skin must re-epithelialize to reestablish the various layers of the epidermis. While the skin is re-epithelializing, it has a very poor barrier function, which results in dehydration, sensitivity, and erythema. The skin feels and looks very dehydrated during this period. With the doctor's approval at the appropriate time after the procedure, the esthetician can help to properly hydrate the skin, reducing the feeling of tightness and easing the rough texture of severely dehydrated skin.

## Ingredients to Help Restore Barrier Function

The substance between the epidermal cells is referred to as the interstitial fluid, intercellular matrix, or cement. This substance is a complex mixture of lipids such as ceramides, sphingolipids and glycosphingolipids, phospholipids, cholesterol, and fatty acids, with hydrating water-binders called natural moisture factors (NMFs) such as sodium PCA. These combined ingredients in the proper proportions can help "patch the mortar between the bricks" in the intercellular matrix, which is essentially absent after laser resurfacing. This helps to reestablish the protective barrier function that keeps skin protected and well-hydrated and will significantly reduce redness following surgery. The use of products and serums based in lipid replacement ingredients, coupled with hydrating ingredients such as sodium hyaluronate, glycerin, or sodium PCA, can help mimic the natural barrier function, resulting in better hydrated, smoother, and more comfortable skin. The serums are often in a silicone base. These products can be lighter weight and much more user-friendly than cumbersome, heavy ointments.

Because freshly resurfaced skin tends to be much more sensitive and reactive than normal skin, it is very important that all products used on post-laser patients be fragrance-free to avoid sensitizing the skin. It is also very important that the products have been properly tested by an independent laboratory for irritancy.

## Treatment Methods

Use of in-office facial treatments can help minimize redness. These treatments involve the use of fragrance-free lightweight hydrating fluids using functional ingredients such as the aforementioned sphingolipids, glycosphingolipids, cholesterol, and phospholipids, along with hydrating ingredients such as glycerin, sodium PCA, and sodium hyaluronate. Light and gentle facial massage with a hydrating fluid, and the use of cold therapy or compresses, along with proper products can help reduce redness in a fairly short period of time. If you are certified in manual lymph drainage, this may be appropriate for post-laser patients. Soothing, nonhardening gel or cream mask treatments are implemented to increase moisturization and help remove dry, dead skin flakes gently. This treatment modality also reduces the appearance of dryness, tightness, and flaking and helps achieve the appearance of skin smoothness.

Proper home care instruction of the patient should include the use of a very mild, fragrance-free, low- or nonsurfactant (one that does not foam much) cleanser, because stronger surfactant cleansers can further irritate and add to the dryness. Use of a well-formulated antioxidant serum may also help soothe the redness and dehydration. Some vitamin preparations may not be appropriate, especially if they sting when applied or increase redness after application.

Routine use of a good hydrator with a concentrated lipid serum eases dehydration and flaking and decreases redness.

This combination of treatment products will also serve as a good pre-makeup treatment, allowing for smoother application of color cosmetics.

**Sun Protection.** Obviously, post-laser patients should have absolutely no direct sun exposure. They should do everything they can to protect their skin from the sun, and it doesn't hurt to remind them that sun is probably the reason they needed the laser in the first place!

Because of the irritancy potential of many absorbing sunscreen ingredients, sunscreen application is usually not advised for the first 18 to 21 days after laser surgery. If any sunscreen is used during this time, it should be a reflecting screen, such as one with micronized zinc oxide or titanium dioxide as an active ingredient.

After the epidermis is reestablished, about 18 to 21 days, the client should be instructed to use a broad-spectrum sunscreen SPF-15 or higher on a DAILY basis. This should be a routine part of their daily care for the rest of their lives. The easiest way to do this is to find a wearable facial moisturizer with a built-in SPF-15 sunscreen or block. Make sure the client understands that a little dab of sunscreen is probably not enough. Instruct the client to apply several dots to the face and neck and massage it in, allowing a few minutes for it to absorb before applying makeup. Don't forget the hands and arms, too—other very vulnerable spots for sun damage and sun-induced aging!

**Milia Formation.** Milia frequently develop during healing of resurfacing procedures. Estheticians are a great help in removing these unsightly cosmetic lesions, which are of much concern to the patient.

Freshly lasered skin is *very* fragile. Do not extract milia unless you have extensive experience in performing milia extraction and have the approval of the referring surgeon.

**Return to Normal Routine.** The client can return to the normal skin-care routine after two to three months. This is, of course, assuming that the client had an appropriate regimen established before surgery. Daily use of a mild effective cleanser, broad-spectrum SPF-15 sunscreen day cream, alphahydroxy acid products appropriate for the skin type, topical antioxidants, and lipid-based hydrators are all helpful in management of the aging skin. There is mounting evidence that these few procedures do help skin look younger and maintain the proper health of the skin.

**Ongoing Care.** The esthetician can help the patient with ongoing care and cosmetic and skin-care needs. Additional skin-care procedures can be added long after the skin has healed from surgery, further improving the appearance of the results of the surgery.

Makeup lessons after the immediate postoperative adjustment period can teach the patient how to best accentuate her new look and detract from any imperfections. The well-trained esthetician can further advise the patient on sun protection and keep the patient abreast of new developments in skin-care, makeup, and plastic surgery techniques that might be appropriate for the patient.

General skin-care instruction and help in selecting the right program for the client are important services, both for the short and long term. The licensed esthetician plays a very important role in management of postoperative cosmetic surgical side effects, health education skin-care instruction, and support for the patient's psyche as the patient returns to normal lifestyle.

## OTHER SURGICAL PROCEDURES

**Liposuction** is the term for surgical removal of fat deposits. The procedure uses a vacuum-like instrument that suctions away fat from areas such as the chin or the cheeks. Liposuction is often also used on the body, such as the hips and thighs. A small incision is made in the skin, and the instrument is inserted into the subcutaneous fat layer, where treatment is administered. Bruising is the main side effect of this procedure. Chin or cheek liposuction is often performed at the same time as a face-lift.

There are no specific additional preoperative or postoperative salon procedures for facial liposuction, except as already outlined for face lift surgery. Treatment of the incision areas should be avoided, and harsh massage should be avoided. Treatment, as always, should not begin until the surgeon approves.

**Implants** are used to improve the cheeks and chin. These are small "sacks" of silicone or saline (saltwater solution) that are implanted in the chin and cheek areas to improve low cheekbone appearance or receding chins. Avoid treating the area immediately after surgery, following the surgeon's recommendations. Implants are often performed at the same time as a face lift.

## Wrinkle Treatments

There are many treatments now available for treating and reducing the appearance of wrinkles. Most of these treatments are **fillers**, which means that they "fill in" the wrinkles being treated. Fillers are primarily designed for individual wrinkles in the normal facial expressions, such as brow wrinkles, forehead wrinkles, nasolabial folds, and crow's-feet around the eyes. Fillers are also used to "polish" results of cosmetic

---

**Liposuction** is the term for surgical removal of fat deposits.

**Implants** are used to improve the cheeks and chin.

**Fillers** are materials used to fill wrinkles and skin depressions by injection or implantation.

## Salon Treatment for Post-Laser Patients

*Before any salon procedure, you must have a direct referral and approval for treatment from the plastic surgeon! Do NOT treat the client without the surgeon's approval!*

1. Have the client complete a health history form, carefully checking for previous allergies, sensitivities, and other contraindications for treatment.

2. Seat the client and carefully examine her skin, *without cleansing first*. There is a chance that the client is not yet ready for treatment, and you must thoroughly examine and check for areas that are still healing. Normally, surgeons will refer the post-laser client around eleven to twelve days after the procedure. Clients should be ready if they have the surgeon's referral. Carefully observe and record areas of redness (erythema), rawness, dryness, dehydration, flaking, and milia. Should you notice any pus or strange-looking lesions, refer the patient back to the surgeon, or call the surgeon for advice.

3. If everything appears normal for postoperative condition, gently cleanse the skin with cool predampened cotton pads with a very gentle cleanser. After cleansing, apply a *nonfragranced* hydrating fluid that contains lipids and hydrating agents such as glycerin, hyaluronic acid, or sodium PCA. The skin should be slightly damp before application.

4. Place the client under (not hot) vapor. Cool steam is preferable. If warm vapor is used, focus it at least 18 inches away from the client's face. The point is to gently moisten the face, not to warm or stimulate it. Vapor should be administered for about five to eight minutes.

5. Gently wipe down the face again with fresh cool cotton pads. Apply more hydrating fluid and gently massage the face in long, gentle effleurage strokes. Do not use any stimulating massage movements. Gentle tapotement (piano movements) is appropriate.

6. Apply more hydrating fluid to ensure the skin is very moist and lubricated. Apply high frequency with the mushroom electrode at a low setting. Use circular movements for about two to three minutes. Stop immediately if the face reddens or if the client complains of discomfort.

7. Once again, apply hydration fluid over the face. Unfold a 4 × 4 gauze square and place across the face. Apply the cryoglobes in gentle circles across the face for about five to seven passes.

8. Apply more hydrating fluid, and then apply a cool wet cotton compress in three strips across the face. Allow this compress to stay on for five to ten minutes.

9. Gently remove any excess fluid with fresh cotton pads. Apply several drops of lipid serum over the entire face.

10. Depending on the redness level, you may apply makeup. However, if the skin is extremely red now or prior to treatment, or if this is the first treatment, it is often best not to apply makeup immediately after treatment. In many cases, it is better to deal with skin care on the first day and makeup instruction the next day.

surgery, improving small areas not affected by the surgery. Fillers are generally injected through an **intradermal** injection. Intradermal means "inside the dermis." The injections are specifically targeted to be deposited in the dermis itself.

**Collagen injections** are the oldest form of wrinkle filler. Commercially known as Zyderm®, Zyplast®, Cosmoderm®, or Cosmoplast®, the collagen in these treatments is obtained from bovine (cow) sources. The wrinkle depression in the dermis is "inflated"

**Intradermal** means inside the dermis, which is where collagen and other filler material may be injected to fill out hypotrophic scars, wrinkles, or pock marks.

**Collagen injections** are procedures performed by a plastic surgeon and involve injecting collagen into depression scars or wrinkles to reduce the appearance of the lesion.

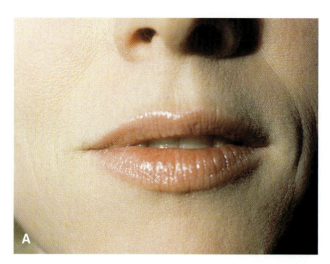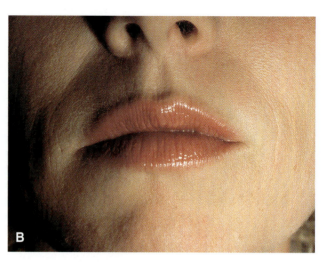

**Figure 22-10** *A*, Note the deep nasolabial folds on this patient. *B*, By injecting collagen, the surgeon achieves a remarkable reduction in wrinkles (Courtesy Kirk Smith, M.D.)

**Fat injections** are filling injections using the patient's own fat to fill depressions and wrinkles.

**Hyaluronic acid** commercially known as **Restylane**® and **Hylaform**®, is a filling material used for correcting wrinkles. Another type of hyaluronic acid is used in moisturizers and other skincare products.

**Botox**® is a drug treatment for wrinkles using a toxin derived from a normally deadly food bacterium. The toxin works by temporarily paralyzing specific muscles that create expression lines.

**Botulinum toxin (BTX)** is the toxin used in Botox®.

with the collagen, immediately reducing the appearance of the wrinkle. Besides the areas mentioned previously, fillers like collagen are also used to treat small hypotrophic (depressions) scars and pock marks (Figure 22-10A and B). Collagen is also injected in and around the lips to add fullness and to improve the outline of the lips.

Collagen injections require a skin test administered before the actual injection to make sure the client is not allergic to the collagen.

Slowly, over a few months, the body absorbs and rids itself of the collagen. Therefore, collagen injections must be repeated every few months.

Besides the potential allergic reaction, other side effects include temporary soreness and lumpiness in the area of the injection, which usually subsides over time. Esthetic treatment should be avoided in the area of the injection for at least one to two weeks. You may treat areas of the face not injected.

**Fat injections** are gaining popularity. The fat used in the injections is "harvested" or taken from other areas of the patient, often obtained from liposuction of the hips, legs, chin, and so on, and intradermally injected, similar to collagen injections. The advantage to fat injections is that there is never an allergy because the fat came from the patient's body. The disadvantage is that fat is absorbed relatively quickly and "overfilling" must take place to make the fat injection results last.

**Hyaluronic acid**, commercially known as **Restylane**® and **Hylaform**®, is another filler used to correct wrinkles. Hyaluronic acid and its derivative, sodium hyaluronate, are used in hydrating products for their strong water-binding capabilities. When injected into the dermis, they also bind water, further helping plump out the wrinkle. Hyaluronic acid injections are absorbed more slowly than collagen injections and are very unlikely to cause allergies.

Gortex® is a synthetic material that has been developed as a filler that is more permanent than collagen. This can be used in lipline or nasolabial injections.

## About Botox®

**Botox**® is a very popular treatment for relaxing wrinkles. Botox® is the commercial name for **botulinum toxin** (also referred to as **BTX**), derived from a toxin from the bacteria *Clostridium botulinum*. This normally dangerous bacterium produces the toxin that causes botulism, a type of often deadly food poisoning. The toxin is obviously very diluted for use in injectables.

Botox® was originally used to treat blepharospasms, or chronic tremors of the eyelid. The botulinum toxin causes paralysis of muscles, and in Botox® this paralysis

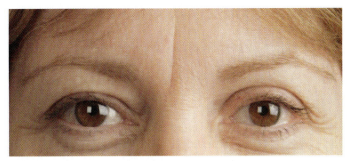

**A** Before

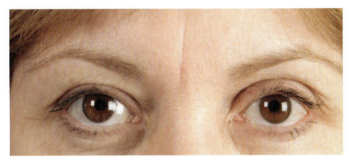

**B** After

**Figure 22-11** Unretouched clinical photos taken before BOTOX® Cosmetic and after treatment with BOTOX® Cosmetic at day 14. Results may vary (Reprinted with the permission of Allergan Corporation. All rights reserved)

is temporary as a result of the dilution of the toxin. When Botox® is injected into a muscle, it causes paralysis of the muscle. In the case of Botox®, this paralysis is temporary, usually lasting a few months.

Intrinsic facial wrinkling is caused from repeated facial expressions. Injection of Botox® into a muscle prevents contraction of the muscle, preventing certain facial expressions, which therefore softens the wrinkle. Botulinum injections are not effective for wrinkles that are not caused by normal facial expressions, such as multiple wrinkles in the cheeks from sun damage.

---

### Home Care for Post-Laser Patients

The first 11 to 12 days are directly supervised by the surgeon.

◆ Days 1 to 5—Antibiotic ointment

◆ Days 5 to 12—Occlusive (petrolatum) applied routinely

◆ Days 11 to 30—Gentle cleanser, soothing antioxidant serum, hydrating fluid, lipid serum

◆ Day 30—Return to normal routine as advised by the esthetician or surgeon

Sunscreen is usually not used until day 18 or until erythema is reduced. Sunscreens can be irritating or sensitizing to freshly lasered skin. Sun exposure must be totally avoided.

These are general guidelines and may vary with the patient or the surgeon.

**Glabella** is the muscle between the eyes that frequently causes expression lines in the forehead area. This area is frequently treated with Botox®.

**Permanent eyeliner** or **makeup** means "tattooing" a permanent eyeline or lipline. It can also be used in the cheek area, and occasionally to help correct dark, flat lesions, such as small, red macules.

Botox® is mainly used on and is most effective in the top half of the face, primarily for the "scowl" wrinkles between the eyes. The muscle injected is called the **glabella**. It is also used to treat forehead wrinkles and crow's-feet wrinkling. Some doctors use it to treat wrinkles in the lower half of the face; however, potential side effects are increased when used in the lower face (Figure 22-11A and B).

Obviously, the main side effect of botulinum injections is the inability to use certain muscles for particular facial expressions. Another side effect, although temporary and not common, is drooping of the eyelids, which is caused when the toxin is accidentally injected into the wrong muscle area.

Botox® injections must be repeated every few months to remain effective. Botox® is also used to treat excessive sweating and migraine headaches.

**Permanent eyeliner** or **makeup** is often performed by plastic surgeons, but in some states is legal for estheticians to perform. The procedure involves a "tattooing" type process that implants small amounts of pigment in the skin. The procedure is often used to create a permanent eyeline or lipline, but it can also be used in the cheek area and occasionally to help correct dark, flat lesions, such as small, red macules. Courses available through many schools teach permanent makeup. Check the laws in your state affecting permanent makeup.

Reconstructive surgery, as previously discussed, is used to help correct skin scars and abnormalities that are caused by accidents, disease, or congenital (birth) defects.

These procedures vary greatly, due to the many differences in the problems being treated. Plastic surgeons often remove facial skin cancers, using their skills to best conceal the demarcations from these treatments.

Often there is no time for pretreatment of these areas. The patient normally sees the esthetician after the surgery has occurred. Often seeking makeup help, the patient is frequently referred by the surgeon for help with concealing scars from the surgery. Sometimes several operations may have to take place to help revise scars from accidents or skin cancer. Makeup help may be required for coverage during and between these operations.

We will not discuss the correction of these types of scars here. The esthetician should take specialty courses in paramedical camouflage makeup in order to help these patients.

## REFERRALS

The plastic surgery candidate will often first seek counseling from the esthetician. Carefully evaluate the client's concerns, and then refer the client to a plastic surgeon. Because plastic cosmetic surgery is an elective procedure, the client will often want to think about the possibility of surgery for some time before proceeding.

You should have brochures available from your referring surgeon that briefly describe the various types of surgery. Plastic surgeons will gladly furnish these at no charge to you once you have established a working relationship. It is best to have relationships with several surgeons. Suggest to the client that they have consultations with at least two different surgeons, to make sure they feel comfortable with the doctor and to see pictures of the doctor's work. Secondly, referring a client to more than one doctor can reduce any liability you might encounter if, by chance, a client has a bad experience with the surgeon.

You should have a working understanding with the plastic surgeon of each other's procedures and needs. Prepare a presurgical and postsurgical brochure discussing esthetic procedures and how they help plastic surgery patients. Work with your plastic surgeon on this brochure, so that both of you are involved and are knowledgeable about typical procedures. When in doubt about treating a cosmetic or plastic surgery patient, always consult the doctor.

Many workshops and classes are available on paramedical makeup and working with plastic surgeons. You should take these courses to best prepare yourself for working with a plastic surgeon.

## TOPICS FOR DISCUSSION

1. What is the difference between cosmetic and reconstructive surgery?

2. What are the various types of physicians who perform plastic surgery?

3. What are some general postoperative skin-care procedures that should be avoided?

4. Why is it important for the plastic surgery patient to have presurgical skin-care treatments?

5. What should the esthetician do when there is a question about a treatment procedure for a plastic surgery patient?

6. Discuss preparing a brochure about esthetic treatment for a plastic surgery patient. Why is it important for both the esthetician and the plastic surgeon to be involved in preparing such a brochure?

7. Discuss the use of surgical lasers for resurfacing. What concerns of the laser patient must be handled by the esthetician?

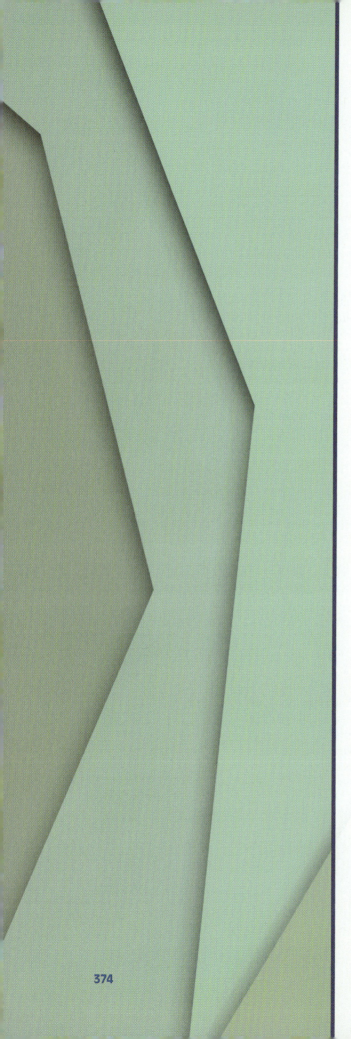

CHAPTER **23**

# Cosmetic Medicine and Medical Relations

## OBJECTIVES. . .

Only a short time ago, estheticians were only beginning to gain acceptance by the medical community. Some estheticians had referral relationships with dermatologists and plastic surgeons, but it was unusual to find an esthetician working in a dermatology office. Now, it seems the norm, rather than the exception—it is unusual to find a dermatology office without estheticians.

The medical community has finally understood the need for esthetics. The reasons for this sudden union are numerous and include the need of the baby boomer client to fight the signs of aging every step of the way.

There has also been a blurring of the line between esthetic services and medical services. Because of advances in technology, such as noninvasive laser treatments, Botox®, and other medical cosmetic services, there are many cosmetic medical services now available that require a doctor to administer or at least supervise. There are also many doctors practicing these services who are not dermatologists or plastic surgeons. There is controversy within the medical community about this issue.

Treating the appearance is also big business. We need to recognize that there is a lot of money in helping people improve their appearance. Many members of the medical community obviously want to cash in on these services.

In this chapter, we will discuss types of esthetic medical services that are offered to clients by medical doctors. These services are not necessarily traditional plastic surgery or traditional dermatological services. We will also discuss how esthetic services and medical services can complement one another and the different types of professional relationships an esthetician can have with a medical doctor.

## HOW ESTHETICIANS WORK WITH PHYSICIANS

Estheticians can provide many services that complement a medical practice. For example, estheticians can provide deep cleansing facial treatments for patients with acne or problem skin clients who also receive medical treatment from a dermatologist. Estheticians can help educate the patient about home care and can help recommend proper home care. They can also teach clients how to cope with the cosmetic side effects of many dermatological drugs.

The dermatologist may refer a client to an esthetician for help in choosing noncomedogenic cosmetics, or they may ask the esthetician to find a cosmetic that will work for a specific client without certain ingredients to which the patient may be allergic. Camouflage makeup cases are often referred by dermatologists.

## MEDICAL TRAINING

Let us discuss the kinds of doctors you may work with and what kind of training they have.

Dermatologists are specialists in the diseases of the skin, hair, and nails. They treat diseases, whereas estheticians treat cosmetic disorders. They study for four years of college and then four years of medical school, at which time they are awarded the Medical Doctor degree (M.D.). Another type of physician is the Doctor of Osteopathy (D.O.). Osteopathic school is very similar to medical school, except that osteopathic physicians traditionally have more holistic training, with emphasis on nutrition, body alignment, and so forth. D.O.s are basically licensed to practice just like M.D.s.

After medical or osteopathic school, doctors generally have a year of internship and then two to four years of specialty residency in dermatology. They train under dermatologists at major hospitals or universities. After all these years of training, they take their board exam in dermatology, administered by the American Academy of Dermatology, the professional association for dermatologists. This special certification is what dermatologists refer to when they say they are board certified.

Dermatologists may also subspecialize in several fields. **Mohs' surgeons** have further specialty training in micrographic surgery, a specialized form of surgery for hard-to-treat skin cancers. Other dermatologists may be dermatological surgeons, specializing in skin surgery, or may practice plastic surgery.

**Mohs' surgeons** are dermatologists specially trained in a very precise form of surgery to remove skin cancers.

Plastic surgeons have four years of college and four years of medical school, internship, and then several years of residency in plastic surgery.

Qualifications for board exams and the different types of physicians who practice plastic surgery have already been discussed in the plastic surgery chapter.

## OTHER DOCTORS

Besides dermatologists and plastic surgeons, there are other types of doctors that estheticians should be acquainted with and be able to refer cases to. Generally, these physicians are M.D.s who are board certified in their various fields of specialty.

Gynecologists specialize in treating women's reproductive and urinary systems and often help women with hormonal disorders. Acne, unwanted hair growth, and hyperpigmentation are all symptoms that can be hormone related.

**Endocrinologists** specialize in treatment of diseases of the endocrine system. The glandular system, if it is diseased, can seriously affect the skin. Thyroid or adrenal disorders, for example, can affect the skin, hair, and nails. **Rheumatologists** are specialists in rheumatoid diseases, including lupus.

**Internists** specialize in the treatment of internal diseases, including heart problems, diabetes, and other internal afflictions. Clients who have body massage may need referral to orthopedic surgeons, neurologists, or chiropractors. Cosmetic dentists, who specialize in the treatment of cosmetic disorders of the mouth and teeth, can also help make the client look better.

> **Endocrinologists** specialize in treatment of diseases of the endocrine system.
>
> **Rheumatologists** are specialists in rheumatoid diseases, including lupus.
>
> **Internists** specialize in the treatment of internal diseases, including heart problems, diabetes, and other internal afflictions.

## WHAT IS "PARAMEDICAL" ESTHETICS?

There has been a great deal of controversy in the esthetics profession about the term "paramedical." This term evolved out of a need for some estheticians to clarify or legitimize what they do.

The truth is that there is no state that recognizes the title "paramedical esthetician." Estheticians who work in medical offices often refer to themselves as "medical estheticians," although there is no official governmental recognition of this term either. Some states do not recognize the esthetician's license when they are practicing in a medical office. Often, the services performed by these estheticians are quite different than traditional esthetic services. These estheticians are working under the doctor's license and, therefore, depending on the individual state law, may perform treatments and services under the supervision of the doctor.

Some estheticians refer to themselves as "clinical estheticians." Although this term is also not officially recognized, "clinical esthetics" infers that the esthetician understands skin from a scientific perspective and understands how to manage the skin using results-oriented approaches. Clinical estheticians often have private practices and may have referral relationships with dermatologists, plastic surgeons, and other doctors.

## COSMETIC DERMATOLOGY AND MEDICAL SPAS

Estheticians can only offer topical, **noninvasive** services. Estheticians are not trained in medical procedures, laser therapies, or injections. These services are said to be beyond the esthetician's **scope of practice**. A scope of practice is the area in which a licensed person has been trained and licensed or certified by the government—in the esthetician's case, the state board of cosmetology. The scope of practice of the esthetician includes services to improve the appearance of the skin but does not include services using instruments or techniques for which they are not trained or are not defined by the law. This means that services that involve treatment below the surface of the skin or on live tissues are **invasive**, considered to be medical treatment, and can only be administered by medical personnel.

> **Noninvasive** describes procedures that do not break the skin.
>
> **Scope of practice** describes services allowed to be performed under a specific license.
>
> **Invasive** describes procedures that break the skin.

When a client requires services that an esthetician is not qualified to administer, doctors can take the client to the next level of esthetic care, whether that might be a Botox® injection or a laser treatment for capillaries.

**Cosmetic dermatology** is a subspecialty of dermatology focusing on appearance-related problems of the skin. The cosmetic dermatologist treats wrinkles and other aging symptoms, scars, hyperpigmentation, telangiectasias, hyperplasias, and any other problem with the skin that affects appearance. They, of course, are also qualified to treat skin cancers, skin diseases, and other dermatological problems.

> **Cosmetic dermatology** is a subspecialty of dermatology treating appearance-oriented problems of the skin.

**Medical spas** are medical offices that may offer traditional spa services and also have medical personnel to offer services beyond the scope of practice of the licensed esthetician (Figure 23-1). Some medical "spas" only offer laser services, Botox® injections, and the like, and do not offer traditional facials, makeup, etc. The medical personnel in medical spas may include physicians, nurses, nurse practitioners, or certified physician assistants. The physician might be a dermatologist or plastic surgeon, but he or she may be a physician who is a family practitioner, ophthalmologist (medical eye specialist), an emergency room physician, or some other type of physician. Because of licensure laws, any medical physician is allowed to administer cosmetic medical services.

Laws regarding medical spas vary greatly from state to state. This is largely because of the "newness" of medical spas. For example, some states prohibit use of a medical laser by anyone except a licensed medical physician. Other states allow nurses to perform laser services. A few states allow estheticians, if supervised by a doctor, to perform certain laser services. Again, the laws vary primarily because medical spas and cosmetic medical treatment are new areas of technology.

Medical spas offer medical services that affect the skin or its appearance. The following lists common services offered by medical spas. This section is intended to be only an overview of these services; it is and not intended to specifically recommend or endorse any of these services.

## Laser Services

There are many different types of lasers used in cosmetic dermatology and by medical spas. Most of these lasers are **nonablative**, which means that they do not destroy or peel the skin to any degree (Figure 23-2A and B, Figure 23-3A and B). They are not the same type of lasers used in laser resurfacing as discussed in the chapter on plastic surgery. Lasers that vaporize or peel the skin are referred to as **ablative** lasers.

Lasers are basically extremely focused, single-colored, polarized light that is beamed through a specialized chamber that contains some sort of chemical. The word laser stands for **L**ight **A**mplification by **S**timulated **E**mission of **R**adiation.

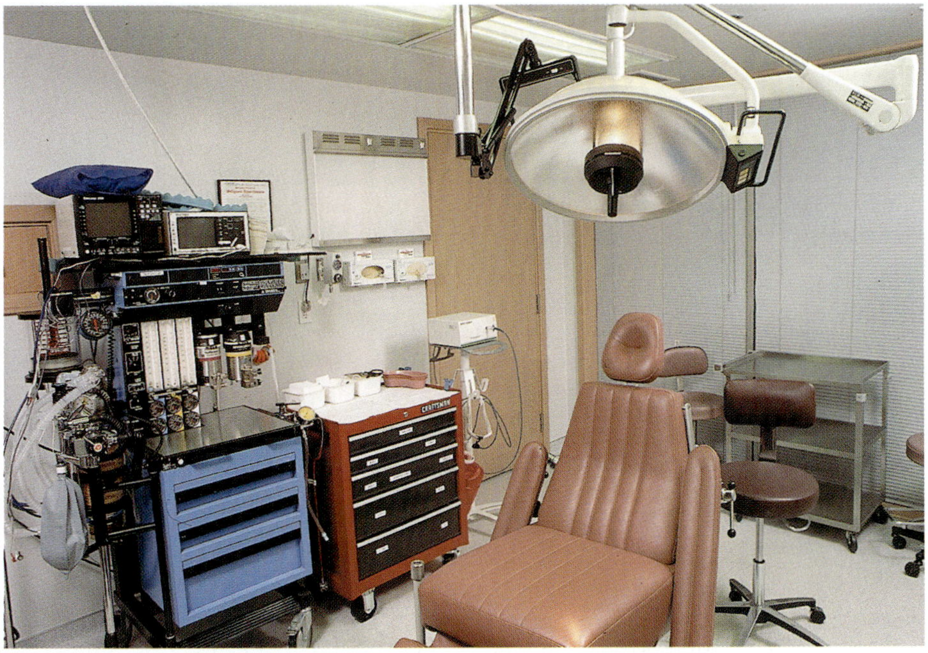

**Medical spas** are spas that offer medical esthetic procedures beyond the scope of routine esthetic services.

**Nonablative** describes a procedure that does not remove tissue.

**Ablative** is a term describing a laser that removes tissue.

**Figure 23-1** Medical spas try to combine the relaxed atmosphere of a spa with medical cosmetic services

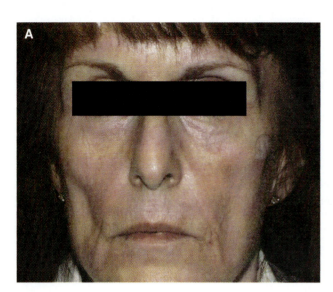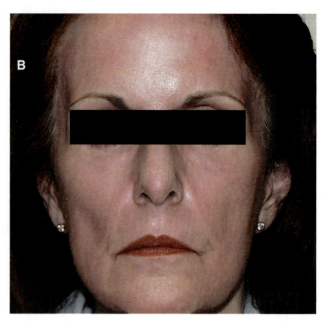

**Figure 23-2** *A*, Aging face. *B*, Aging face resurfacing with nonablative laser (Photos provided by Judith Crowell, M.D.)

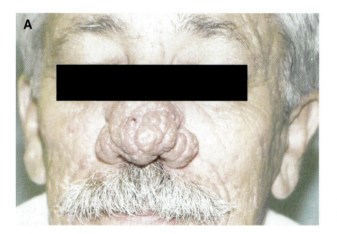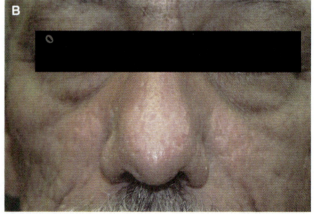

**Figure 23-3** *A*, Rhinophyma. *B*, Rhinophyma after laser treatment (Photos provided by Judith Crowell, M.D.)

**Coherent** describes extremely concentrated light.

What differentiates one laser from another is the specific wavelength of the light, the type of material in the chamber through which the light is beamed (such as Nd:YAG, which stands for neodymium:yttrium aluminum garnet), the color of the laser light, and what type of material within the specific type of laser will absorb the laser light. The light is extremely concentrated or focused, referred to as being **coherent** light. Specific lasers can focus on specific tissue (for example, blood vessels) without affecting surrounding tissue. Lasers often work by slightly injuring a specific tissue, depending on the body's healing mechanisms to respond, and this response is what creates the desired effect of "repair."

Some lasers can work on different problems. By varying the wavelength, the laser can focus on blood vessels (telangiectasias), hyperpigmentation (lentigenes or melasma), or other problem areas.

# Laser Hair Removal

Laser hair removal involves the use of a laser to remove unwanted hair for long periods of time. This is particularly effective for large areas of dark hair, such as backs and legs, but laser hair removal is also used on the face.

The laws regarding this area vary from state to state. Some states allow estheticians or electrologists to perform laser hair removal, although most states require some form of medical supervision.

# Spider Vein and Capillary Removal

Using a specialized laser, telangiectasias or spider angiomas are treated, the blood supply to the area is cut off, and the telangiectasia disappears. The laser creates heat in the blood vessels, causing it to dry up, and the vessel is eventually absorbed by the body. This type of laser service may be very helpful for patients with rosacea and persons with vascular birthmarks.

# Hyperpigmentation Treatment

Hyperpigmentation treatment is specialized laser treatment that focuses on treatment of hyperpigmented areas, melasma, and sun-related freckles and splotches.

# Intense Pulsed Light and Foto Facials®

Intense pulsed light (IPL) is a type of very strong light therapy that uses a powerful, very focused light to treat telangiectasias and hyperpigmentation (Figure 23-4). IPL is not technically a laser because it contains multiple colors of light. Several treatments are often required. IPL is also sometimes promoted as a treatment for wrinkles and as a way to improve skin surface smoothness. Effectiveness for wrinkles varies. IPL works best for telangiectasias, solar freckles, and other hyperpigmented areas.

# Radio Frequency Skin Tightening

Thermage® is a trademarked name for a medical procedure using radio frequency heat energy to stimulate collagen production and tighten fibrils, resulting in skin tightening. Results vary, and it generally takes at least a month to see results after treatment. Several treatments may be needed.

Another new similar technology is known as **electro-optical synergy (ELOS)**. ELOS uses a combination of light and radio frequency energy. ELOS is used for tightening, hair removal, telangiectasias, and hyperpigmentation.

Skin tightening does not produce the same effect as a traditional surgical face lift. It does not remove excess skin, nor does it alter the muscle structure like a surgical lift.

One drawback of radio frequency treatment is that it may produce more pain than other procedures.

**Electro-optical synergy (ELOS)** is a medical technique of treating cosmetic disorders using a combination of light and radio frequency energy.

# Other Services Offered by Medical Spas

**Botox®.** Botox® injections are often administered in medical spas. Botox® injections are used to treat wrinkles caused by repetitive facial expressions, especially in the forehead and brow furrow. For more information on Botox®, see the chapter on treatment of the plastic surgery patient.

**Wrinkle Injections.** Cosmetic fillers, such as hyaluronic acid injections (Restylane® and Hylaform®) (Figure 23-5A and B), collagen injections (Cosmoderm® and Cosmoplast®) (Figure 23-6A and B), calcium hydroxyapatite (Radiance®), and other materials are used to fill wrinkles. See the chapter on treating the plastic surgery patient for more information on cosmetic filler injections.

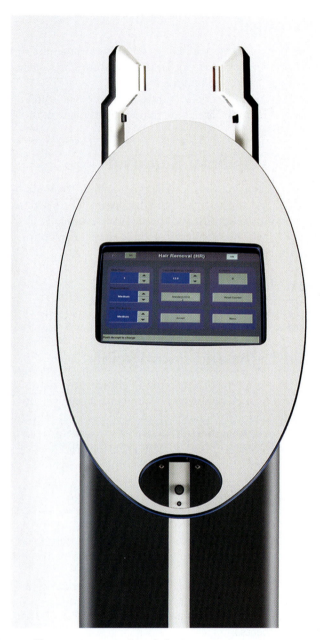

**Figure 23-4** Ellipse Intense Pulse Light System (Photograph Courtesy of Candela Corporation, Wayland, Massachusetts.)

## ESTABLISHING A RELATIONSHIP WITH A DOCTOR

Choosing doctors for referral is a very important decision. You want to establish relationships with the best doctors for your clients. You also may want to choose a doctor who does not compete with you by offering traditional esthetic services. If you are in private practice as an esthetician, it is usually the best business practice to choose a doctor for referral who does not have estheticians on staff. This way you and the doctor can refer to each other, knowing that neither professional is directly competing with the other.

Many doctors employ estheticians, and this is another opportunity you may want to consider. If you work for a doctor, you may offer traditional esthetic services,

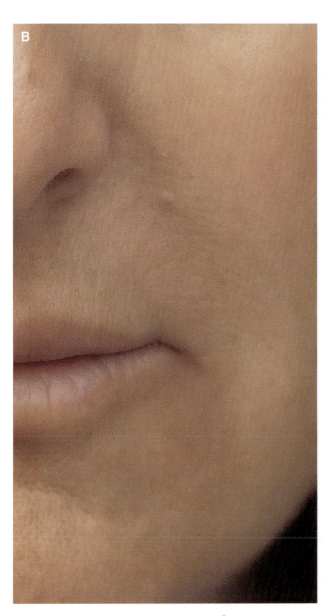

**Figure 23-5** *A*, Prominent oral commissures. *B*, Same patient after injection with Hylaform® (Reprinted with permission from Inamed Aesthetics.)

but you may also assist the doctor with other cosmetic medical services. Depending on your state laws, you may be able to offer other services under the supervision of the doctor.

It is important to check out the credentials of the doctor with whom you may be working or referring. Board certification in dermatology or plastic surgery is an important consideration, although there are many medical spas that are run by doctors who are not dermatologists or plastic surgeons. The reputation of the doctor within the community is a big factor to consider. If you have numerous clients who have good experiences with a certain doctor, that doctor may be a good contact. If you have a friend who is a doctor, ask him or her about the reputation of the doctor you are considering working with.

You also want to choose to refer your clients to a doctor who administers a lot of these services. Some doctors offer cosmetic treatment as a side service, and these

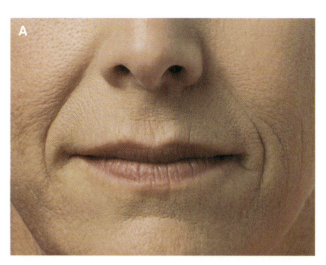
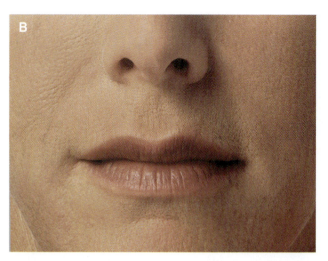

**Figure 23-6** *A*, Nasolabial lines. *B*, Same patient after injection with Cosmoplast® (Reprinted with permission from Inamed Aesthetics.)

doctors generally do not have as much experience as those who perform these services all the time.

The doctor you wish to work with may have similar questions for you. If they are reputable, they will only want to refer to estheticians who are highly qualified and take good care of the patients they refer for esthetic treatment.

Physicians are often not familiar with esthetician training. You should prepare a complete résumé listing all your credentials. You should list all academic esthetic training, specialties you may have, and any additional degrees you may hold. If you hold a specialized diploma or certification from a recognized organization such as CIDESCO, EstheticsAmerica, BABTEC, or ITEC (see the chapter on the scientific approach), make sure you list this, along with a short explanation of the certification, because the doctor may not be familiar with esthetics board certifications. Specifically list if you have real clinical training or advanced training in the sciences.

List all your work experiences, any professional organizations to which you belong, and any special awards in the esthetics field. Make sure your résumé looks very professional. It may be beneficial to contact a résumé service organization to help you write your résumé.

## WHAT DOCTORS LIKE . . . AND DON'T LIKE

Doctors have very serious, scientific training. They generally do not have much training in artistic fields and are not always well-acquainted with special techniques in the esthetics field. Be specific about what kind of special training you have had. Doctors are trained in the scientific method—make sure you read the chapter on the scientific approach. This will help you better understand why doctors are sometimes skeptical about estheticians.

Sometimes it may seem that doctors do not care much about esthetics. Often a doctor is more concerned about a patient's medical condition than about a cosmetic problem. Medical concerns outweigh cosmetic concerns. In other words, a physical reaction is more important than how something looks. If a patient has skin cancer, for example, getting rid of the cancer outweighs how the skin will look after medical treatment. Ideally, of course, both factors will be taken into consideration, but the patient's life and medical condition are always first!

Doctors in general are impressed with estheticians who have a good working knowledge of dermatology and how the human body functions in general. It helps to have additional training in other medically related fields. Estheticians who are also nurses, for example, often do very well working with dermatologists. If you have a good background in a science-related field, it will help you greatly when communicating with physicians. Doctors also appreciate it when an esthetician takes a scientific approach to cosmetic treatment. Examples of this are practicing clinically, using sterile techniques, using time-tested methods, and respecting when a client needs dermatological care, rather than esthetic care.

The biggest dislike of dermatologists, and doctors in general, is unscientific, "miraculous" approaches to beauty. If you make exaggerated claims or always tout the latest "miracle" treatment, you will not get much respect from the medical community. "Natural" treatments also raise medical eyebrows. There are advantages and disadvantages to using "natural" products. As one prominent dermatologist said, "Tuberculosis is natural, and so are scorpions!" For more information on why "natural" is not always best, read the chapter on sensitive skin.

The bottom line is that most doctors are honest with patients and expect the same from you. They know that neither of you can perform miracles. Be honest with your medical colleagues. Admit when you don't understand something. And don't act as if you are the dermatologist's equal. You are in entirely different, related fields.

## YOUR FIRST CONTACT WITH A DERMATOLOGIST

Call and make an appointment with the dermatologist to talk. Tell the receptionist who you are and briefly explain why you would like to talk to the dermatologist. If the receptionist is hesitant about making the appointment, leave a message for the doctor to call you. If the doctor returns your call, ask for an appointment to come by and talk.

Remember, not all doctors understand what estheticians do. Briefly explain what services you perform and your particular specialties. Bring your résumé. You may want to bring a book with you to show what kind of education you have had.

Ask if the doctor has any particular specialties and suggest working with you. Relax and get to know the doctor as a person. You will often find you have more in common than you think.

Ask the dermatologist for any patient brochures distributed in the office. Familiarize yourself with these brochures and any other patient education materials the doctor uses routinely. This will acquaint you with the doctor's techniques and may also give you an idea of how you could fit into the practice.

Invite the doctor to visit your salon. Offer a free treatment, and after the treatment offer some free samples of products. Do everything just as you normally would. Tell the doctor that you will act as if he or she were any other client. This way the doctor will see how you really work. Most dermatologists are actually very impressed with a good facial treatment. You might also offer a free treatment to the doctor's nurse or assistant. They often are involved with patient education in the office.

After you get to know the doctor you may ask if you may observe some procedures. Spending a day with a dermatologist is a truly enlightening experience. You will see cases you never see in the salon, and you will leave with a better understanding of medicine in general.

Don't forget that the interview is also a great opportunity for you to see how you feel about the doctor with whom you are meeting. Is he or she friendly and warm? Does he or she have a holistic approach to medicine? Does he or she already have a working understanding of esthetics? All of these factors will help indicate a successful medical referral situation.

# DOCTORS' CONCERNS

## Allergies

Have a good understanding of how allergies develop and how irritation occurs. Dermatologists see a lot of allergic reactions and a lot of contact dermatitis. Be knowledgeable about common cosmetic ingredient allergies and patch testing. Ask the doctor to help you understand the method of allergy testing.

## Comedogenic Cosmetics

Comedogenic cosmetics is an area where you can really win a dermatologist over. If you have a good understanding of comedogenicity and acne, you can provide an excellent service to the dermatologist, helping patients find noncomedogenic, nonacnegenic cosmetics and skin-care products.

## Rosacea and Sensitive Skin

Many patients are diagnosed with rosacea, and many people have sensitive skin. Having a good knowledge of rosacea management and sensitive skin is very helpful to dermatologists.

## Sun Damage

Dermatologists are impressed if you have a good knowledge of skin cancer and sun damage. They will be equally unimpressed if you offer tanning sessions in your salon!

## Electrolysis

Here is another excellent service for esthetic referral. Dermatologists see a lot of cases of unwanted hair that may be a result of another medical condition. Electrolysis is generally very well accepted by dermatologists and doctors in general.

## Camouflage Makeup

Doctors very often refer patients for help with camouflage and corrective makeup. It is important for you to be well versed in corrective makeup techniques and clinical camouflage makeup. Doctors will frequently refer patients with scars or birthmarks, accident victims, post-skin-cancer treatment patients, and patients with disfigurements for help with makeup. Do not be discouraged if this is all they refer at first. Eventually, one of those patients will have skin-care treatments and will return to the doctor with glowing results and comments.

## Extraction

Dermatologists often refer patients for treatment of comedones. They are often already treating the patients with other prescription drugs. Knowing how to treat these patients will help you prove yourself to the doctor. Discuss your extraction techniques with the doctor and set up a list of rules for various types of patients.

## Skin Care Management for Dermatological Drugs

Tretinoin (Retin-A, Renova®, azelaic acid (Azelex®), adapalene (Differin®), and other prescription topical drugs are often prescribed by dermatologists. These and other topical drugs can have side effects on the skin and often make the skin more sensitive to some cleansers, cosmetics, and other skin-care products. You should be familiar with management of clients being treated with other drugs that can affect the skin, what ingredients and products should be avoided, and which are unacceptable treatments for sensitive skin. Helping clients find suitable products while being treated with these drugs is an important part of a clinical skin-care practice.

Patients taking Accutane® are another group who need help with extra gentle skin care. See the chapter on acne for more information.

## Seborrheic Dermatitis and Other Inflammations

The doctor will be interested in how you deal with the patient who has a history of seborrheic dermatitis or other types of dermatitis. Some forms of skin-care products and treatments can aggravate seborrheic dermatitis. In general, stay away from fatty moisturizers, aggressive cleansers, and fragranced products.

## Learning More about Dermatology

Perhaps you are lucky enough to have attended a school that has a lecturing dermatologist on staff. This type of learning experience is an extremely valuable preparation for working with a dermatologist. Try to take continuing education classes with dermatologists or take classes that address some of the pertinent topics we have discussed as being important issues to them. Read all that you can, obtaining brochures and purchasing dermatology textbooks to study on your own. There are several condensed versions of these types of texts, and a variety of good books are available, written in easy-to-understand language, that discuss common dermatological problems.

Some pharmaceutical companies are progressive enough to offer training to allied health professionals, including estheticians. Many of these programs are new, and more will, no doubt, be offered in the future. Many of the esthetician's journals offer regular interviews with medical experts and frequently contain articles about the subjects we have discussed. Taking a course in medical terminology is also a good idea so you will better understand medical language.

## HOW TO REFER A CLIENT

When you notice that a client has a problem that needs referral, tell the client to call your referring dermatologist for an appointment. Send the dermatologist a referral slip about your client, why you are referring the client, and what services you have been performing to help the client. Make arrangements with the dermatologist to have him or her send you a reply referral letter letting you know what their diagnosis was and what treatment they have prescribed. In this letter they will tell you what should be done in the salon as a follow-up. Occasionally, a dermatologist will tell a client not to have esthetic services for a period of time. This should be explained in the doctor's letter, as well as the reason for this recommendation. Sometimes, particularly if the patient has minor skin surgery, or has recurrent dermatitis or a communicable disease, it is necessary to discontinue esthetic treatment.

## SOME COMMON PROBLEMS

Many estheticians have discussed problems they have in their relationships with dermatologists. Many of these are caused by miscommunication between the doctor and the esthetician. This is why it is so important to have an open line of communication with the dermatologist. We will discuss some of the most common complaints estheticians have about dermatologists and the common problems dermatologists have with estheticians.

## Why Do Dermatologists Only Recommend Certain Product Lines?

Just as you are educated about certain product lines, dermatologists receive training about certain products. Drug companies sponsor product knowledge classes and workshops, just as cosmetic companies do. So it is only natural that the doctor recommend familiar products. An esthetician would not recommend unfamiliar products either.

Doctors recommend what is widely available to their patients. They also recommend products they know their patients can afford. Dermatologists are particular about many allergy-causing, comedogenic, or irritancy-inducing chemicals used in cosmetics. Therefore, it is important that you have products available that meet these standards. You should try to have available moderately priced, noncomedogenic, hypoallergenic cosmetics that are as frangrance-free as possible. Dermatologists are concerned about allergies, and fragrances frequently cause allergies. This does not mean that this type of product is all you should carry, but you certainly should have a specialty line available for this type of client. Furnish information to dermatologists about your products, and furnish them with some sample products to try themselves.

## Why Do Dermatologists Always Recommend Soap and Water?

Soap and water are readily available to most patients in all income groups. Soaps that dermatologists recommend rarely cause allergy problems. Soaps are more rinseable than many cleansing milks, an important factor in treating skin problems. Talk to the dermatologist about recommending rinseable "soapless" soaps, which have the same rinseability as soap but without the residues and possible higher pH. Again, you should have this type of product available, and it should be fragrance-free.

## When I Send a Client to a Dermatologist, the Client Doesn't Come Back to the Salon!

This could result from different situations. First, get the doctor to agree to send you a referral letter letting you know about the client's progress; if esthetic treatment should be discontinued; and, most importantly, why.

Occasionally, a client will find that the visit to the dermatologist solves the problem and simply elects not to return to the salon at that time.

Occasionally, you will discover that you are working with an "esthetician basher"! The best way to deal with this kind of doctor is to find another doctor whom you can work with.

Again, you may want to choose to refer to a doctor who does not have an in-house esthetician, rather than to a doctor who does. You may risk losing a client to the doctor's esthetician.

## Dermatologists' Problems with Estheticians

Here are some common complaints dermatologists have about estheticians.

**The Esthetician Is Not Scientific.** To fully understand this, please read The Scientific Approach chapter. Many products on the market were developed based on anecdotal evidence, which is not scientifically sound. If you use and recommend products with exaggerated claims, or that have no scientific basis, this is a problem for many dermatologists. The solution to this problem is to carry products that are as scientific as possible and that do not make unbelievable claims.

**The Esthetician Uses Products That Are Too Heavy or Comedogenic.** Both of these are "no-nos" with dermatologists. As previously discussed, carry a good line of lightweight, fragrance-free, noncomedogenic cosmetics.

**Patients Complain That the Esthetician Is "Hard-Sell."** An esthetician should never take a "hard-sell" approach, no matter what kind of client you are dealing with. Carefully evaluate each client's individual needs, as well as lifestyle, budget, and skin-care needs. You should let the doctor know the range of what your products cost so they can brief their patients.

Some patients simply cannot afford esthetic services. Medical doctors see patients with serious medical problems, many of whom may not be able to afford esthetic services. Try your best to help these patients find an affordable product that they can use at home, even if they don't visit regularly for services.

## WORKING WITH THE PLASTIC SURGEON

Plastic surgeons are generally easier to work with than dermatologists. Cosmetic surgeons have clients who can afford elective cosmetic surgery. These clients can usually also afford esthetic services and more upscale products.

Because plastic surgery is often elective, plastic surgeons are more interested in esthetics, due to the artistic aspects of their specialty. They are interested in having their patients look as good as possible. Esthetic services "put the icing on the cake" by accentuating their work. Good skin care and proper makeup really enhance a good cosmetic surgery procedure. You should establish a relationship with a plastic surgeon and have an understanding with the surgeon about treatment procedures so that you both know what to expect from one another.

The bottom line is that good communication and a healthy respect for each other's professions is the key to a successful working medical relationship.

## TOPICS FOR DISCUSSION

1. What are some services that you can provide to the dermatology patient?
2. What type of conditions might you refer to the dermatologist?
3. Discuss a physician's training.
4. Discuss scheduling a first-time meeting with a dermatologist.
5. What are common communication problems between estheticians and dermatologists?
6. Discuss some ways to improve relations between the esthetics and medical communities.
7. Discuss how to choose the right doctor to whom you can refer clients.

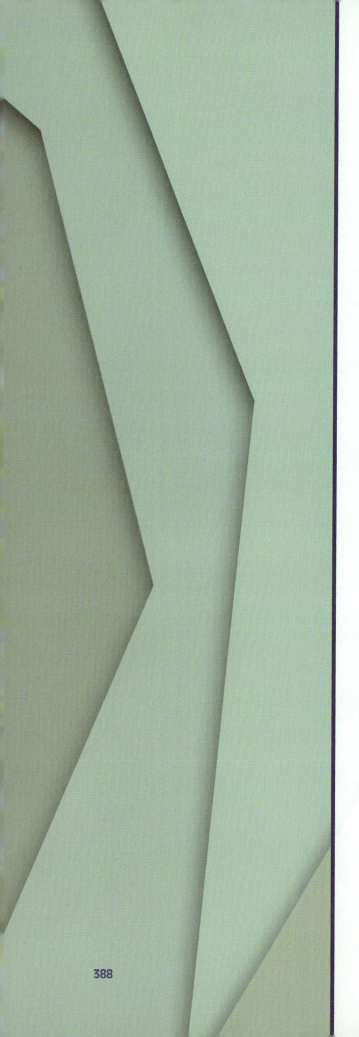

# CHAPTER 24

# The Scientific Approach

## OBJECTIVES. . .

Improving your education is a vital part of professional growth. Setting standards and learning to evaluate new developments is an essential part of any profession.

In this chapter we will discuss the need to be scientific in your approach to the practice of esthetics and the many educational opportunities that are available for advancement in the profession of esthetics.

Esthetics, like other health-related fields, is not an exact science. Too many factors are involved to determine the exact cause of a skin problem or to suggest an exact solution to a skin problem. So many factors are involved in any treatment involving the human body, whether the treatment is esthetic or medical. Therefore, estheticians can only give a "best guess" opinion about skin conditions and what they recommend to help.

We can, however, make an educated guess, taking the time to learn as much as we can about the human body in general and the skin in particular.

# THE SCIENTIFIC METHOD

The **scientific method** refers to the experimental technique of developing a hypothesis, or idea, based on available information. After the hypothesis is established, the method involves testing the idea and interpreting and publishing the results of the experiment. Let's look at an example. Years ago, doctors observed that certain keratolytic agents helped to peel the skin. They knew that many forms of acne were essentially caused by dead cells building up and clogging the follicles. It made sense that a keratolytic agent applied to the skin of acne patients would help loosen and remove dead cell buildup, opening the follicle and therefore increasing the oxygen content of the follicle canal. They also knew that acne bacteria could not survive in the presence of oxygen. They assembled a group of acne sufferers and experimentally applied keratolytic agents routinely to the skin of these patients. They tried to control the patients' other habits. In other words, if some of these patients were using special soaps, or vigorously scrubbing the skin, this could affect the results of the study. Factors that can affect an experiment are called *variables*. If there are too many variables in a study, it is hard to determine what causes changes that occur in an experiment.

In order to see if other factors caused changes besides the keratolytic agents, these scientists assembled a **control group**, a group of acne patients who did everything the same as the experimental group but did not apply the keratolytic. Instead they were given a product that looked the same as the keratolytic product but that did not actually contain the keratolytic. Such a product is called a **placebo**. Scientists observed that the group of acne patients who used the product with the keratolytic experienced marked improvement in their acne, whereas the group who applied the product without keratolytic had no improvement.

This method of research showed that keratolytics can help acne patients. The scientists carefully observed the number of acne lesions present on all of the patients' faces before and after the experiment. They carefully calculated the percentage of decrease in acne lesions of the group using the keratolytic and compared it to the control group. Then they applied specially designed mathematical formulas to measure the differences they observed. Using this type of mathematical calculation is called **statistics**. If there is a measurable difference in factors before and after the experiment, as there was in the group using the keratolytic, the results are said to be statistically significant. The scientists then published the results of their study, and the theory of using keratolytics to help acne eventually became standard practice.

This is a very simplified example, but it illustrates the scientific method. Other factors can influence a study. The number of subjects (patients) studied is an important factor. If too few people are studied, the study will not be significant. If the study does not take place over a long enough period of time, the study will not be significant. Research like this takes a lot of time and money. Drugs may be tested for years and years before being released. Side effects and possible dangers of using the drug must also be studied. If a drug helps a certain condition, but at the same time hurts another area of the body, it often cannot be practically used. Cosmetics generally have less research performed on them than drugs. The main reason for this is money. It is very expensive to perform complicated research studies. Also, as we learned in the chapter on claims in cosmetics, if a cosmetic manufacturer makes a claim that it affects anything but appearance, it is considered a drug and is subject to governmental regulations that require much more research. This is why doctors often consider the need for cosmetic treatment to be questionable. Cosmetics are generally not tested nearly as extensively as drugs and therefore are not as scientifically sound as pharmaceuticals, according to many scientists.

Research on cosmetics is often performed on the ingredients rather than the product itself. The active agent is tested in the laboratory to determine its benefits, and then it is mixed with a usable vehicle, such as a cream or lotion. More and more

**Scientific method** refers to the experimental technique of developing a hypothesis, or idea, based on available information. The hypothesis is tested and, interpreted, and results are published.

**Control group** is the group in an experiment that does not change behavior.

**Placebo** describes a substance used in an experiment that does not contain the ingredient thought to achieve a change.

**Statistics** are precise mathematical measurements of changes in an experiment.

cosmetic companies are testing their products and measuring improvement in the subjects' appearance.

If a product contains ingredients that are thought to be beneficial for the skin, this theory is called *anecdotal*. Anecdotal evidence is based on observation and theory, but the theory has not been thoroughly scientifically tested, as we discussed earlier. This doesn't mean that the product has no beneficial cosmetic effects; it simply means that the results and use are based on anecdotal, rather than scientific, findings.

An example of anecdotal information is the use of plant extracts and essential oils. There has been some scientific research in the use of these extracts, but not enough to establish scientifically significant findings for all of the many extracts that are used in cosmetics. Pharmaceutical companies frequently use chemicals that are actually extracted from plants, but the chemicals are isolated and pure, rather than using the entire extract, as many cosmetic companies do.

This brings up the subject of "natural" versus "synthetic." Natural cosmetics are regarded by some estheticians as superior to "chemicals." But plant extracts are nothing more than a group of different chemicals, because all materials on earth are made of chemicals! This is the main, and justified, argument against "natural" products. As we discussed in the chapter on sensitive skin, if a person experiences an allergic reaction to salicylic acid, it is easy to determine that the person is allergic because salicylic acid is used as an isolated chemical. But if a client has an allergic reaction to a product containing sweet birch extract, a plant source for salicylic acid, it is hard to determine if the client had a reaction to salicylic acid or to one of the many other chemicals that comprise sweet birch extract.

This example is why dermatologists are often skeptical about the use of plant extracts and essential oils in cosmetic products. In general it is accepted that the fewer and more isolated ingredients that are used in cosmetics, the less potential there is for allergic reaction.

## EVALUATING PRODUCTS

When you talk to a manufacturer about a new product or line of products, you should try to establish how scientific the research has been on the products. Ask many questions. Has the product been evaluated as thoroughly as possible? Do their claims sound believable? Or are they using "puffing" descriptions? **Puffing** refers to using complicated descriptions of the products to describe their effects on the skin. Some companies have excellent products and still use "puffing" because they are attempting to avoid making drug claims. If a company claims that a product has an effect on the functioning of the body, it is making drug claims.

What is the company's approach to skin care? Are formulations based on current research and do they use techniques that have been time tested? What are their developer's credentials? If they make claims for hypoallergenicity or noncomedogenicity, how are the products tested?

You must have a sound background to be able to ask good questions and evaluate a product. How do you prepare so you know what questions to ask? There are many things you can do to improve your scientific approach to skin care.

## Go Back to School

Take some courses in chemistry, biology, and other sciences at your local community college or university. Start with beginning level classes. Many estheticians go back to school for additional classes and even degrees. A college degree in a related field such as health, chemistry, nutrition, or biological sciences is very helpful in the practice of esthetics. Many very successful estheticians have degrees in other related fields. You don't have to give up your practice to expand your education. More and more colleges

**Puffing** is a term used to describe the way some companies make their products sound better than they are.

offer night or weekend classes for working people. Some major universities now offer special two- to five-day classes in cosmetic sciences. One of these is the University of California at Los Angeles. For further information on this program, contact UCLA Extension.

## Read Your Journals

You should subscribe to every journal in the beauty business. Contacts for magazines are listed in the bibliography section of this book.

These journals contain a wealth of information, including information about the many products available to estheticians. Many excellent estheticians write for these journals, describing their good and bad experiences. There is so much you can learn each month from reading these magazines.

## Buy Any Book You Can about Skin

Visit your bookstore every month and purchase any new books about skin or health. Visit your college bookstore and purchase beginning level textbooks in anatomy, chemistry, biology, and other subjects related to esthetics.

An extremely important learning source is trade shows! You will meet and learn from some of the top estheticians, dermatologists, chemists, and researchers in the industry.

Stay for the whole show, and attend all the classes you can. You will learn a lot from your fellow attendees. The fellowship and learning experience has no price and is an extremely valuable learning tool. But you won't meet them if you don't go to the shows!

While at the shows, talk to the exhibitors and speakers and see from whom you feel you can learn the most. Ask if they offer additional training or classes. Make arrangements to attend classes offered by these specialists. Get on their mailing lists so you can receive a calendar of upcoming events or speaking engagements.

Three types of classes are generally offered at trade shows.

General education is taught at a "main stage" routinely throughout the convention. This is included in your admission fee. Usually held in a large ballroom, speakers discuss their specialties, or there are panel discussions. These lectures are usually less than an hour each.

Manufacturer education is offered in private classrooms. This is where the manufacturers teach you about their products. Obviously, manufacturers want you to buy their products after the classes. This is an excellent opportunity to evaluate new products. Remember, these lectures are usually commercial, but they are still a great way to learn more about your profession.

Workshops and seminars are often offered after the main convention. These are usually referred to as post-classes. Post-classes usually carry a separate fee and allow you to spend two or more hours with an accomplished speaker. If you read journal articles that you like or find helpful, the authors of these articles may be featured at trade show post-classes. The education in these classes is often called generic, meaning that it is not commercially product oriented. Spending this kind of time with a top esthetician is by far the best learning experience you can have.

## Regional Seminars

Most skin-care companies have educational programs available, both product classes and general advanced esthetics classes. These classes often last a day or more and are offered frequently. Of course, this involves traveling to the city where the seminar is held, but you will usually find it very worthwhile.

## Clinical Skin Care

As we have discussed previously, clinical skin care is a results-oriented program approach to esthetics. This combines a thorough assessment of the particular client's needs and a step-by-step plan of action, based on scientific treatment methods, and individualized home care, based on performance ingredients.

The profession is taking a turn toward clinical approaches, and although there will always be a need for relaxation therapy facial treatments, many estheticians are interested in offering clinical care, which is for many estheticians more challenging and rewarding.

## Advanced Schools and Training

Basic skin-care training, in general, does not offer enough hours or the specialized instruction necessary for advanced clinical skin care. It is up to the individual esthetician to decide what type of practice he or she wishes to pursue. It is often necessary to look for schools or programs that offer advanced specialty classes.

Fortunately, more of these specialty programs are now emerging. These programs offer one- to five-day intensive learning sessions, often with well-known skin-care experts. To find more about these types of graduate programs, look for information in skin-care journals.

## Join Your Professional Associations

EstheticsAmerica is the esthetics division of the National Cosmetology Association (NCA). If you are a licensed esthetician and you join the NCA, you are a member of EstheticsAmerica. EstheticsAmerica sponsors national seminars that offer both business and technical classes and education.

EstheticsAmerica is the United States chapter of CIDESCO International, the oldest and best-established esthetics organization in the world. CIDESCO helps to set standards for the industry and administers the CIDESCO International Examination, a board certification exam for estheticians. In many countries, estheticians attend schools that have been accredited by CIDESCO and are eligible to take the exam upon graduation. There are now several CIDESCO accredited schools in the United States. For graduates of schools that are not accredited, CIDESCO offers the "Three Year Exam." This means that if you have graduated from a licensed esthetics school, have practiced as a licensed esthetician for three years, and complete a special intensive training program through CIDESCO, you may take the exam. The exam is difficult, and you should plan on several months of preparation for the test. If you pass the test, which is both written and practical, you are awarded the CIDESCO International Diploma. Estheticians who pass the exam are called CIDESCO Board-certified estheticians. The CIDESCO diploma is recognized as the highest earned title in the world for estheticians.

For information on NCA, EstheticsAmerica, and CIDESCO programs, contact NCA at 401 North Michigan Avenue, Suite 2200, Chicago IL 60611. In the United States, call 866-871-0656 or 312-527-6765, or visit the NCA Web site at ncacares.org.

The American Association for Esthetics Education (AAEE) is an organization dedicated to providing specialized advanced education for estheticians. It offers continuing education credits for some states and offers regular specialty seminars and classes. Contact AAEE at 401 N. Michigan Avenue, Chicago, IL 60611. Call 1-800-648-2505 or 312-245-1570, or visit the AAEE Web page at isnow.com.

Probably the biggest function of the professional organizations is serving as legislative watchdog for the profession. This helps prevent deregulation and helps ensure safety and standards for public health. Most professional organizations also offer special seminars, conventions and congresses, magazine subscriptions and journals, special insurance programs, and many other benefits.

Strive to obtain the highest credentials you can. There are three special secrets to being a great esthetician. You must receive the best education possible. You have to communicate well with people. You have to, most of all, love your profession!

## TOPICS FOR DISCUSSION

1. Describe the scientific method.
2. What does *statistically significant* mean?
3. What kind of factors can affect a study?
4. What is the difference between scientific and anecdotal evidence?
5. Discuss how to evaluate products.
6. Why is it important to read and subscribe to esthetic journals?

# BIBLIOGRAPHY AND RECOMMENDED READINGS

Bark, J. (1989). *Retin-A and other youth miracles*. Rocklin, CA: Prima.

Baumann, L. (2002). *Cosmetic dermatology*. New York: McGraw-Hill.

Bevan, J. (1979). *The Simon and Schuster handbook of anatomy and physiology*. New York: Simon and Schuster.

Boyd, A. (1998). *The skin sourcebook*. Los Angeles: Lowell House.

Brinker, N., & Chihal, J. (1997). *1000 questions about women's health*. Arlington, TX: Summit.

Brown, G. (2005). *About face*. New York: Ballantine Books.

Chase, D. (1989). *The new medically based no-nonsense beauty book*. New York: W.W. Norton.

Chihal, J., & London, S. (1999). *Menopause: Clinical concepts*. Durant, OK: EMIS Medical.

Desowitz, R. (1987). *The thorn in the starfish*. New York: W.W. Norton.

Dwyer, J. (1990). *The body at war*. New York: Mentor Books.

Fitzpatrick, T., Johnson, R., Wolff, K., Polano, M., & Suurmond, D. (1997). *Color atlas and synopsis of clinical dermatology*. New York: McGraw-Hill.

Flandermeyer, K. (1979). *Clear skin*. Boston: Little, Brown.

Fulton, J. (1984). *Dr. Fulton's step-by-step program for clearing acne*. New York: Barnes & Noble Books.

Gerson, J. (1999). *Standard textbook for professional estheticians*. Albany, NY: Milady.

Goldberg, D., & Herriott, E. (2003). *Light years younger*. Herndale, VA: Capital Books.

Goodman, T., & Young, S. (1988). *Smart face*. New York: Prentice-Hall.

Gray, H. (1995). *Gray's anatomy*. Philadelphia: Running Press.

Haberman, F., & Fortino, D. (1983). *Your skin*. New York: Berkley.

Irwin, B., & McPherson, M. (2002). *Your best face*. Carlsbad, CA: Hay House.

Johnson, B., Moy, R., & White, G. (1998). *Ethnic skin*. St. Louis, MO: Mosby.

Jovanovic, L., & Levert, S. (1993). *A woman doctor's guide to menopause*. New York: Hyperion.

Jovanovic, L., & Subak-Sharpe, G. (1987). *Hormones—the woman's answer book*. New York: Fawcett Columbine.

Kaiser, J. (1999). *Healing HIV*. Mill Valley, CA: HealthFirst Press.

Leffell, D. (2000). *Total skin*. New York: Hyperion.

Lowe, N., & Sellar, P. (1999). *Skin secrets*. London: Collins & Brown.

Michalun, N. (2001). *Skin care and cosmetic ingredients dictionary*. Albany, NY: Milady.

Milady. (2003). *Milady's standard: comprehensive training for estheticians*. Albany, NY: Milady.

Otto, J., & Towle, A. (1993). *Modern biology*. New York: Holt, Rinehart & Winston.

Perricone, N. (2000). *The wrinkle cure*. Emmaus, PA: Rodale Press.

Pugliese, P. (2001). *Physiology of the skin II*. Carol Stream, IL: Allured Publishing.

Pugliese, P. (1991). *Advanced professional skin care*. Bernville, PA: APSC.

Schoon, D. (1994). *HIV/AIDS & hepatitis*. Albany, NY: Milady.

Scott, A., & Fong, E. (1998). *Body structures & functions*. Albany, NY: Delmar.

Steigleder, G., & Maibach, H. (1984). *Pocket atlas of dermatology*. New York: Thieme.

Stoll, D. (1994). *A woman's skin*. New Brunswick, NJ: Rutgers University Press.

Teaff, N., & Wiley, K. (1996). *Perimenopause—preparing for the change*. Rocklin, CA: Prima.

Turkington, C., & Dover, J. (1996). *Skin deep*. New York: Facts on File.

Warshofsky, F. (1999). *Stealing time*. New York: TV Books.

Winter, R. (1999). *A consumer's dictionary of cosmetic ingredients*. New York: Three Rivers Press.

Wolfe, D. (1988). *Introduction to college chemistry*. New York: McGraw-Hill.

## PERIODICALS

*American Spa*
One Park Ave.
New York, NY 10016
212-951-6600

*Cosmetic Dermatology*
26 Main St.
Chatham, NJ 07928-2402
800-480-4851

*Dayspa*
7628 Densmore Ave.
Van Nuys, CA 91406-2042
818-782-7328

*Dermascope*
2611 N. Beltline Rd. Suite 101
Sunnyvale, TX 75182
800-961-3777

*Les Nouvelles Esthetiques—American Edition*
3929 Ponce de Leon
Coral Gables, FL 33134
800-471-0229

*PCI (Progressive Clinical Insights) Journal*
484 Spring Ave.
Ridgewood, NJ 07450-4624
201-670-4100

*Skin, Inc.*
362 South Schmale Rd.
Carol Stream, IL 60188-2787
630-653-2155

*Skin and Allergy News*
12230 Wilkins Ave.
Rockville, MD 20852
800-654-2452

# INDEX

Hydration means water is added, 116
  aging skin, 142
  night creams, 161
  oil skin, 148
  sensitive skin, 198
Hydrocortisone is a hormone that helps relieve inflammation and skin irritation, 105, 199
Hydrocotyl (*Centella asiatica*) is part of a patented botanical complex that helps to improve the appearance of elasticity, 143
Hydrophilic ingredients, or "water-loving" ingredients, attract and bind water, 124, 136
Hydroquinone is an active topical ingredient that inhibits the production of melanin. It is used melanin suppressants, 105, 147, 294
Hydroxyl radical is a very destructive form of free radical, 37
Hyfrecator is an electric needle used by a physician to remove small growths or treat certain vascular skin lesions, 103
Hygiene. *See* Cleaning
Hyperpigmentation refers to any condition that has more than a normal amount of melanin, 94, 293
  aging and, 286
  AHA peels, 316, 333
  birth control pills and, 72
  characterization, 88
  laser surgery and, 366
  laser treatment, 379
  lightening treatment, 164–165
  post-inflammatory, 88
  sun-induced, 293
  treating, 294–295, 322–323
Hyperthyroidism is a condition in which the thyroid gland secretes too much thyroid hormone, 75
Hypertrophic describes a raised scar above the skin's surface, 89
Hypertrophy is thickening of tissue, 94
Hypoallergenic cosmetics are cosmetics that have generally been manufactured without the use of certain ingredients that are known to frequently cause allergic reactions, 174, 185
Hypopigmentation refers to any condition that has less than a normal amount of melanin, 94
Hypothalamus gland controls some involuntary muscles, such as the muscles of the intestines that help move food through the gastrointestinal system, 61
Hypothyroidism is a condition in which the thyroid gland secretes too little thyroid hormone, 75
Hypotrophic describes a depressed scar, 89

Idebenone is a very powerful antioxidant, 319
Immune describes the body's defense against disease and inability to contract an illness due to excellent function of the immune system, 33
Immune system is the body's mechanism for fighting disease, 33
  allergies and, 183
  antibiotics and, 38
  communication, 34–35
  complexity of, 32
  components of, 32–34
  free radicals and, 37–38
  function of, 32
  slowing of, 36
  vaccines and, 38
Immunity, natural, 33
Immunity, skin's role, 39–40
Immunoglobulins, or Igs, are antibodies that protect against specific invaders, 33
Immunosuppression refers to the slowing of the immune system, 36
Impaired means there is damage in the barrier function of the skin, 11
Impetigo is a bacterial skin infection resulting in weeping sores, commonly seen in children. It is characterized by large, open weeping lesions, 44, 52, 94
Implants are used to improve the cheeks and chin, 368
In vitro refers to scientific testing that occurs outside of a living organism. It has not been tested on a live specimen, 176
Infections. *See also* specific types
  AIDS-associated, 52–53
  common bacterial, 94–96
  fungal, 21, 96
  localized, 20–21
  opportunistic, 46
  viral, 96–100
Infectious diseases are highly contagious diseases that can easily be transferred to another person, 44
Inflammation. *See also* Dermatitis
  acne-associated, 225
  knowledge of, 385
  subclinical, 37
Inflammation cascade is a series of biochemical reactions that lead to production of self-destruct enzymes that damage the skin, 141, 181, 310
  chronic inflammation and, 181–182
  effects of, 310
  occurrence, 181
Inflammatory acne is flares of acne without comedones, and can result from hormonal flares or acnegenic products causing follicle irritation, 251
Inflammatory means swollen and red, 216

Inflammatory mediators are chemicals released by irritated cells that alert the immune system to the irritation, 181
Ingrown hairs, 84
Intense pulsed light is a powerful medical light treatment used to treat pigmentation, vascular lesions, and aging skin, 103, 379
Intercellular cement is the cushion of lipid substances between the cells of the corneum that keeps the skin from dehydrating and helps protect the skin from irritative substances, 11, 128
Interleukin is present in the cytoplasm of T cells and is released as an alarm system when the T cell is alerted to a foreign body, 35
Internal phase is the dispersed part of the emulsion, 125
International companies, 176
Internists specialize in the treatment of internal diseases, including heart problems, diabetes, and other internal afflictions, 376
Interstitial fluid is the fluid between the cells, 11
Intradermal means inside the dermis, which is where collagen and other filler material may be injected to fill out hypotrophic scars, wrinkles, or pock marks, 369
Intravenous drugs, 46
Intrinsic aging is the part of the aging process that is due to the actual passing of the years, wearing out the body, and hereditary factors, 281
Invasive procedures are procedures that enter the body, 22, 376
Ionic bond is the bond of two ions joining to form a molecule, 109
Ionized is a substance that has been charged by changing its atoms to ions, 116
Ions, or charged atoms, are the resulting atoms with new charges when atoms "steal" or "give away" electrons to each other, 109
Iontophoresis uses electrical current to polarize preparations into the skin, 17
Irritancy potential is the tendency of a substance to cause skin irritation, 192
Irritant contact dermatitis (ICD) is inflammation resulting from a substance that is irritating skin, 183
Irritants are substances that can inflame the skin, 184
  avoiding, 319
  causes, 184
  testing, 193

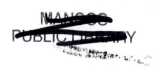